The Heart Doctors' Heart Book

THE AUTHORS

MARSHALL FRANKLIN, B.S., M.D., D.A.B.I.M., F.A.C.A.

Director Cardiac Catheterization Laboratory, Director Cardiac Rehabilitation, Associate Director of Cardiology, Norwalk Hospital, Norwalk, Connecticut
Associate Attending in Cardiology, St. Joseph Hospital, Stamford, Connecticut
Associate Attending in Medicine, Stamford Hospital, Stamford, Connecticut
Attending in Surgical Cardiology, White Plains Hospital, White Plains, New York
Lecturer in Cardiology, The Mount Sinai Hospital and Medical Center, New York City, New York

MARTIN JOEL KRAUTHAMER, B.S., M.D., D.A.B.I.M. (CV), F.A.C.C.

Co-Director Section of Cardiology, Associate Attending in Medicine, Stamford Hospital, Stamford, Connecticut
Director Coronary Care Unit, Associate Attending in Cardiology, Norwalk Hospital, Norwalk, Connecticut
Associate Attending Division of Cardiology, Department of Medicine, St. Joseph Hospital, Stamford, Connecticut

A. RAZZAK TAI, M.D., D.T.M.&H., M.R.C.P., D.A.B.I.M. (CV)

Chief of Cardiology and Senior Attending, St. Joseph Hospital, Stamford, Connecticut
Associate Attending in Medicine, Stamford Hospital, Stamford, Connecticut
Attending in Cardiology, Norwalk Hospital Norwalk, Connecticut
Consultant in Cardiology, Wyckoff Heights Hospital, Brooklyn, New York
Assistant Attending in Medicine, Greenwich Hospital, Greenwich, Connecticut
Director, Cardiac Rehabilitation Program, New Canaan (Connecticut) Y.M.C.A.

OTHER BOOKS BY ANN PINCHOT

Hear This Woman!
Hagar (with Ben Pinchot)
52 West
Jacqueline Kennedy: A Biography
On Thin Ice
The Man Chasers
The Movies, Mr. Griffith and Me (with Lillian Gish)
Weep No More My Lady (with Mickey Deans)

The Heart Doctors' Heart Book

Marshall Franklin, M. D.,
Martin Krauthamer, M. D.,
A. Razzak Tai, M. D.,
and Ann Pinchot

Illustrations by Mary Baukus, R.T.

Photographs by Nick Scutti

GROSSET & DUNLAP
Publishers New York

Published simultaneously in Canada
Library of Congress catalog card number: 73–15131
ISBN 0-448-11524-7

Printed in the United States of America

FOURTH PRINTING

Authors' note: All names have been changed to protect the privacy of our patients with the exception of those listed in the acknowledgments. None of the medical procedures described in this book should be undertaken except under the direction of a general physician.

The illustrations in this book are, of course, diagrammatic, and are not meant to be realistic drawings of the heart and circulatory system.

To all our patients

This book would not exist if not for Sue Pinchot, with love from her mother and her three heart doctors.

Acknowledgments

In preparing this book, there have been many people who have assisted us, from the girls in the office who fixed us uncounted numbers of tunafish sandwiches, to those who transcribed tapes and typed.

In particular Miss Margaret Lidy, Mrs. Marion Murphy, and Miss Rosemary DeAngelo from our office in Darien; Mrs. Jeanne Williams, Norwalk Hospital and Mrs. Betty Meany, St. Joseph Hospital.

To the catheterization teams at Norwalk, St. Joseph and Stamford Hospitals. To the nurses in the ICU/CCU, general nursing floors and Emergency Rooms of these three hospitals.

To Norman Brady, Administrator of Norwalk Hospital, Sister Daniel Marie, Administrator of St. Joseph Hospital.

To Dr. L. L. Brock, Medical Director, Exercise Equivalents, Colorado Heart Association, for the chart, Appendix C.

To the physicians who have expressed confidence in our work.

We would like to thank the following people who have contributed material to the book:

Mrs. Rebecca Marcus, R.N., B.S.N., Instructor in Coronary Care Nursing.

Physicians Michael Zales, M.D., John Sacco, M.D. and Eugene Wrona, M.D.

Specifically to patients John Ready and his wife, Carroll, and Kenneth Wachter and his wife, Mary, who tell the stories of their heart attacks in their own words.

Our thanks to all those physicians and researchers who developed the equipment and concepts we apply to patient care today. And a special thanks to F. Mason Sones, Jr., M.D. and Earl K. Shirey, M.D. for developing coronary arteriography and simplifying so many of the cardiac catheterization procedures we use today.

And finally to our wives and families for bearing with us through long hours of taping, and working, and midnight sessions, and for relaying messages, and for their constructive comments, and most of all, for their support.

Our deepest thanks to our editors, to Grace Bechtold and to Lee Schryver for the endless hours of patient and constructive work.

Contents

PART V

WHAT THE PATIENT DOES

Preface

Twenty-five years ago knowledge of cardiology was uncertain—both for the doctor and his patient. Our forebears simply did not understand the nature of heart problems, and in their lack of knowledge created a folklore largely dedicated to futility and inaction.

During the past generation, specialists in many fields—with insights and interests in physiology, psychology, radiology, photography, and other technical fields related to the medical profession—have created methods of solving heart problems which were simply insoluble a few years ago.

Although these developments have brought us beyond all previous hopes in effective diagnosis and treatment, they have also produced a credibility gap which is extremely difficult for the patient with heart disease and those who love him to understand.

During the past generation, those of us who have been preoccupied with developing better techniques for diagnosing and treating organic heart disease have been upbraided by many people who don't know the facts in this book.

I must tell you that we today who wear white coats live in an incredibly disciplined and sophisticated medical environment. And that environment greatly enhances the survival of heart victims and the chance to return to a full life.

Doctors Marshall Franklin, Martin J. Krauthamer and A. Razzak Tai, through their thoughtful and warm contributions to this book, have done much to quell the vague and nameless fears generated by ignorance. I sincerely hope that those of you or your family who are stricken by the worst scourge of our century will read it, gain insight, and cooperate more knowledgeably to live effectively beyond your expectations.

F. Mason Sones, Jr., M.D.
Chairman, Department of Cardiovascular Disease and the Cardiac Laboratory
The Clinic Center
Cleveland, Ohio
November, 1973

PART I

THE HEART DOCTORS AND THE HEART CARE UNIT

Chapter 1

Our patients and our group

The heart is a pump.
The heart has four chambers.
The heart is nourished by the coronary arteries.
The heart is a generator, with its own electrical system.
The heart gives warning.

You are listening, but do you hear? Communications are often short-circuited. Fear, anxiety, tension are all road blocks which keep the news—even comforting news—from coming through. Heart patients in particular have a tendency to listen to the physician without really hearing or absorbing his advice. And there is some reassuring advice for those who want to keep their hearts healthy.

We are cardiologists. We do everything we can to prevent heart disease. When it occurs, it is our job to treat it, to arrange for surgery if needed, and to devise the routine and life style that will help the heart patient live as rich and full a life as his damaged heart will allow.

Our offices look out on the Darien railroad station. Darien is an affluent suburban community, and a high percentage of its male population commutes daily to Madison Avenue and Wall Street in Manhattan. From six o'clock in the afternoon on, we get a full view of well-dressed commuters getting off the express from Grand Central and shuffling off to their parked cars. The younger men manage to retain some of their bounce. But many of the middle-aged men share a weary dispirited lag that the Bar Car hasn't eased.

All three of us were working late one evening, sorting color slides and dictating case histories when the doorbell rang. Office hours were long over. It was nearly nine and Dr. Tai, who was on call, was picking up his satchel to leave for the hospital.

He opened the door. Framed in the doorway was John C., a former patient. Although the October wind was sharp, his top coat was unbuttoned and his right arm sagged with the weight of his brief case. He looked at us with pain-filled eyes.

"John, come in," Dr. Tai said. "Is something wrong?"

"I just came back from a week's business trip," John said, his voice hoarse with fatigue. "I've got pains across my chest. The pills didn't help, I took some on the train. I want you to take a look at me and tell me if I'm going to live to get home."

He did live.

Dr. Tai drove him to the hospital and after giving him emergency care, put him in the Coronary Care Unit. This time, John didn't make a fuss when the nurses took his blood pressure every two hours, and when he was plugged into the oscilloscope which monitored his heartbeat.

John had fortunately been listening with the third ear, that subconscious warning signal that primes us when something is going amiss in our bodies. Oddly enough, John had a similar premonition before his first heart attack, four years ago. "I felt something was wrong. Like a terrible cloud hanging over me. I felt I was going to die—"

This was his second heart attack—myocardial infarction, in the medical world. We charted the damage to his heart by means of cardiac catheterization and gave our verdict—he would have to retire from his pressure-cooker job. We told him that this heart attack was not an isolated incident from which he would recover and go back to his previous life style. He was one of the unlucky ones. At first, he wouldn't believe us. But we finally convinced him.

To the patient, a heart attack is often an acute illness and not regarded as a sudden valley in the continuing panorama of chronic heart disease. To the doctor, it is an immediate clinical manifestation of a disease process that started long before the heart attack actually occurred, and will continue after it.

If a heart condition isn't serious or advanced, we encourage the patient to live a normal and unrestricted life. In John's case, this was impossible. He was obliged to retire from commuting, high-pressure business lunches and flights back and forth across the Atlantic with no respect for the jet lag.

"It's unsatisfactory," he grumbled about the less demanding part-time job he took in a nearby town. "But it's the *least* unsatisfactory."

It was a severe adjustment, both fiscal and emotional, but his wife assured him that she would rather be a modestly affluent wife than a rich widow. It was actually tougher for John to readjust than for his wife. But a man with a severely scarred heart must make a choice.

The New York Heart Association (see Appendix A) would classify John C. as functional Class III: "Patients who are restricted by symptoms, so that less than ordinary activities, even minor ones, produce discomfort. They are, however, comfortable at rest."

The last tests showed that John's heart condition is stable.

We are cardiologists, physicians who care for heart disease patients. There are three of us, and we have a partnership and share offices. Because of the great advances in diagnosing heart trouble, and because heart conditions are by far the greatest health threat in American life, we are a growing specialty.

We are not heart surgeons. If, by examination, we discover the patient requires surgery, we explain his condition to him and his family doctor. We are always honest about any danger involved in surgery, and we carefully explain the risks, helping the patient to make his own decision. Patients who need heart surgery we recommend to outstanding heart surgeons in the country.

As heart specialists, we handle many cases that never reach surgery. Our work generally begins when the family doctor examining his patient finds something amiss, something that affects his heart. Or when his patient is suddenly felled by a heart attack.

If the problem is just developing, we help before it becomes serious. We run a series of tests to pinpoint any problem. If the patient has had a heart attack, with his doctor, we direct his critical care in a Coronary Care Unit of a hospital. We aim to make precise diagnosis and recommendations. When the patient returns to his family doctor, both he and the physician are informed about the condition of his heart, and the physician is in a position to give him better care.

Our practice is primarily hospital oriented. Our examination of a patient goes far beyond the general examination of the family physician. We are heart detectives, tracking down through tests of all kinds—including those using sophisticated equipment—what may be wrong with a patient's heart.

We use cardiac catheterization, and greatly expanded tests, which give us a map of the patient's heart, and that map is the guide by which the surgeon operates when it is necessary.

Let's describe cardiac catheterization. This is an overall term for a number of tests explained in detail in chapter 15.

Briefly—in a cardiac catheterization, a tube is inserted in a blood vessel of the arm or leg, and passed into the heart. Dye is injected through the catheter, allowing us by means of the most sophisticated still and action photography, to make a map of the patient's heart as the dye outlines each of the blood vessels. This is how we discover whether there is a narrowing in any of the coronary arteries, which may be a prelude to a heart attack, or whether there is trouble in any one of the valves which govern the circulatory system's blood flow, and whether a problem requires surgery.

It is a very sophisticated procedure, performed with special equipment in the radiology or cardiology division of a hospital, where every safeguard is at hand in case of any possible emergency.

All patient records are kept in our offices. This routine dates back to 1964, when Marshall Franklin first started his private practice. Marshall Franklin was one of the first cardiologists to set up a catheterization laboratory in a community hospital, in Connecticut.

After we see patients in our office, we give them a verbal report. We dictate reports to the referring physician, providing him with a written record of the consultation, including our opinions and recommendations.

We use a kind of question and answer form for patients who may not quite understand their situation.

"Take a sheet of ruled paper," we tell the patient. "On the left side, ask your questions. Leave enough space on the right side for our answers."

We take care of this in our office, and it works out well. If we had to dictate answers for every question that would come up in an individual case, we would get bogged down in overwhelming paperwork.

We snatch some time in the office to discuss each other's patients and their management, especially when we are following many sick patients all at the same time. At night, we have a three-way telephone conference which often runs two hours or more. We have a telephone adapter in each of our homes, allowing us to talk simultaneously as if we were in the same room.

Each of us has participated in designing, setting up and managing coronary and intermediate care units in the hospitals we service. This includes ordering and testing very expensive equipment.

We join in vital cardiac training programs with physicians, nurses and technicians in various hospitals, such as teaching Cardio-Pulmonary Resuscitation for ambulance corps, police and firemen. We lecture to various service groups—Rotary, Kiwanis, Lions, Exchange Clubs—on the recent advances in heart disease, because the knowledge explosion in cardiology is fantastic. It is important that the layman understand that today we can lower the killers—cholesterol and triglycerides—(see chapter 11), control high blood pressure and diabetes, fight obesity. This book tells the story in full.

Patients say:

"I've got chest pains. Indigestion, maybe. How can I be sure it isn't my heart?"

"My family doctor said even if I cut down on cholesterol, my body will make more. I'm the type. So why should I be miserable and deprive myself of steak and French fries?"

"Isn't this cholesterol bit part of growing old? It's natural for the heart to give out when you're old. You gotta die of something. So what's the big deal?"

"Doc, you say, Angie, stop smoking. Don't eat pasta. So

look at my neighbor. Kept his weight, no cigarettes, no beer. So last week, I went to his wake."

"What can one do with heredity like mine? My grandfather died at 40. So did my father. I may as well live it up while I can."

"You say a woman's estrogen hormones protect her heart? What happens after the change of life?"

"What the hell are you doctors doing with all the contributions for the Heart Fund? Why can't you find a simple formula to cure us of heart disease?"

The questions come from all our patients. The man sent to us for a checkup that may or may not indicate heart problems, the woman in the flush of her menopause, bewildered by the hormones that are making a battleground of her body, the anxious family and friends.

The cardiologist can use the newest weapons on hand, which weren't known even five years ago. He can keep up with new inventions that make yesterday's techniques obsolete. But his patient must listen to the answers.

Never before has so much been written about the heart. We are in the midst of a heart disease epidemic. This year, more than a million Americans will be stricken with heart attacks and about 675,000 will die, nearly half before they reach a hospital. Who of us has not had at least one member of the family or a friend touched by coronary heart disease? And if you are now 40 years old, your life expectancy is actually no greater than that of a man or woman who managed to reach the same birthday in 1900. To many of us between the ages of 25 and 65, death is apt to come not through guns, car smashups, or other accidents, but through diseases of the heart.

Our contemporary American life style has contributed to the state of our arteries. The young man lolling before his television screen, a can of beer and a cigarette by his side, knows the score of the Dallas Cowboys, but as for his cholesterol level, forget it. And Sunday, after no exercise all week, he stands in line for a couple of hours to tee off, plays a frustrating eighteen holes in the midday sun, rewards himself with several martinis and a high cholesterol dinner. He ends up fatigued, sowing the seeds of future disease in his coronary tree.

"It's as if we're all thumbing our noses at nature," a patient told us recently, "saying, 'It can't happen to me.' "

It can—and is more likely to happen to some people than others. You inherit a certain risk factor for coronary disease if other members of your family have died of it at an early age, in their 30s or 40s.

You inherit a risk factor if your family has a tendency to high blood pressure.

You are in the "Danger, watch it!" area if your blood tests show lipid (fat) abnormalities, such as high cholesterol and triglycerides.

You may be in for trouble if you are considerably overweight. An overweight person must carry extra pounds all day long, forcing the heart to do more work. Returning to normal weight can be the deciding factor in success or failure of a program aimed at decreasing the frequency of anginal episodes, and lowering blood pressure.

You may be more vulnerable to coronary heart disease if you have gout or if you are a heavy cigarette smoker. And if your job is sedentary. And if you are subject to strain and emotional tension in your business or private life.

Ten years ago, we knew little about risk factors. Today, we can pinpoint them.

If you happen to have two or more of them, you and your physician should embark on a regime to help counteract any future dangers. This won't guarantee you a cardiac-proof old age. But it will stave off the factors that seem to bring on heart attacks. And even if you should have a heart attack, your chances of surviving and living a reasonably normal life are considerably enhanced. Tests have shown that people who begin to take care of themselves early in life have many more years free of coronary distress than those who ignore the risk factors. Their attacks, if they do happen, are less severe. Recovery chances are much more optimistic.

If you already have a heart condition, other diseases may aggravate it. You are vulnerable to future risk if there is *diabetes mellitus* in your background. A slow thyroid is a hazard because it may exacerbate the heart condition. On the other hand, an overactive thyroid makes the heart work harder and faster, and in a patient with arteriosclerosis, we want to reduce the work load. Proper thyroid medication can make management of the heart problem easier.

The list is long. Gall bladder disease can trigger anginal episodes. Lung problems make heart disease more difficult to treat. Of course, these additional situations do not occur in every patient, but when they are pinpointed and helped, both patient and doctor feel better.

Anything that causes the heart of a patient to work harder increases its need for nourishing blood. Emotional upsets, fatigue, too much exertion, excessive food, sexual intercourse, cold weather, can all precipitate angina. It makes sense then, for the patient not to tackle two or three of these hazards at one time.

In summary, we recommend that our patients do not make love out of doors in a blizzard after a seven-course steak dinner at the end of a hard work day.

Prevention for everyone

Okay. The doctor has told you that it is arteriosclerosis. Hardening of the arteries. What about the future? Is it going to get better—or worse? What about those narrowings? Must they continue to deteriorate?

We cannot answer these questions which are put to us so often, but some others we can. Arteriosclerosis is a chronic disease. Like arthritis. Or diabetes. Once the individual has it, it doesn't go away. The narrowings that already exist cannot be dissolved by any techniques known today. There have been reports that they have lessened, but these are so rare that they are medical curiosities.

Can we help prevent arteriosclerosis in the heart as well as in other places in the body? We do know what the risk factors are, and the chapters that follow give the salient facts about how to eliminate them. In addition:

Check up on blood pressure. If it is elevated, the doctor can help you bring it down by medication and proper diet.

Avoid tension.

Get adequate rest and relaxation.

A physical conditioning program with aerobic exercise is necessary. Continue, even if it is hard in the beginning.

Plan on living. We sometimes meet people who have emotionally geared themselves to die. Each day they live deepens their depression. Therefore, we say, don't plan on dying, because if you do, and live, you're in real trouble.

The person with no heart problem may not be interested in such a rigorous program. But he may feel differently if he has a heart attack later in life. Although we can guarantee nothing, prevention is a good bet. We try to follow these precepts ourselves. With considerable difficulty, we may add.

So we must try to keep every heart muscle fiber we were born with. Each is priceless. We feel modern methods allow us to anticipate a heart attack in many patients. Modern treatment can relieve symptoms and for many, avert heart damage.

Sometimes, after the three of us have spent a week in Emergency Rooms, Coronary Care Units, making rounds, dictating patient reports, and consulting, we feel like the old Puritan preacher, Cotton Mather, who hurled thunderbolts of Thou Shalt Nots at his sinning congregation.

We check our patients with careful clinical followups, with treadmill exercise electrocardiograms, so that early deterioration may be detected before it causes trouble. When a patient has suffered damage to one surface of his heart, he won't be able to tolerate damage to another surface as well as if his heart were normal. What we tell the patient in the most diplomatic way is simple. Look, friend, your heart is scarred, but you survived. It's not what it used to be. But it's still got plenty of mileage left, provided you treat it right. And that usually means a new way of living.

If he accepts the suggestions and goes on the program we've arranged for him, we're inclined to be optimistic about his chances.

Bob A. was typical of our cardiac patients. He recovered from a massive myocardial infarction with the kind of depression that is usual in coronary victims. His first thought was: "My life is over."

Even after he was convinced that his heart muscle was stronger than he thought, the other problems loomed up, equally frightening.

"This new way of life you talk about," he said to Dr. Krauthamer, who sat on his bed, talking to him. "What about my obligations to my family?"

"You'll meet them. Modified to accommodate your new life style."

"What about sex? I'm only 43. And my wife—"

"Listen, Bob. When you are able to climb two flights of stairs, you'll be ready."

Patients are inclined to fall into a post-coronary depression for several reasons. One is that they fail to realize that modern techniques can help almost all patients. The majority can return to a nearly normal life. We have found that once a patient understands, he tolerates his condition more easily.

This book can be a guidebook for the heart. It is not intended to replace or alter the physician's advice. A heart patient's best friend is his competent family physician. Each heart varies in some degree; it is important for the patient to have the attention of a doctor who is thoroughly familiar with him.

Chapter 2

Is this a heart attack?

CHET L.:

He was very much like other middle-aged executives who boarded the commuter train every day. At 7:05 that Tuesday morning in April, Chet L. parked his small foreign car opposite the railroad tracks and sprinted across the cracked asphalt to the station. He could count on the express being at least fifteen minutes behind schedule, which gave him time to grab a cup of coffee and a Danish at the station counter. He ate standing up, exchanging small talk with fellow commuters, men like himself who had begun to ride earlier trains in order to get a seat for the fifty-minute ordeal to Manhattan. He gulped the coffee, strong and bitter, and ignored the Danish after the first bite. He lit a cigarette, his fifth since getting up. The men packed around him in the stuffy old station had, for all their good suits and topcoats, the commuter syndrome—they were puffy-eyed from lack of sleep, slightly paunchy, and restless with the energy of profitable time schedules.

The express straggled in. No seats unless you sprinted up front. Chet dashed to the first car, already foggy with cigarette smoke, and grabbed a single seat facing backwards, which he detested. He lit a cigarette from the stub of the other. The Danish lay just below his esophagus, a heavy lump, pressing against his breastbone. He should dispense with his topcoat. It was a burden. But he was content just to sit.

Steam was billowing from the radiators. When it was zero outside, it was scarcely warmer than that in the coaches. But on a warm spring day, they blasted you with heat. He lit a fresh cigarette, drawing the smoke deep into his chest and exhaling, as though to fumigate the miseries that assailed him. Whenever he had time for morning coffee at home, he took a couple of pep pills, which helped him through the first hours. But this morning Jane had overslept. The PTA meeting at the Country Day School had dragged to midnight. There was the drive for the new gym and while the Board of Trustees didn't exactly blackmail you into an overgenerous contribution, it was made damn clear that you'd better come across.

He folded the *Times* to the sports page. Just holding the page triggered that twinge in his left arm. Bursitis, probably. Chet was never one for doctors. Last time the executives of his company were screened for health check-ups, he was in Milan on business, and he never bothered to see the doctor. He didn't believe in giving in to himself.

As a rule, he welcomed a busy schedule, and today was going to be hectic. His new assistant, John Blaek, the whiz from the Wharton School of Business, was in the wings, waiting for his big chance. The ride into Grand Central Station tired him, and he was glad to let the crowd precede him. He swallowed a couple of aspirin at the office, but the ache in his shoulder persisted. It was an effort to breeze through the morning meetings with his usual aplomb. During a couple of pre-luncheon double Scotches, he gave an ad agency fellow the bad news that the agency was fired, and felt heartsick himself.

The 2:30 session with his boss dragged. The Old Man never let you forget he started the company during the Depression with nickels and dimes, and he expected the company to show good news on the right side of the ledger, period.

Chet listened with the expected deference. Instead of speaking up, showing facts, he let his superior cow him, and returned to his office frustrated, drained, but reminding himself objectively that $35,000-a-year jobs weren't exactly around these days.

John Blaek was getting ready to leave. His face was gelatinous with sympathy.

Chet was getting his papers together for a meeting with a potential customer. Suddenly, the air seemed too oppressive—he could scarcely breathe.

"John, I have Ed Meadows coming to the Yale Club at 5:30 for drinks. Sit in for me, will you. I forgot I had another appointment."

"You okay?" John asked, taking the papers Chet gave him.

"Sure, I'm okay. What could be wrong?"

"Well, you look bushed."

"I guess I am."

Chet left his office shortly afterwards. He flagged a cab, although it was only four blocks to Grand Central. His weariness couldn't be blamed on spring fever or middle age. This was different, a feeling that something was about to happen.

Even before the diesel engine carried them out of the tunnel into the sooty twilight of Harlem, he began to feel pain. He couldn't blame it on bursitis any longer. He lay back in his seat.

A pincer tightened around his chest. The trip seemed endless. The nausea rose. He took an antacid and chewed it. The heavy pain was high up, like a band gripping him. Finally, the conductor was collecting tickets which meant the station was just ahead.

I've got to hold on, Chet thought. He tightened his jaw and suddenly the pressure on his chest was so excruciating that he didn't have the breath to cry out. The pain was too awful to bear.

A police car was patrolling the station area, so when the conductor and a fellow commuter helped Chet off the train, the police didn't wait for the ambulance but drove him quickly, red lights flashing, to the Emergency Room of the local hospital. A chill wind was blowing, but he was sweating heavily, and his face was gray.

So much in life depends on being at the right place at the right time. The best place for someone with a heart attack is in the Coronary Care Unit, with emergency aid at hand.

Chet was aware of being in a room where many things were happening at once, a stretcher and nurses and a young man in a white coat working on him.

"Are you allergic to any drug?" the man asked, and after Chet shook his head, he felt the prick of a needle, and the fellow said, "You'll feel better in a few minutes."

Another nurse was taking his blood pressure, there were bottles beside the stretcher and an oxygen mask over his face. He was trying to answer the doctor's questions. He had no cardiac history, but he was too weary to answer any more, and they found Jane's number (in case of Emergency) and his family doctor's, and the pain was drifting away, leaving him free but attached to tubes and wires.

When he opened his eyes again, he was in another room. A nurse was wrapping his arm in the blood pressure cuff, watching the mercury.

"Again?" he said, nearly in a whisper.

"Again." She was short, plump and cheery. "Welcome to CCU."

He looked puzzled.

"Dr. Franklin will be here any minute."

DR. FRANKLIN:

What are the symptoms of a heart attack?

Discomfort in the chest. A pressure sensation that varies from a squeezing to an oppressive pain. It may spread to shoulder, arm, neck or jaw. Sometimes, it is accompanied by perspiration. Patients describe it as a cold clammy sweat. They may feel sick to their stomachs. Sometimes shortness of breath is present. Those who have experienced it cannot always describe what they feel, but they know it is serious. It is like nothing the patient has ever known before, a feeling that something cataclysmic is happening. Even when there are few other symptoms, that sense of doom is often there.

What should you do if you think you're having a heart attack? Take no chances! Get to a hospital any way you can, as fast as you can. Have someone call the police or your doctor. Some towns now have mobile coronary ambulances, equipped for the emergency.

Suppose it's in the middle of the night? It doesn't matter. Get help fast. Don't imagine it is indigestion or "something else." Don't be a "nice guy." If you can't reach your doctor, or an ambulance, call the police. *Victims brought to the hospital by ambulance or car immediately after they feel the attack stand a far better chance of surviving than those who wait.*

The only way to reduce mortality from heart attack (myocardial infarction) is to shorten the time span from the moment the person first feels his chest pains and the time he receives initial medical care.

The chief problem is the patient's delay in summoning medical help. Researchers have found that most people who become aware of chest pains seek non-medical advice for "indigestion." They get irrelevant remedies, and the delay is considerable. And often fatal.

The patient who already has had one heart attack takes even longer to seek medical help. Does that surprise you? Denial is so strong in those with heart disease. The delay in one study ranged anywhere from one hour to six.

Fortunately, on-the-spot resuscitation of cardiac arrest victims is being taught throughout the country at Heart Association chapters. It would be wise and life saving for at least one member of each family to know how to perform cardio-pulmonary resuscitation (CPR).

Here is a resume of the steps for emergency resuscitation of a cardiac arrest victim outside the hospital. *Caution:* the following should be undertaken only by those who have completed an approved course in CPR.

1. Check pulse, pupils, and breathing. If there is a pulse and victim is breathing, do nothing except get the victim to the hospital as fast as possible. Check the size of the pupils. Right after cardiac arrest, pupils are dilated. Once adequate resuscitation starts, they shrink.
2. If no pulse or breathing, thump the chest.

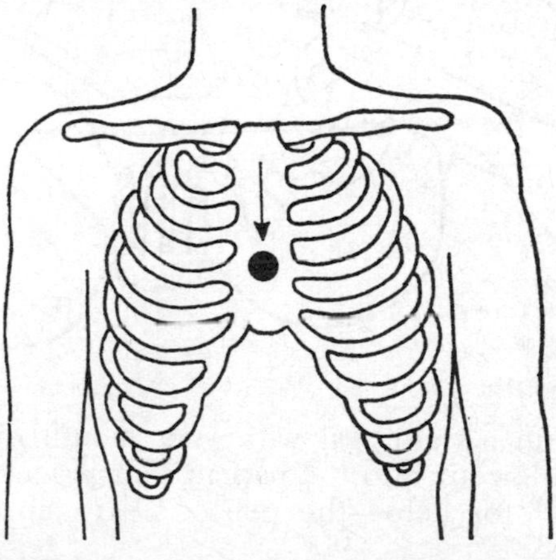

Thump the chest.

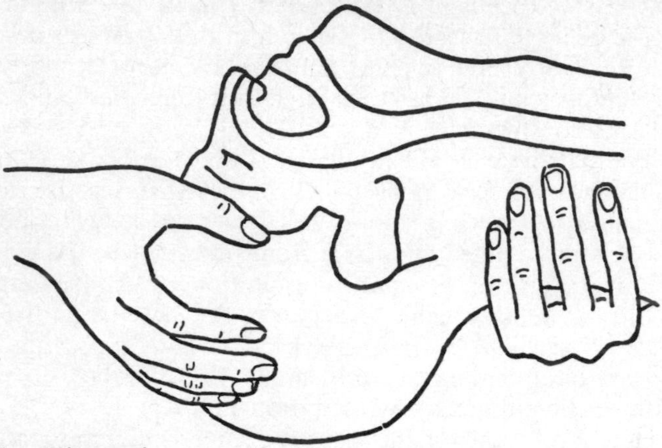

Extend the neck.

3. Immediately check the mouth, clear it of any sputum, object, or false teeth. Once it is clear, pinch the nostrils and extend the patient's neck.

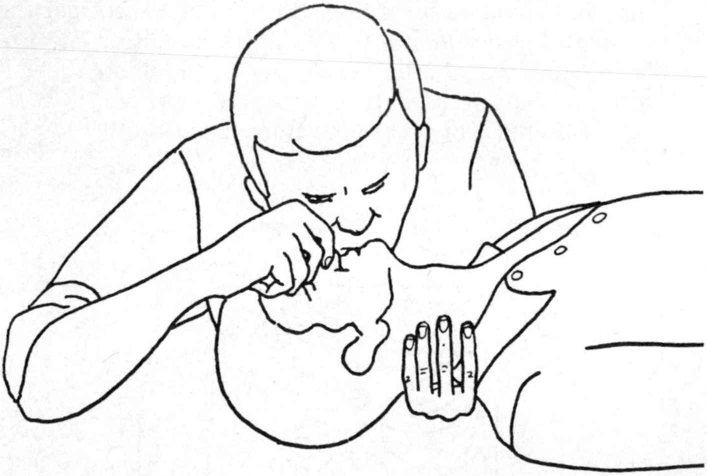

Blow into mouth.

4. Form a tight seal with your mouth over the patient's. Blow air into the patient's air passage.

5. Call for help—the police department or fire department.

6. If you are alone with the patient, compress the chest five times with the heel of your palm placed low on the breast bone and one hand over the other. The chest should be depressed for at least 1½ to 2 inches, once per second. Then shift your position—extend the patient's neck, form a tight seal and again blow air into the mouth. The rate is five compressions to one breath.

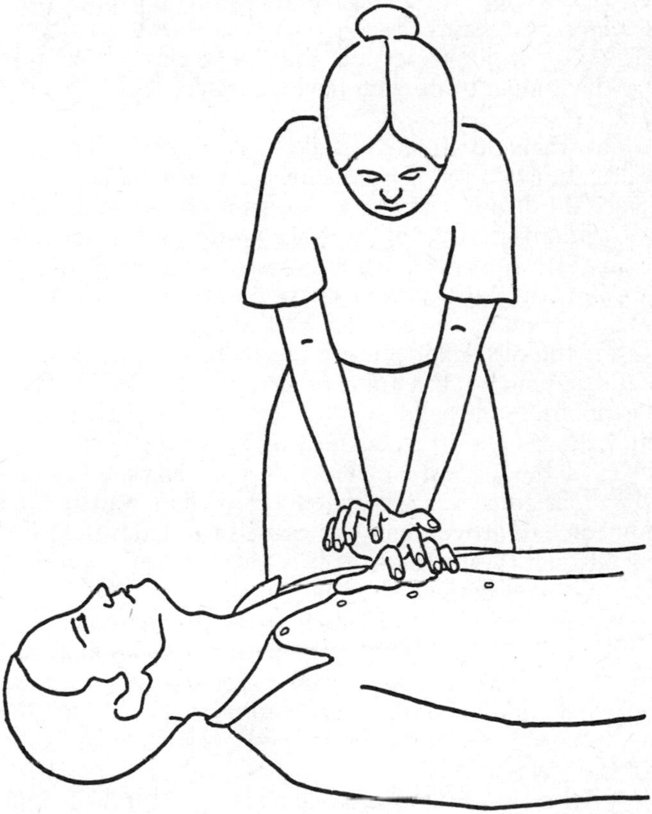

Compress the chest.

Or if you have another person to assist, you should begin chest compression while your assistant performs mouth-to-mouth breathing.

7. Get an ambulance and transport the patient to the hospital while maintaining external cardiac compression and resuscitation. It is important not to stop these two efforts.

Mobile coronary care

Why do so many people with heart attack die suddenly?

A research team working on autopsies of victims discovered that a clot was found in the artery in only 8 to 18 percent of the cases.

It is now thought possible that 85 percent of the people who die suddenly do not have complete blockage of the blood vessel.

Why then do they die suddenly? Probably because of electrical instability of the heart. This means that after the attack, the heart beats in a disorganized fashion. It beats so irregularly that it isn't able to pump blood. Emergency Rooms of a hospital have equipment to regulate the wild beat, but often the patient doesn't arrive there in time.

The researchers believed that the dying heart might be saved if the physician could bring these life-saving facilities to the patient at the time of catastrophe. Electric shock (via defibrillator paddles) applied to the patient's chest could change the irregular beating to a regular rhythm. In this case, the patient's chances of survival would be good.

Precious time was lost when the patient waited for the ambulance to arrive, then was carried to the hospital Emergency Room. With traffic as it is today, even an ambulance has a problem getting clearance on the road. The research teams came to these conclusions: From the time the patient called his doctor to the time the patient was brought to the Emergency Room, a significant amount of precious time elapsed. A mobile coronary care ambulance could eliminate the doctor's delay, the Emergency Room delay and the admissions delay.

An Irish physician originally set up the first mobile coronary care unit with monitoring equipment, and physicians as part of the ambulance corps.

This is how it works: Members who ride the coronary ambulance are trained in CPR and care of the cardiac patient. The team answers an emergency call, arrives at the patient's house or wherever he happens to be stricken.

Before moving the patient, the team attaches electrodes to his chest, an electrocardiogram (ECG) monitoring his heartbeat is transmitted constantly to the hospital's Coronary Care Unit, where a nurse or doctor will interpret it on a monitor.

If the electrocardiogram is stable, showing no electrical alteration of activity that might be life threatening, the patient will have an intravenous started, he will have oxygen available and will be transported to the hospital. If there are signs of an imminent catastrophe, such as heart failure, cardiac arrest, appropriate medications can be given to the patient while he is still in the ambulance. The Mobile Coronary Care Unit is a tremendous step forward, and such units exist in many cities today.

A number of patients in a special study were later interviewed in the hospital. Between 50 to 75 percent had gone to their physicians two weeks before their attack and complained of not feeling right. When the doctor found nothing wrong in an electrocardiogram (and it was invariably normal), the patient began to feel like a hypochondriac.

In Seattle, the University of Washington has expanded the lifesaving facilities in its football stadium. It has been found that the excitement of a football game may trigger heart attacks in spectators. To give instant first aid, security officers and ushers bring the heart victim to one of four first aid stations, staffed by a physician and Red Cross volunteers, trained in cardio-pulmonary resuscitation. A fan known to have a cardiac condition is urged to check in before the game. The stadium and Red Cross have achieved an extraordinary record there.

The time will come when this type of emergency first aid will be available in all public places: sports arenas, planes, commuter trains and large offices and factories.

In many cities, emergency service personnel are being trained in cardio-pulmonary resuscitation, especially policemen and firemen, many of them volunteers or members of an auxiliary force.

Public awareness, however, remains the key to survival.

Ten years ago, even if you reached the hospital in the first hour after your heart attack, you still had a 30 percent chance of dying. Today, if you get to a hospital quickly, the mortality risk is only 15 percent.

This miraculous improvement is due to the Coronary Care Unit. Those patients now saved might a decade ago have developed a sudden fatal chaotic heart rhythm. This danger is greatest just when the heart attack occurs and in the first hours afterwards. Today, if it happens in the hospital, it can be treated, in some cases even prevented.

Chapter 3

Coronary care

CHET L.:
A hand-printed sign is pasted on the glass panel of the swinging door that leads to the Coronary Care Unit:

IMMEDIATE FAMILY ONLY. TWO TO A BEDSIDE. FIVE MINUTES.

It was quiet in the big room where Chet lay. Chet found it peaceful, except for the nurse who checked his blood pressure every two hours and watched the monitor beside him. She noted whether he was sweating, chilled, or short of breath. She asked questions: Do you have any chest pains? Did you have a bowel movement?

If there was one thing Chet detested, it was the bedpan. To him it was the final humiliation, a regression to infancy. So he was allowed, after 24 hours, to use the commode by his bed, but it was the only activity allowed him. His diet was a far cry from his business lunches. On the first day, juice, jello, and broth. It didn't matter, he wasn't interested in food.

The technician came every day with a machine and took his electrocardiogram (ECG). A portable X-ray unit was trundled in. The nurses lifted him up the first day so the technician could slide the X-ray plate underneath his body.

When it was quiet in the ward, the nurses stopped by to talk and answer questions, and he learned a good deal about the Coronary Care Unit. There were six beds here, separated into private cubicles, radiating around the Central Nursing Station, like the spokes of a giant wheel. Each patient's cubicle was glassed in, with provisions for drapes or blinds to come down over the glass.

Every bed in the Unit was occupied. Its patients seemed plugged into the world of tomorrow. After Chet had been wheeled up to the Unit, he was transferred to a bed. Two nurses shaved small areas of his chest which were then washed with an aromatic solution. Adhesive electrodes were attached to his chest and led to a television-like oscilloscope displaying his electrocardiogram. Chet noted that his electrocardiogram, together with that of the other patients, was transmitted to the Central Nursing Station, where doctors and nurses could constantly observe them on a battery of identical monitors there.

DR. KRAUTHAMER:
In the Coronary Care Unit, the vigil for coronary patients goes on 24 hours a day. It is a vigil composed of tubes and wires that draw their findings from the patient's body and translate them into signals at the bedside and the Central Nursing Station. The patient's heartbeat is each nurse's responsibility. The patient will never have a more dedicated guard.

Round-the-clock monitoring of sick hearts makes it possible for the staff to foretell an approaching crisis by the action displayed on the monitor. And to treat it swiftly if it does occur. It is possible for a doctor or nurse, simply by pressing a button, to print out tracings of any unusual heart action that is seen on the monitor.

Electrocardiographic events can also be recalled by a recorded storage system. If a serious irregularity of heartbeat occurs, the cardiologist wants to be able to study it in detail as well as to see what preceded this crisis. The memory system makes this possible. Each patient's oscilloscope also has an alarm system. If no heartbeats register on the oscilloscope screen for a number of seconds, the alarm triggers a bell and a paper tape writes out the ECG. A nurse hurries to the patient.

The alarm also goes off if the patient's heartbeat climbs *above* a certain rate, or falls *below* a certain rate. When the alarm sounds, the memory system freezes, preserving 20 to 60 seconds before the alarm has sounded. In this way, the doctor can play back what happened before and study it.

All kinds of other equipment are carefully arranged around the Coronary Care Unit. Defibrillators, those miraculous heart restorers. A portable image intensifier (special X-ray unit) for inserting pacemaker wires into a patient's heart. Equipment for monitoring the pressure of the central venous and arterial system. Pulmonary equipment to help the lungs. And medications at the Central Nursing Station.

The Coronary Care Unit is kept at a comfortable temperature by climate control. Some hospitals permit music for its tranquilizing effect on cardiac patients. Richard Rodgers is preferable to Mick Jagger.

The Coronary Care Unit was devised by Dr. Hughes Day in the early 1960s, and in most hospitals, coronary equipment and care is centralized in a separate unit. Accident victims or other seriously ill patients will be admitted to a separate Intensive Care Unit. In some other hospitals, the two are combined.

In CCU, the patient is examined by an intern or resident at least twice daily, and also by his own physician. Other doctors often make rounds, one in charge, designated by the Chief of the Unit. Not every physician is equally conversant with the problems a heart attack can engender. Physicians who care for CCU patients have special training in coronary care. Only by cardiology training and working in CCU can this experience be gained. Many doctors, to preserve the integrity of private practice, have donated their time to pick up the fine points of cardiology, which will be helpful to them even in general practice. Some physicians without training in coronary care, often ask a cardiologist to assume the care of their heart attack patient until he is out of danger and leaves CCU.

CHET L.:

The heart patient, like Chet, lying in the womb of his bed, is apt to feel isolated, helpless and terribly alone. Particularly if the nurse screens him off when another patient is being attended.

"When can I get out of here?" is a familiar cry in Coronary Care.

"Another 24 hours," said Dr. Franklin, who had just read Chet's most recent ECG and checked on his X-rays. It looked like a normal recovery from a myocardial infarction. X-rays were taken to determine if there was enlargement of the heart or evidence of heart weakness, which would be indicated by pulmonary congestion—backing up of the blood into the vessels of the lungs. But Chet was free from this danger. His blood tests were returning to normal. His spirits were pretty good, too.

Much better than during the first couple of days. In the beginning, they kept him sedated because of anxiety and pain. He was aware of much movement around him, but he was far out on his own hazy planet. But he knew he'd had a heart attack. Struck by a coronary thrombosis, he wanted to live. Desperately.

Time counted in commuter trains, business offices, private luncheon clubs, stockholders' meetings.

Time counted differently in the Coronary Care Unit, where you were swathed in sheets, poked with needles, hooked up to oxygen and monitors, like a mechanical man. Chet did as he was told by the cheerful nurses, and he drifted in and out of a light sleep, and sometimes Jane was at his bed, trying to look calm, but with panic in her set face, like the pictures of wives in the Accident and Health Insurance ads.

It was peaceful in the Unit at the hours between dusk and dark. The nurses made their rounds, bringing fresh water, letting down the backrest so the patients were ready for the night. The night nurse came to his bedside with medication. Chet had been watching the oscilloscope screen. It seemed to hold a special fascination in the darkened room. He could not take his eyes away from the jagged pattern of his heartbeats across the monitor's face.

Ellen, one of the younger nurses, had told him that some men with engineering backgrounds liked to play games with their monitors. They could change the pattern on the oscilloscope with muscular movements.

"One of our patients, a real pugnacious fellow, said, 'You think you're all so smart. Well, I can change the tracing and you won't even know what's going on.' "

She added that some doctors take this as a sign the patient is getting better, although others feel it is part of the denial syndrome. ("You see, there's nothing wrong with me.")

Some actually believe that the oscilloscope is making their heart go. If the tracings on the machine cease for a few seconds, they are convinced their hearts have stopped beating, even though they are breathing normally.

DR. FRANKLIN:
The cardiologist looks on the CCU nurse as his partner. On other nursing floors, the nurses aren't allowed to give the patient medication without the doctor's written or telephoned permission. The CCU nurse has considerably more authority, since there is more danger of a catastrophe (such as a cardiac arrest) in this Unit than anywhere else in the hospital. She is expected to follow the protocol for taking care of the patient under these circumstances, since the balance of life at these rare moments is so delicate that a few minutes spent in tracking down a resident or a doctor might determine whether or not a life is saved.

To the cardiologist, the management of the cardiac patient without the Coronary Care nurse is impossible.

Coronary Care nurses are specially trained. They exercise both nursing skills and an instinct for warm communications with their patients. They read electrocardiograms, give medicines intravenously, use the defibrillator paddles.

What are their qualifications? How are they chosen?

They are all graduate nurses and mostly on the young side, perhaps a year or two out of training, comfortable with their medical-surgical training, but not content to rest on their knowledge.

"The girls who are taking courses for Coronary Care work are a fantastic group," says Rebecca Marcus, herself a registered nurse and an in-service instructor at a local hospital. "They are the most motivated individuals I've ever met. They feel that everything we say to them is gospel, because a single fact may save a patient's life. They study unbelievably hard."

The typical Coronary Care nurse isn't afraid of modern techniques and new equipment; as a matter of fact, she is attracted to them. She is chosen for CCU because of her interest in the work. She may come to the courses with some apprehension but with an awesome sense of responsibility. She feels that she is going to learn to save lives. She has both pride and fear: that she must live up to whatever goal she has set for herself, but may not be able to.

"The art of nursing has nearly been lost for various reasons," a head nurse said recently. "We have to recapture it in Coronary Care. A nurse makes patients feel better, and by making them feel better, she feels better. There should be a bond between nurse and patient, almost a psychic feeling that fortifies the patient's will to live."

However, as the nurse becomes involved in the healing process, it can be painful for the patient. He looks to her for comfort, but she gives him injections or an exhausting treatment. In the very process of helping him recover, she has to cause him some discomfort.

ELLEN R., Coronary Care Nurse:
She was on the general nursing staff for two years before deciding to try out for the Coronary Care Unit. A graduate of a fine nursing school attached to a university hospital, she was young (22), personable, conscientious and dedicated. Her only problem in dealing with severely sick patients was her own fear of death.

Instructors explore the area of fear with the nurses. In discussion groups, nurses are made aware of what the patient may be feeling if he thinks he faces death. The young nurse must gain a profound empathy with the cardiac patient, to understand the frustrating problems of a man or woman cut down in the prime of life, at the height of his career, concerned that he may not be able to continue his role. It's difficult for her to understand what a crisis this is for him in every aspect of his life. In CCU, the nurse must spend a good deal of time with her patient. She talks to him; she attends him. The mere presence of the nurse makes the patient feel good. This is the mystique of the nurse.

It is always important for the nurse to know what the physician has told the patient. Good communications between patient and nurse is important, because of its importance to the patient's recovery. And this is a goal toward which doctor and nurse work as a team. If the nurse knows what the doctor has told his patient about his condition, it makes her lot easier. She doesn't have to be quite so cautious when she talks with the patient.

Patients are often given American Heart Association booklets, and nurses discuss the information with them. These booklets become a point of reference and reinforcement.

Why did it happen to me? Is it apt to happen again? How can I avoid a next time?

The cardiologist's advice is vital, and the nurse's approach helps make the difference in the patient's reaction to the attack.

The patient's emotional defense is frequently denial. Often a negative kind of denial. *I will not take medicine. I did not have a coronary. There is nothing wrong with me. I don't know why I'm here.*

The nurse finds this sort of negative behavior hard to accept because she wants to help the patient. Sometimes she has to restrain him physically as he tries to get out of bed.

"One way of helping the patient," Ellen says, "is to go back over what happened to him. '*Why did you come here? You had a pain, right? Did the doctor tell you what might be causing this pain?*' If he will only admit it may be 'my heart' you can begin to work with him. Sometimes I will say, '*Look, if you had a broken arm, you could put it in a cast and it would mend. You can't put your heart in a cast. The only way to mend your heart is to rest it. Then you can use it again.*' "

Ellen says: "I think we're all aware of the fact that a heart patient goes through many phases, almost like Shakespeare's Seven Ages of Man. There is the shock of a heart attack, the sense of helplessness, like an infant, the feeling of inertia and despondency, a kind of *I'm doomed* attitude. And then, gradually, a feeling that the end of the world hasn't come, that he is recovering."

Sometimes he decides prematurely that he is well enough to go home. He simply will not accept the limitations on what he can do. One patient told Ellen, who was giving him a shave, that when he felt better he would shave her legs for her.

"When they start kidding us," Ellen says, "or complaining, we know they are improving."

A beautiful process of education goes on in the hospital, between patient, nurse and family. The gap in patient-family relations is bridged by the nurse. Sometimes the nurse is asked, "How can the family help?" The nurses like to meet the patient's family because it gives them insight into the patient. Then they try to reassure the family, knowing it's an alien, frightening world to them. The nurse feels more comfortable once she knows what the physician has told the family about the patient's condition. It's important to relate the patient's progress to them. For instance, that he had his lunch sitting up in a chair and stayed there for a half hour. They all look so eagerly for small signs of progress and are so encouraged by them. If they look worried, the nurse often spends time reassuring them.

The nurse is particularly alert to the wife's behavior. If a couple has been married long, they know each other well. If the wife is upset, the patient will sense her mood and his condition is apt to deteriorate. The nurse can tell if there is disharmony between husband and wife by watching the monitor and the cardiogram strips. Should the patient become upset, the nurse will manage to get the person who upset him out of the Unit quickly, but smoothly. The staff has tremendous anger toward anyone who gives grief to the patient and puts him in jeopardy.

When a wife's presence is beneficial to the patient, the nurse may allow her to sit at her husband's bedside, not talking, just to be there.

DR. FRANKLIN:
Four days after his heart attack, Chet was moved from the Coronary Care Unit to the Intermediate Care Unit.

Intermediate Care is a new and growing concept in progressive patient management. It is a kind of half-way house between Coronary Care and general nursing care. Here, there is still special equipment and trained personnel, but each nurse cares for more patients. The patients walk around. ECG monitoring continues, but via telemetry—the patient carries a small portable radio-transmitter which sends his ECG to a central monitoring station. If something goes wrong, a nurse checks on the patient immediately.

Each morning, the world was new for Chet. His simple privileges gave him enormous satisfaction. He again learned the satisfaction of shaving and feeding himself.

He was learning what a complex and fascinating organ his heart is.

"You're making progress, Chet," Dr. Franklin told him. "We'll let you sit in a chair today. Try it for fifteen to thirty minutes, twice, maybe three times."

"Oh, I can do better than that," Chet said.

Yet after fifteen minutes, his bed looked inviting. When the nurse asked later in the afternoon if he'd like to sit up again, he said, "No, thanks." That night, he was severely depressed.

Yet the next day, fifteen minutes wasn't so much. He remained in his chair for the full thirty minutes, pleased with himself. On the third day, he was sitting up three times without any problems. We were pleased, then.

He was also warned never to strain himself while having a bowel movement and put on a laxative program. He felt more comfortable and less tired. It was an important factor in his recovery. On the ninth day, he was given bathroom privileges. He still washed and shaved himself in bed.

The second week marked another stride forward, as he was moved to a general nursing floor. He was now allowed to get out of bed more often, to move around the pleasant private room.

Physicians often vary in their recommendations. Some mobilize the patient the second day after his attack. Others may hold off until the end of the third week. Even when the patient is on the general nursing floor, he is watched carefully for any signs of recurrent chest pains.

We are familiar with Chet's personality type. Our practice has included the care and follow-up procedures for a staggering number of executives, men in their mid-40s, or early 50s, at their peak of productive powers, caught by a heart attack.

Yet it may not happen again. It is difficult to prognosticate, but the person who follows his doctor's advice about rest, exercise, diet, takes his prescribed medication, and modifies his life style, has a good chance to avoid new attacks.

The problem is that most men of Chet's nature and temperament return to the old job.

We believe that Chet will follow prescribed medical orders, at least in the beginning. He was a cooperative patient. No matter how many inner conflicts he might have experienced, he is a sensible, disciplined man, unlike other patients who promise everything and return to their old self-destructive patterns. They end up with recurrent symptoms and often second heart attacks.

But even the most disciplined patient will grow lax sometimes. If he is feeling well, he is apt to cheat a bit at first, later a little more, especially if there are no repercussions. It's human nature. As doctors, we counsel and advise. But in the end, it is up to the patient. He can save himself if he has a goal—to survive.

Chapter 4

Cardiac crisis

ALEX W.:

He is the theater critic for a major television network, and he came into Coronary Care the day Chet left. The nurses often listened to his 11:00 P.M. report in the Nurses Room. They consider him attractive, with a kind of Peter O'Toole élan. He is witty, without the stinging attitude of some of the lesser critics. So the nurses were all excited when he was brought into the hospital one afternoon.

It was Sunday in early August. Alex and his wife left Larchmont for a sail on Long Island Sound with a couple of friends. The men were fishing, and Alex's wife had just opened the thermos of Bloody Marys when Alex had a strike. His battle with the 15-pound bluefish shattered the calm of the Sound.

As he was reeling in his trophy, he wrenched his shoulder. For an excruciating moment, he thought he had dislocated it, as the pain shot up into his neck and jaw. A couple of aspirins and a Bloody Mary didn't help. Nedda, his wife, insisted on putting in at the Cove. At the marina, a police car was cruising along the boardwalk, and the officers drove Nedda and Alex to the hospital.

"It's nothing much," Alex said to his friends in a whisper, as he was helped into the car. He was conscious throughout the ride.

Dr. Tai, who was on call that day, had already been summoned. The officers had radioed ahead to the hospital. Electrocardiogram and tests confirmed an acute heart attack.

During Alex's first night in CCU, Dr. Tai checked him twice and assured Nedda that her husband's condition was stable.

The following three days proved uneventful. Alex was making progress. He no longer needed a blood pressure check every two hours; he was able to sit on a chair by the bed. He was well enough to be transferred to Intermediate Care.

The next morning, Alex looked pale and restless. Ellen, the nurse, noticed he was rubbing his chest, though there were no changes on the monitor. She knew from experience that you had to drag symptoms from a male patient.

"You look a little uncomfortable," Ellen said. "Is anything bothering you?"

"Not a thing," Alex said politely.

She didn't have much to go by because he wouldn't complain. Few of the male patients did.

The nurses from Intermediate Care often visited the CCU and were always helpful in making the transition smoothly.

"Are you sure I'm ready to leave here?" Alex asked. He felt safe in CCU.

10:45 A.M. Time for Alex's transfer. He tried to joke with Ellen as she got him ready. She was helping him with his robe when it happened. He suddenly gasped, color drained from his face, and his breathing stopped.

"Code 99," Ellen cried out. "*Code* 99."

DR. TAI:

Crisis is a way of life in a hospital. The staff is accustomed to life and death situations, to perilous moments when the balance is in jeopardy and no one knows, in spite of will, medications, instant help, how it will come out.

"Code 99" is the emergency signal at two hospitals where we practice. As it goes out over the loudspeakers, fear and tension are conveyed, not by the disembodied voice, but by the call itself. Somewhere in the hospital, a heart has suddenly stopped beating. The patient is in cardiac arrest.

The call over the loudspeaker is a summons.

Alex lies on the bed, pale and without pulse. There are

four minutes in which the blood circulation must be restored or the brain suffers irreparable damage. Ellen makes a fist and thumps his chest. A strong thump. Sometimes it is enough to start the heart's action. Not now.

Meanwhile the cardiologist, anesthesiologist, a therapist from Respiratory Therapy, converge on the Unit. One of the Coronary Care nurses wheels over the "crash cart" of medications that the cardiologist might need. The defibrillator unit to shock the dying heart back to life is waiting.

A few moments have sped by. The tall rangy young man who is a respiratory therapist begins the mouth-to-mouth resuscitation, keeping sequence in time with the external cardiac compression. The anesthesiologist inserts a tube (intubates) into Alex's throat to keep the breathing passages clear.

Dr. Tai comes racing into the Unit. He looks at the monitor and takes the defibrillator paddles from the nurse—the paddles have already been moistened with conductive jelly—and with the staff out of the way, he gives Alex an electric shock. The other measures are resumed immediately after the shock: external cardiac compression, breathing by the anesthesiologist's bag attached to the tube in the windpipe. The staff tense and intent, willing the heart to begin its normal rhythm. ECG electrodes on Alex's chest conduct the heart's electrical impulses and display it on the oscilloscope.

Three and a half minutes. Alex's heart has taken over. It is beating on its own, a normal beat, no longer reacting wildly.

We had set up a whole protocol for such an emergency, and they had started at the top with the first action and going on down the line. The protocol is a kind of recipe for treating a classic heart arrest.

ELLEN:

"We did it!" She was glowing. She was sitting in the Nurses' Room with Bette, the licensed practical nurse, and Steloff, the resident. Everything had gone off like an exquisitely mechanized watchworks.

"Even Dr. Tai couldn't find fault this time," Steloff

said, a bit smugly. Dr. Tai is a perfectionist. "It's a life you're dealing with," he always reminded them. "A human being."

Later, Ellen went over to Alex's bed to remind Nedda, his wife, that her time was up.

And that's when Nedda looked at her husband with something like awe tinged with fear and whispered, "Alex, you're like Lazarus . . ."

Alex grimaced and turned his head away.

DR. TAI:

The two most important catastrophes that require urgent attention are:

1) Ventricular tachycardia—a form of very rapid heartbeat (see page 61).

2) Ventricular fibrillation—a chaotic, disorganized heart action.

Cardiac arrest, such as Alex's, is usually due to ventricular fibrillation.

In ventricular tachycardia the patient may feel a pounding in his chest. Symptoms vary, depending on the type of heart disease he has. The heart is racing, so there isn't enough time for the heart chambers to fill with blood, nor enough time for it to be pumped to maintain circulation. The patient may begin to suffer chest pains, faint or go into congestive heart failure with fluid building up in the lungs.

What is the treatment?

a) Medication given intravenously.

b) If the patient is in dire trouble with rapidly falling blood pressure, electric shock to the heart is indicated. Should the patient be partly awake a rapidly acting sedative is given first.

This rapid heartbeat often leads into the irregular heart action known as ventricular fibrillation. Or fibrillation may occur spontaneously. In either case the patient is unconscious because there is no effective output of blood. The heart muscle is disorganized and writhing. Every individual muscle bundle of the heart is behaving like an anarchist. There is no flow of blood to the brain.

No time for hesitation. The defibrillator.

How the defibrillator works

The defibrillator is a machine which can be operated from a wall socket but is frequently operated by battery. The decision on how much electrical energy to use rests on the flawless judgment of the person applying the defibrillator. There are two metal paddles, about five inches in diameter. They are usually of polished stainless steel with insulated handles to protect the doctor or nurse applying them from shock.

The two discs are placed firmly on the patient's chest, one over the breast bone, the other to the left of the left nipple. Once applied, and with no one touching the patient, the signal is given. *Fire!*

A button is pressed.

The electrical discharge passes from one paddle to the other, through the heart. The heart stops. The heart doesn't beat at all. For a few seconds. The doctors and nurses are waiting, breathless themselves, for the heart's own natural pacemaker to take over. It is a tense moment.

Then the heart recovers.

This is what happens:

The electric shock causes all the heart's muscle groups to discharge their energy at once. Now the heart's own pacemaker has its chance to send an impulse down and reactivate the heart's beat normally.

If the heartbeat is very rapid, but with harmonious activity, one shock of the defibrillator, discharging the heart's electrical activity all at once, may be enough to cause this focus of rapid activity to grow quiet long enough for the heart's own pacemaker to take over.

Because the patient is seriously ill, there is always a chance that the heart may not respond. If the heart's pacemaker doesn't take over, other procedures for a heart that isn't beating must be instituted. Defibrillation should be performed only by those trained in cardio-pulmonary resuscitation (CPR).

ALEX W.:

"I had a bad dream," he said later, when night was gentle and the Unit dark and protective. Nedda leaned down to kiss him but the oxygen tubes which were restored to his nostrils blocked her.

Denial.

It had not happened to him. It hadn't happened to him. He filed the statement in the computer of his mind, and nothing they would say or his wife would say could shake him. He was angry when Nedda came for her visit, leaned down and kissed him and said, awed and grateful, "Lazarus . . ."

There had been cardiac arrests in CCU during his stay, but they had nothing to do with him. He had simply fainted and everybody got shook up.

When one of his team at the television network dropped in and tried to question him about how it felt to die and live again, Alex wanted to toss him out of the room. His visit made the oscilloscope run away like crazy, and the nurse, Ellen, came in and asked the visitor to leave. Then Nedda tried to talk with Alex about his resuscitation, but he brushed her off.

One afternoon, when he was finally transferred to Intermediate Care, Ellen dropped by for a visit. It was that moment of quiet in the afternoon, visitors gone, before the nurses came around with pre-supper medications. Alex was so glad to see Ellen's bright, cheerful face that he felt his eyes brim over.

"It's good for you," she said, handing him a tissue. "We had one patient here a while back who kept saying to himself, 'Let go and let God.' You know, after a while, it got to us, too."

"I have dreams," Alex said. "I dream I died."

"Look," Ellen said, "it would be surprising if you didn't have dreams. Or nightmares."

When a patient was obliged to remain in Coronary Care a long time, it is usually a big psychological setback for him. He may become lethargic as well as depressed, or even develop a psychosis.

A week later, when he was transferred again, this time to the general nursing floor, Alex was nagging at Dr. Tai. "Look, I'm okay. When do I get out of here?"

ELLEN:

Her friends often asked questions about her work. "If a

patient has a cardiac arrest, do you tell him about it afterwards?"

"Well—" she usually hedged, "we may say he fainted or his pulse increased, and we used an electrical means of stabilizing his heart."

The patient usually accepted the explanation. Alex wasn't the only one who dreamed he had died. Other patients described it as a floating feeling or Other World feeling. Nine out of ten patients who had experienced cardiac arrest had psychological problems that involved fear of dying and death. When they were asked to draw sketches of what they felt, one patient drew a setting sun, another the crash of a plane.

PART II

HEART DISEASES

Chapter 5

The heart's wonders

DR. TAI:
The heart is a pump:

The heart is a muscular pump; its job to supply a flow of blood to the body and to the body's vital organs.

Blood, that miracle fluid, performs a series of tasks such as supplying oxygen, removing carbon dioxide, supplying the tissues with nourishment, carrying hormones to the proper parts of the body, equalizing the temperature of the body, and sending out metabolic building blocks for growth and repair.

If something goes wrong with the heart, the blood may not circulate as it should.

If the blood flow to the brain is cut off for three to five seconds, the result is a feeling of light-headedness. Within ten to twenty seconds, unconsciousness will occur. Deprived of circulation for four minutes, brain damage will occur, although other cells in the body can survive for as long as thirty to fifty minutes without blood.

Decreased blood flow to the kidneys interferes with function there. If the kidney doesn't receive enough blood at the proper pressure, it cannot make urine adequately to carry off waste products. These then build up in the blood stream and have, in turn, harmful effects.

No part of the body can perform well without adequate blood supply. Though blood may be well oxygenated in the lungs, it may not be delivered from the heart adequately to the body. In addition, slow flow allows waste products to build up in the tissues, causing the muscles to tire more easily. The skin grows cool and moist. Fatigue is more apparent.

Many of the things that go wrong—and that we cardiologists must detect and remedy are revealed in this book.

We hope it will help every patient and his family to understand the heart's wonders.

How much pumping does the heart actually do?

Each beat pumps two ounces of blood; a teacupful every three beats; five quarts every minute. Seventy-five gallons every hour. And the average heart beats 100,000 times a day.

It pumps enough blood to fill a gasoline tank four times every hour. And this is only to keep the machinery of the body at an idling rate as we sit or sleep.

During strenuous activity, such as jogging or playing tennis or swimming in competition, the heart pump may approach fourteen barrels an hour.

During a person's average nine-to-five working day and his routine home life after business hours, the heart pumps about seventy barrels.

In a 70-year life span, that comes to nearly eighteen million barrels.

The heart has four chambers:

This remarkable pump has two sides and four chambers. The sides are separated from one another by solid muscular walls.

Each side contains a collecting chamber called an *atrium*, and a pumping chamber called a *ventricle*. The atria receive blood and the ventricles pump it.

The walls of the atrial chambers are thin. As they are only collecting centers and though they contract, they do no hard work. The ventricles are the main pumping chambers of the heart. Their walls are several times thicker than those of the atria.

The right-sided heart chambers are separated from their left-sided partners by the *inter-atrial septum* (wall) and the *inter-ventricular septum*. During the normal development of the heart in the fetus, there are openings in these walls which close by the time of birth.

It takes only three to five ounces of blood to fill each chamber.

Between each atrium and its ventricle lies a valve made of thin pliable tissue leaflets. They open wide to allow blood to pass without obstruction and then close completely to avoid backward leakage as the blood is pumped onward. They are flaplike and cannot support themselves.

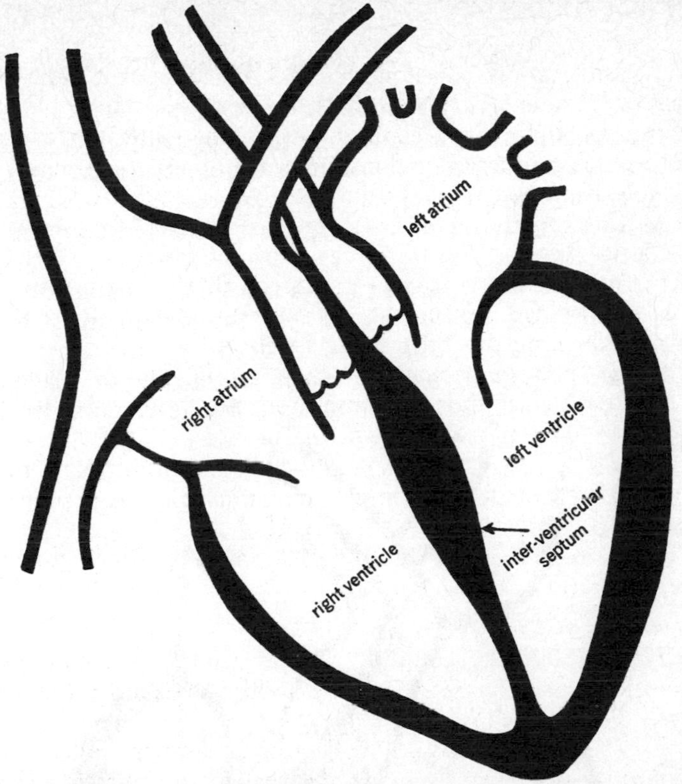

The heart has four chambers. Two of them are the atria (entrance chambers) and two are the ventricles. The atria are separated by a wall, an inter-atrial septum (not shown, as it lies behind the arteries). The ventricles are separated by the inter-ventricular septum.

They are called *atrio-ventricular* valves. A famous physician described them as being soft as silk and strong as steel.

The one on the right side contains three leaflets and is called the *tri-cuspid* valve. The one on the left has two leaflets and is called the *mitral* valve.

There are also valves at the exit of each ventricle—the right ventricular valve is called the *pulmonic* valve; and the left ventricular valve is called the *aortic* valve.

The combined action of the valves and pumping chambers insures a one-way flow of blood.

The action sequences on each side of the heart are the same. The atrium fills the ventricle while it is relaxing and its pressure is low (diastole), across the open atrio-ventricular valve. The atrium contracts, delivering as much blood as the ventricle will accept. It primes the ventricle for its upcoming contraction and an increase in pressure (systole).

Now the concert of motion begins.

As the ventricle contracts, pressure begins to increase inside it. As the pressure in the ventricle rises, the leaflets of the atrio-ventricular valve are forced to a closed position. The ventricular pressure equals and surpasses that of the atrium, keeping the valve leaflets tightly together.

If not for its moorings by strong tissue threads (*cordae tendinae*) to mounds of muscle on the ventricular walls

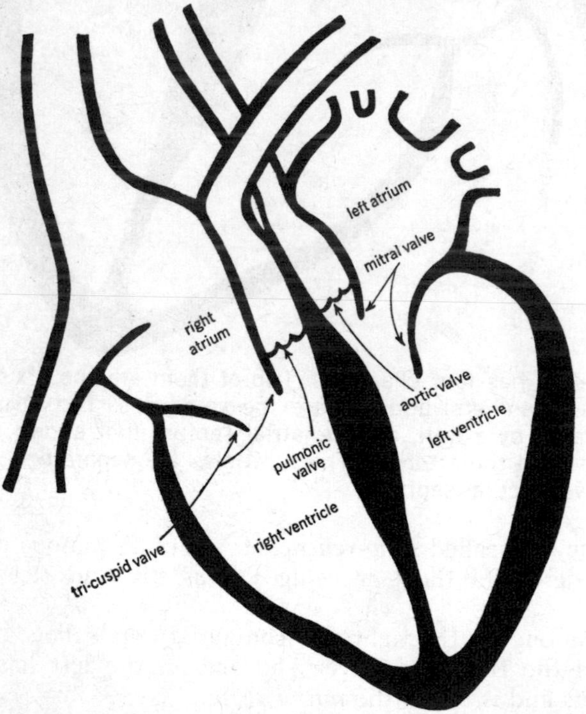

The valves

The entrances and exits of the ventricles are guarded by thin, strong, pliable floodgates—the valves. The atrio-ventricular valves guard the entrance: the tricuspid valve on the right, the mitral valve on the left.

Arterial valves guard the exits: pulmonic on the right, aortic on the left. The action of the ventricles controls the opening and closing of these valves.

(*papillary muscles*), these valves leaflets would flap backward into the atrium, causing leakage of blood. When normal, they slam closed, pulling at their moorings, but never leaking.

Here is a moment of dramatic wonder, just before the ventricle empties:

For a brief pause in time, when both ventricles are entirely filled with blood, all four valves are closed. The two atrio-ventricular valves are closed because the ventricular pressure is now higher than the pressure in the atrium. At the same time, the pressure in the ventricles is still less than the pressure in the arteries which is holding the arterial (exit) valves shut.

Each ventricle continues to contract with no change in

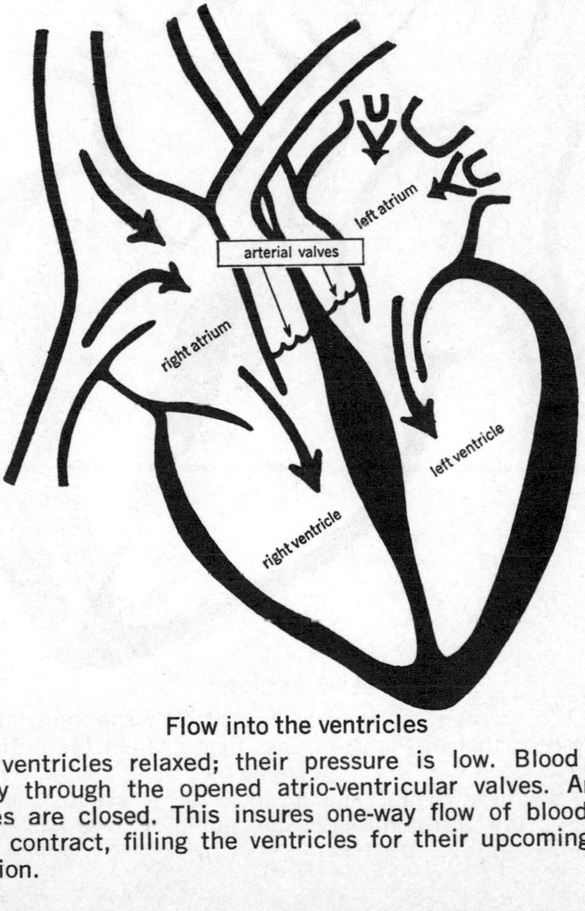

Flow into the ventricles

The ventricles relaxed; their pressure is low. Blood flows freely through the opened atrio-ventricular valves. Arterial valves are closed. This insures one-way flow of blood. The atria contract, filling the ventricles for their upcoming contraction.

the volume of blood it contains. This brief moment is called "isovolumic contraction." It ends when the ventricular pressure equals and then surpasses that of the exit arteries. The arterial valves are then thrust open and the blood from the ventricles is ejected across the now open valves into the arteries.

The pressure continues high while the ventricular chamber becomes smaller and smaller as the blood empties into the artery. Finally, it is over. The ventricle has completed its contraction, has nearly emptied itself.

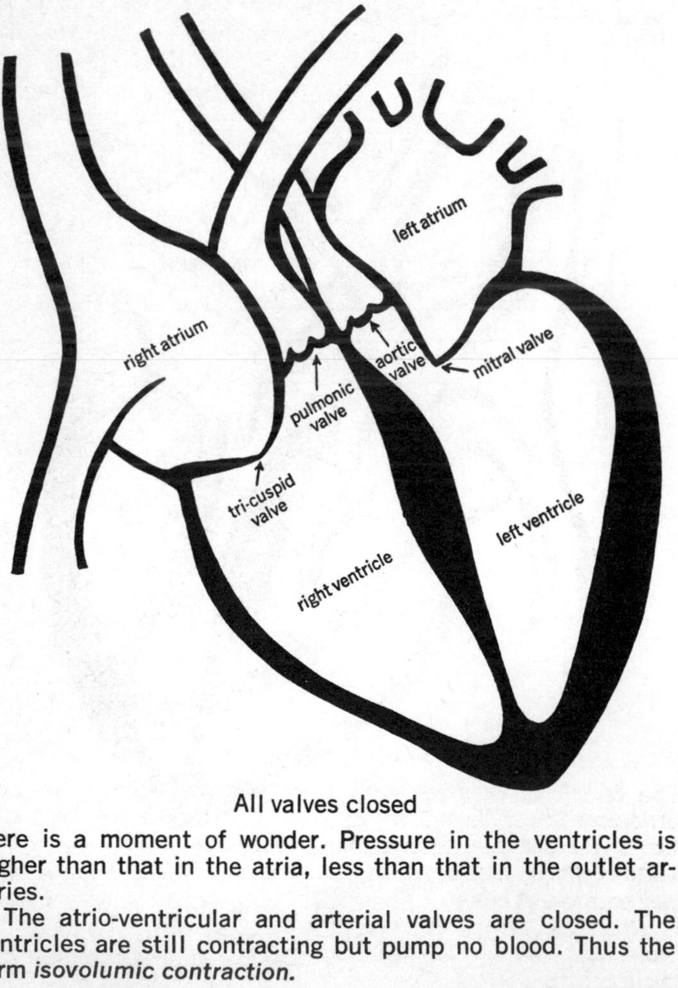

All valves closed

Here is a moment of wonder. Pressure in the ventricles is higher than that in the atria, less than that in the outlet arteries.

The atrio-ventricular and arterial valves are closed. The ventricles are still contracting but pump no blood. Thus the term *isovolumic contraction.*

Now, like a spent warrior having thrust his last, it relaxes, suddenly and completely. The pressure in the artery drops, forcing its valve to close. Cup-shaped, it supports itself. Again for an instant, the ventricle finds itself a "closed chamber," neither filling nor emptying during "isovolumic relaxation." Ventricular pressure decreases and falls below that of its atrium, which has been filling with blood, on standby, for the completion of the ventricular contraction.

Now, the atrio-ventricular valve opens and the atrium empties its contents into the ventricle, filling it, as the cycle repeats itself again and again.

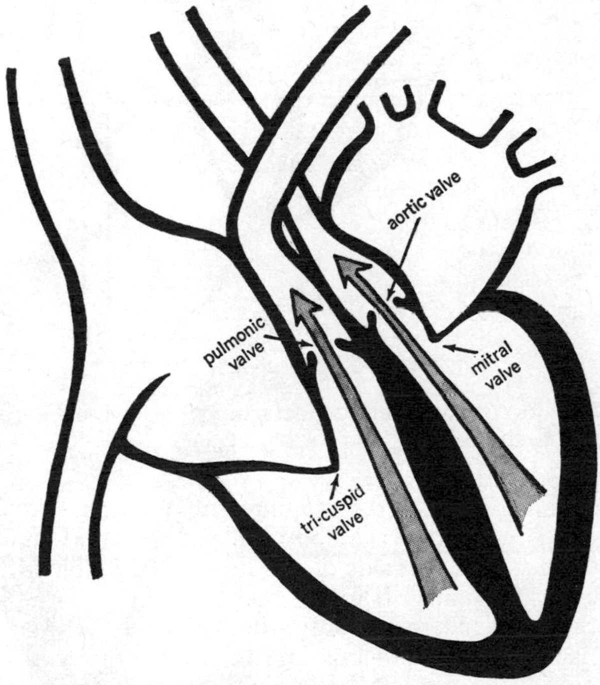

The ventricles pump

The ventricles contract, forcing arterial valves to open and atrio-ventricular valves to shut. This pumps blood into the lungs (via the pulmonary artery) and into the body (via the aorta) without leaking backward into the atria, insuring one-way passage of blood.

When the ventricles finish contracting, the arterial valves close and the atrio-ventricular valves open. The heartbeat cycle begins again.

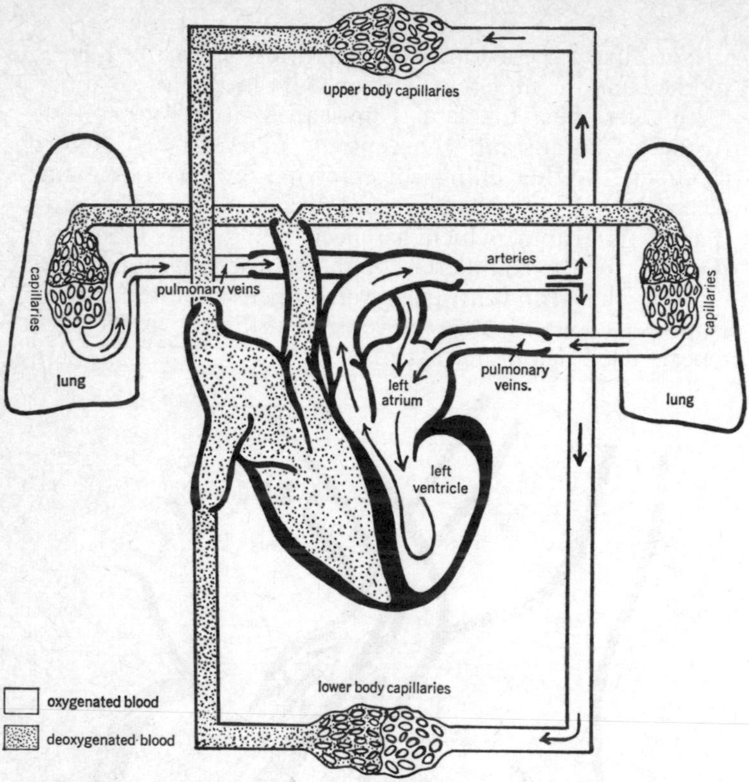

The left side of the heart collects blood from the lungs and pumps it to the body.

Each side of the heart has a different function. The right side of the heart collects blood from the body and pumps it to the lungs. The left side of the heart collects blood from the lungs and pumps it to the body.

Pumping blood *to* the entire body, as the left ventricle does, is a more difficult task and requires more work. The left ventricle, as a result, has the thicker and stronger wall. It usually generates about five times as much pressure as the right ventricle. It pumps the same amount of blood as the right ventricle but at a higher pressure. In fact, it is the power of the left ventricle that helps to maintain your blood pressure. If your blood pressure happens to go up, the left ventricle will have to work even harder to meet this additional load.

The blood isn't pushed out of the ventricles the way a

piston compresses air and gas mixture in a car. Ventricular muscle is arranged in a spiral around the heart chamber and wrings itself out when it contracts. Both ventricles contract almost simultaneously. An equal amount of blood is expelled by each. This has to be, in order that the flow to the lungs is the same as the flow to the body. If not, there would be an imbalance of volume in the circulation. The body couldn't function.

Blood from the body tissues returns to the heart by way of veins. They start as small vessels but join together as they near the heart, much the way the Ohio, Missouri and Red rivers come together to create the Mississippi.

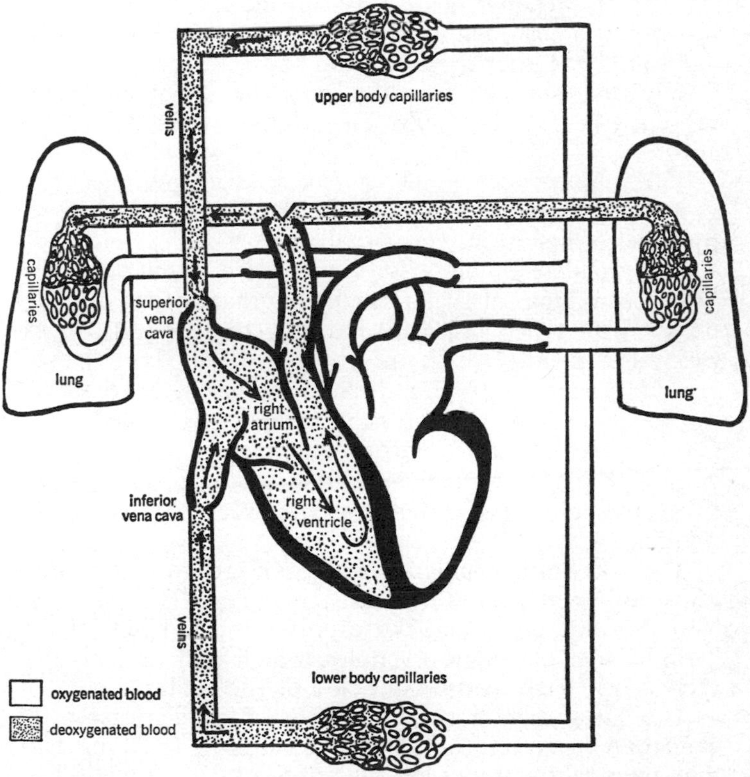

The right side collects blood from the body and pumps it to the lungs.

The large veins of the body join together to form two larger veins that go into the heart: one receiving the blood from the head and arms, the other collecting from the lower parts of the body.

These are the *vena cavae.*

The one that comes from the upper part of the body is called the *superior vena cava,* and the one from below the *inferior vena cava.*

These vena cavae bring their blood to the right atrium.

From this point, the blood passes through the tri-cuspid valve, which opens allowing the blood to pass from the right atrium to the right ventricle. This occurs just after the right ventricle has completed its previous contraction and emptied itself. During the next contraction, the right ventricular pressure again goes up, closing the tri-cuspid valve, and then opening the pulmonic valve. The blood flows to the pulmonary artery and to the lungs.

The arteries branch from the aorta, the largest and toughest blood vessel in the body. The arterioles branch from the arteries.

These blood vessels get smaller in size but greater in number as they get farther from the heart and closer to the tissues they ultimately supply.

The smallest blood vessels are called *capillaries.* The body has millions of them, usually in groups called *capillary beds.* The arteries and veins are only the conduits, or expressways. Capillary beds are where all the body exchanges take place: oxygen, food, and essential substances are picked up and delivered, while waste products are carted away. Capillary vessels are so narrow that blood cells must flow through them in single file and their walls are so thin that substances can freely interchange between the blood and tissues.

These delicate capillaries are protected from the high pressure in the arteries by muscular pre-capillary arterioles. Without this protection the capillaries would burst.

Capillaries empty into venules, which lead to veins that carry blood back to the right side of the heart.

The lungs have a similar system of capillaries for the exchange of oxygen and carbon dioxide in the lung sacs. The pulmonary arteries are the arteries to the lungs. These arteries divide and subdivide into multiple smaller and smaller vessels.

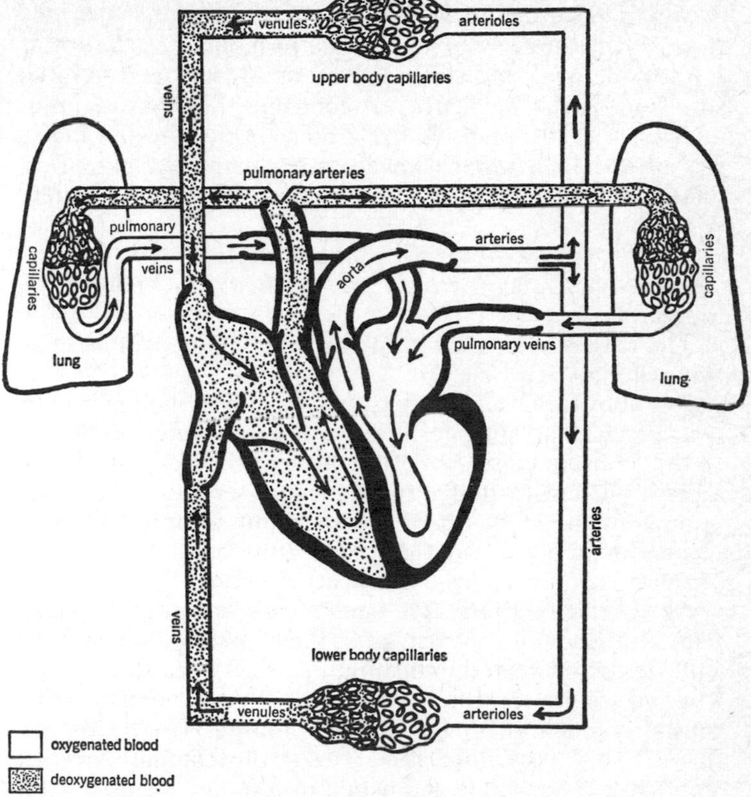

The circulation

The exchange of oxygen and carbon dioxide takes place in the lungs across the thin walls of the capillaries.

The "impure" blood takes up oxygen from the air passages of the lungs and releases the carbon dioxide. From there, the carbon dioxide is exhaled. The oxygen-rich blood now flows through four large veins into the left atrium of the heart.

The "oxygenated" blood then passes across the mitral valve into the left ventricle from which it is pumped across the aortic valve into the aorta.

This completes the cycle of circulation.

DR. FRANKLIN:
The heart is nourished by the coronary arteries:

When the heart propels blood from the right atrium through the lungs to its final thrust of blood into the aorta, it has done work and expended energy. It has used oxygen, sugar, and other nutrients. To continue this life-sustaining activity, the heart muscle itself must be fed by the blood stream or it will suffer damage and a part of it may even die. It must be nourished so it can continue to feed the rest of the body.

The heart is fed by the coronary arteries.

These small blood vessels are the first two branches of the aorta.

The aortic valve sits within the aorta at its point of exit from the left ventricle.

Just above the valve leaflets, less than one inch from the heart, are the openings of the two coronary arteries. Before fresh blood can be sent to other parts of the body, the heart takes a portion as its fee for transport services. The heart pumps five to six quarts of blood in one minute. Close to one-half pint (5%) of this blood runs back through the coronary arteries to feed the heart muscle.

The coronary arteries are small. They are slightly wider than the lead in a pencil, and they quickly branch into tributaries that keep diminishing in size. When the heart is working vigorously, the flow through the coronary arteries can be as much as three pints in a minute. The reason for this extraordinary blood flow is that the coronary arteries aren't stiff. They dilate and widen in response to the heart's call for more oxygen as its work load increases.

Anything that narrows the coronary arteries or interferes with their ability to expand can decrease the supply of blood to the heart.

This will interfere with the heart's ability to function: at first, under stress, either physical or emotional, because that is when the heart needs extra oxygen and nourishment; and later even under lighter loads.

The heart muscle needs this blood to survive. A severe decrease in coronary flow can cause pain (angina). Total absence of flow in a coronary artery can damage or cause death of a piece of heart muscle (heart attack or myocardial infarction) (see chapter 6, "Angina, the Vital Warning, and Coronary Heart Attack").

There are two coronary arteries: the right and the left.

Shortly after the left coronary leaves its point of origin in the aorta, it branches into two main divisions. So doctors frequently talk of the "three" coronary arteries: 1) the right coronary artery, 2) the left anterior descending, and 3) the left circumflex.

Each in turn branches into innumerable vessels, creating

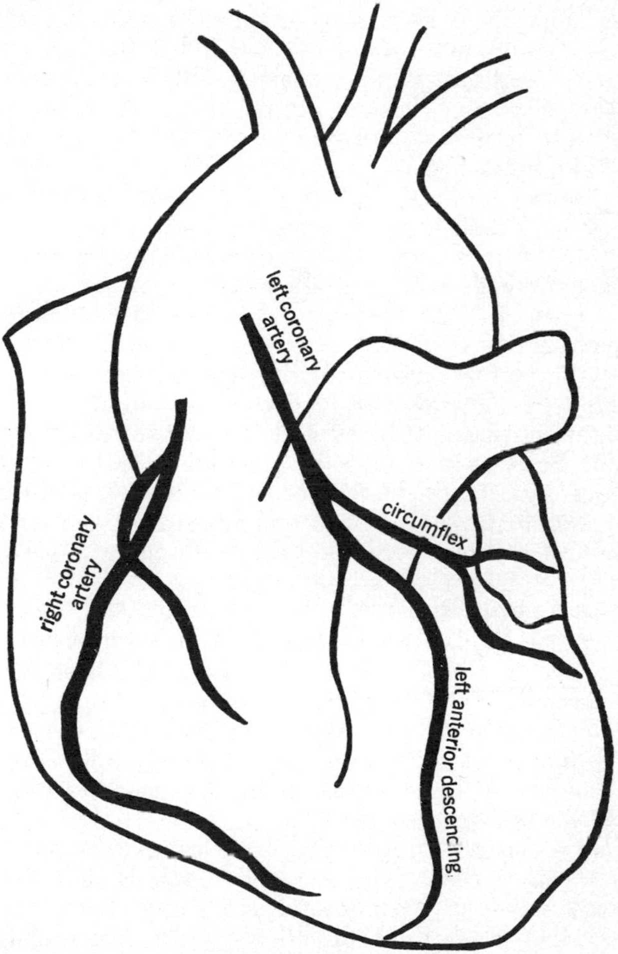

Arteries of the heart

Coronary arteries supply the life's blood to the heart. These arteries originate from the aorta.

a capillary network that surrounds and nourishes each heart muscle cell.

The initial portion of the coronary artery runs on the surface of the heart. But its branches burrow into the heart muscle. As the heart contracts, these branches are caught in a squeeze play. Very little blood can flow through the coronary artery during this contraction phase of the cardiac cycle. The major flow through these blood vessels comes during the relaxation phase. Fortunately, about two-thirds of every heart beat is spent relaxing. The heart is contracting or generating pressure during one-third of the cycle. Beat, rest, rest, beat, rest, rest.

When rapid heartbeat (tachycardia) occurs, more time is cut out of the resting phase than the contracting part of the cycle. This causes a relative decrease in coronary flow. It is one of the reasons a very rapid heartbeat is dangerous for anyone with cardiac problems. Especially, if the rapid beat continues for a long time (see chapter 8, "Short Circuit of the Heart").

As you perform during the day, waking, bathing, eating, walking, the energy expended calls for variations in the amount and speed of blood sent out by the heart.

The heart muscle alters its commands to the coronary arteries to match the body's needs. The miracle of the heart is the automatic second-by-second adjustment and readjustment. All within a very fine tolerance limit.

The heart's by-pass system

Remember, the heart is nourished by the coronary arteries. If any one of them is blocked, that part of the heart it feeds will die (heart attack).

Heart muscle without oxygen can live only for twenty to forty minutes. If another nourishing blood supply can reach the endangered heart muscle in time, it can be saved.

Where can this new blood supply come from?

Nature has the answer. The heart grows new blood vessels in some people. These are small vessels that connect one coronary artery to another. If one coronary artery is narrowed, then blocked off, the other can feed the threatened heart muscle by way of the bridging blood vessel.

These new blood vessels are called *collaterals,* and they grow only when there is a need for them. When a coronary

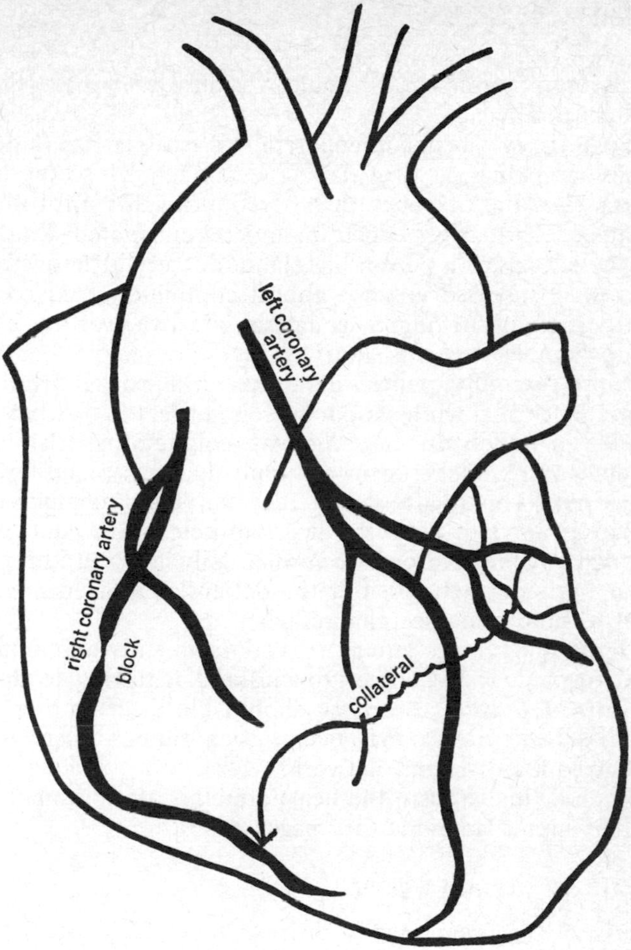

Collaterals

artery slowly narrows, a piece of heart muscle is gradually deprived of oxygen-rich blood. That means progressive strangulation of a piece of the heart.

This slow starvation seems to work as a prod to stimulate the collaterals to develop and grow. They are partial substitutes for what has been lost. Unfortunately, not every person with a narrowed coronary artery (arteriosclerosis) develops collaterals. We believe their growth may be encouraged by exercise and hampered by tobacco. But we really aren't sure. Some people who are lucky have them. Others don't.

Sometimes we explain collaterals to patients as a kind of disability policy.

It's the kind of policy that pays no benefits until illness or an accident strikes. Then it's much appreciated. You see, the collaterals, if a person has them, do very little until the narrowed, diseased vessel is almost completely blocked off. Until then, the bridging collateral sits by, waiting. Then the payments (benefits) start.

Most disability policies don't pay the patient the full salary he earned while working. You get less than what you made on the job. In the same way, collateral vessels, being rather small branches, cannot supply as much blood flow as a normal coronary artery. But they can supply enough oxygenated blood to keep the heart muscle alive. And often enough to allow reasonable normal daily activity. For some even strenuous activity. But the patient may need medication to help him (see chapter 16).

Sometimes the collateral network is an early one, not yet well formed. It has some growing and maturing to do. If the diseased coronary artery should close off during this time, a heart attack may occur, even though there is an undeveloped collateral network.

Should this happen, the heart attack is often a small one rather than a large one (see pages 71–74).

DR. KRAUTHAMER:

The heart is a generator, with its own electrical system:

Lub-dup, Lub-dup, the beat of the heart, slower at night when you are sleeping, faster by day as the legs eat up pavements or the bus door shuts before you can board it. Fast or slow, that beat matches its activity to yours. As long as the heart is healthy, it keeps on going without a pause, speeding up and slowing down according to the body's signals.

The heart has its own electrical system which does two jobs:

1. Insures a heartbeat; and
2. Organizes pumping action of heart muscle.

A special group of cells (pacemaker cells) regularly produce a "spark" to initiate each heartbeat. Another group of cells (conduction cells) rapidly distribute this impulse to the heart muscle. They do this in a manner that coordinates the heartbeat in an efficient pumping action.

No muscle of the body can work (contract) without an electrical impulse to start it off. In many parts of the body (arms, legs, for instance), this is accomplished by an impulse traveling to the muscle from the central nervous system (brain or spinal cord).

The heart is independent. It has its own natural pacemaker region that causes it to beat.

In the right atrium (the collecting chamber on the right side), at a point where it is entered by one of the large veins returning blood to the heart (the superior vena cava), is the *sino-atrial node*. This is the heart's natural pacemaker.

It is a small area, invisible to the naked eye. Under a microscope, a scientist can differentiate this piece of the heart from the surrounding heart muscle. Here the triggering impulse starts on its trip through the four chambers of the heart.

The natural pacemaker can be influenced by nerves that reach the heart.

Also by substances in the blood stream (hormones).

But these outside influences only modify or alter the heart's own basic, independent rhythm. The heart, through its own generator, will always try to return to its basic pattern of beats, ranging from 60 to 100 per minute. Only with a continual outside stimulus will a healthy heart maintain a more rapid or slower rate.

If you are in good shape, your heart rate will go up as you exercise. But it will slow down again as soon as you stop, and within a few minutes, it will return to the resting rate. How much time it will take depends on: 1) how vigorous the exercise was, and 2) your physical condition.

As soon as the interfering factor (which in this case was normal—exercise) is removed, the heart tries to return to the rhythm of the natural pacemaker.

Other stimuli are also received by the pacemaker—for example, fever or excitement—so the heart rate is actually determined by multiple factors, all screened and balanced by the sino-atrial node. Your heart's mini-computer.

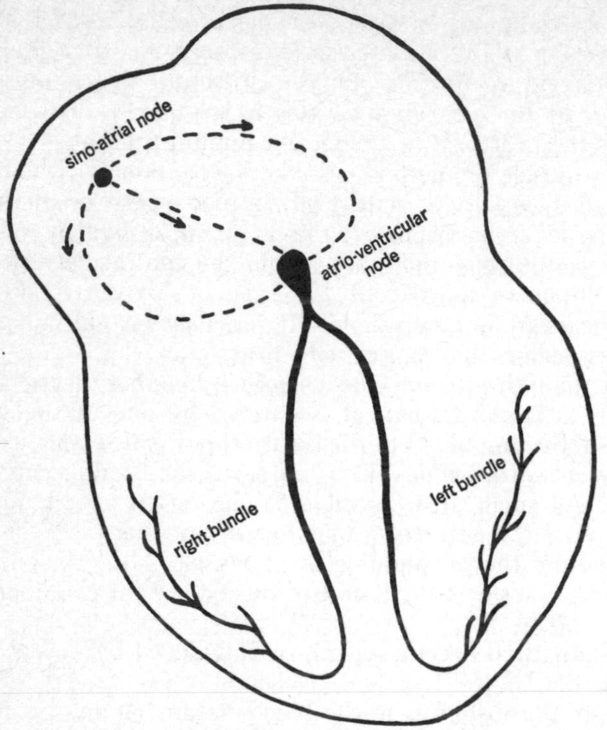

The natural pacemaker

Electrical impulse is generated in the sino-atrial node. It is transmitted through fleshy wires across the atria (upper chambers) to the screening station—the atrio-ventricular node.

The impulse then travels through another set of fleshy wires, called the right bundle branch and the left bundle branch, in the right and left ventricles.

Finally the impulse passes to the ventricular muscle by the H-P system. Thus the message is sent to the chambers to contract in sequence.

Proper timing of the electrical impulse is essential for coordinated heart action.

The pacemaker cells have fired. The sino-atrial node has passed the impulse along. The electrical signal spreads from the S-A (sino-atrial) node to the adjacent muscle cells of the right atrium where it is located. The impulse moves quickly along fleshy wires (conduction cells) stimulating one muscle cell after another. Like a falling row of dominoes, each cell triggers the next in line. Once a number of cells are stimulated, the signal spreads as a "wave" of electrical energy. Just like the ripple from a pebble dropped in a pond, it radiates from the sino-atrial node through both the right and left atria.

Each muscle cell, as it is stimulated, starts to contract. At three feet per second, the signal is quick enough to pass completely through both upper chambers in time for all the muscle cells to participate in an organized atrial contraction. But the impulse reaches the ventricles before the atrial chambers have finished their job. It would move into the ventricles too quickly, if not checked. Yet, if it went any slower in the atrium there would be disorganized contraction of the atrium. The first atrial muscle cells would finish contracting before the entire atrium was activated.

Nature has solved this dilemma rather simply. The upper (atrial) and lower (ventricular) chambers are electrically isolated from one another, the only passage between them through a special way (delay) station. Called the *atrio-ventricular node* (A-V node) as distinguished from the S-A node, this is another area of special heart cells. This is the electrical entrance to the ventricles.

Electrical impulses travel in the A-V node slower than anywhere else in the heart. Eight inches per second, a snail's pace compared to the impulses in the atrium where they go almost four times as fast.

After the delay in the A-V node, at the electrical entrance to the ventricles, there is need for a telegraph system to speed the signals on their way. Another group of fleshy wires, the *His-Purkinje* (H-P) system, does the job well, conducting impulses faster than any other heart structure. Thirteen feet per second. Four times faster than in the atrium and twenty times faster than in the A-V node. This rapid delivery system allows the ventricular muscle fibers to work together in an organized manner.

The His-Purkinje system has a second function. It is not only a conducting system. It also acts as a "fail-safe pacemaker." The S-A node impulses "turn off" the H-P pacemaker unless the S-A node impulses fail. Under these conditions, the H-P system "escapes" and takes over until the S-A node impulse returns again. If it weren't for this, some afflicted people would die (see chapter 8, "Short Circuit of the Heart").

The electrical signal passing through the muscle of the heart is recorded by the electrocardiogram (ECG), which indicates whether all is well or not. The ECG accurately inscribes the "current" as a series of waves or deflections from a baseline.

Many years ago the "squiggles" or waves recorded by the ECG machine were named:

The small "P" wave is created by the atria's thin walls. The thick ventricular walls generate the large "QRS complex." There are other waves on the cardiogram. The "T" wave, for instance, is produced by the recovery of the ventricles after they contract.

Measurements are made of their heights and duration (width). Different contours of a P wave or QRS complex can be very important in the diagnosis of heart disease.

Though not infallible, recording the heart's electrical activity is one of the simplest, safest and most informative ways we evaluate the heart. A more accurate check is made by the "stress" cardiogram, taken during physical activity (see chapter 14, "Testing, Testing").

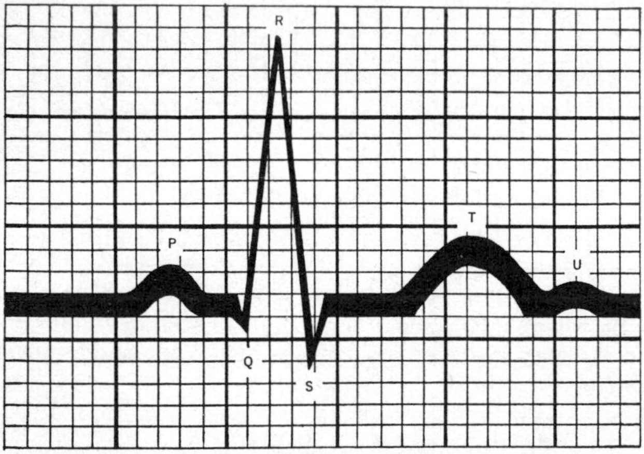

Normal electrocardiogram

The P wave is produced by electrical activation of the upper chambers (atria). The QRS complex is produced by electrical activation of the pumping chambers (ventricles). The T and U waves indicate recovery of the ventricles.

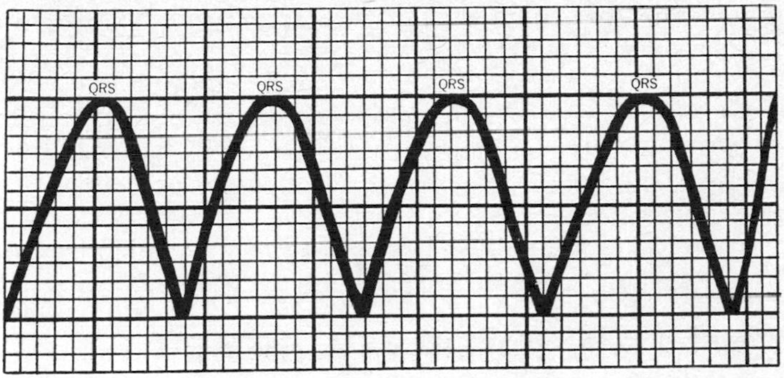

Ventricular tachycardia

Each wave is a wide, abnormal QRS complex. The rate is rapid—150 beats per minute.

Proper emergency treatment is essential, since ventricular tachycardia can progress to ventricular fibrillation (see page 36) and death.

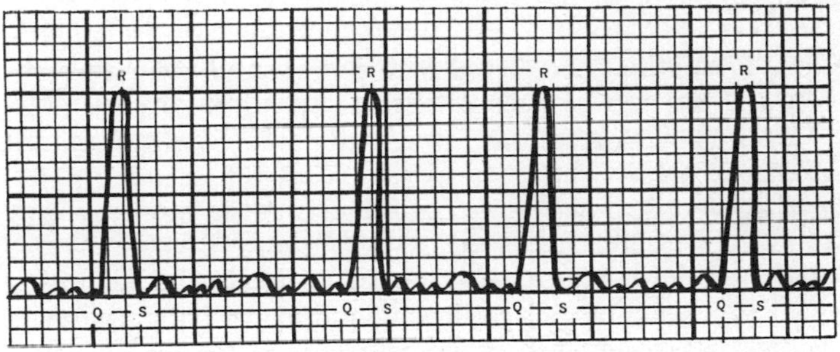

Fibrillation

Irregular heartbeat due to lack of organized activity in the upper chambers (atria) shown by the wavy baseline.

The fine fibrillatory waves from the atria are seen in the area between the QRS complexes.

No P waves are seen, as the atria are not functioning normally.

Chapter 6

Angina: the vital warning and the coronary attack

DR. FRANKLIN:
Angina is the cry of the heart.

A classic description was published by Dr. William Heberdon in 1818. Like many things that are old but beautiful, it has been copied and paraphrased but still stands as a landmark in medical description:

> They who are afflicted with it are seized while they are walking (more especially if it be up a hill, or soon after eating) with a painful and most disagreeable sensation in the breast which seems as if it would extinguish life, if it were to increase or continue; but the moment they stand still, all this uneasiness vanishes.
>
> In all other respects, the patients are, at the beginning of this disorder, perfectly well, and in particular, have no shortness of breath, from which it is totally different. The pain is sometimes situated in the upper part, perhaps in the middle, sometimes to the left than the right side. It likewise very frequently extends from the breast to the middle of the left arm. The pulse is, at least sometimes, not disturbed by this pain, as I have had opportunities of observing by feeling the pulse during the paroxysm. Males are most liable to that disease, especially such as have passed their fiftieth year.
>
> After it has continued a year or more, it will not cease so instantaneously upon standing still; and it will come on not only when the persons are walking, but when they are lying down, especially if they lie on their left side, and oblige them to rise up out of their beds.

What is angina?

It is the cry of the heart for more oxygen. In more than 90 percent of patients, the cause of angina is narrowing of the coronary arteries which feed the heart. They have become narrowed by arteriosclerosis (hardening of the arteries), the fatty buildup or "rust" of the blood vessels.

Angina and a heart attack are *not* different diseases. They are the different stages of the same disease.

Coronary heart disease is a progression. First, the coronary artery starts to narrow down. Then the narrowing becomes bad enough to decrease blood flow to the heart muscle, causing angina—chest discomfort on exertion. Extreme narrowing often brings on heart damage. When the artery is blocked completely, cutting off all blood supply, the heart muscle then dies. This condition causes the severe chest pain of the heart attack.

Not all people experience both symptoms. One patient may develop angina that lasts for years without culminating in a heart attack. Another may have a full-blown heart attack, without ever experiencing the warning chest symptoms until the severe pain of the dying heart muscle sends him to the hospital.

Many potential victims practice denial by saying: "My friend, John, dropped dead of a heart attack a week after he had a checkup and his doctor gave him a clean bill of health. His electrocardiogram was normal. So why should I bother with an examination?"

It's much like the woman with a little lump in her breast. It's only a tiny lump until the doctor examines it, calls it a tumor and asks for a biopsy. In all likelihood, it's merely a cyst, but the doctor is playing it safe.

The same general theory goes for the businessman. The chest pain which hit him while he was walking back to the office after a rich lunch is indigestion, until his doctor tells him otherwise. Not that he checks with a doctor until there is an emergency. Why bother?

The ostrich-in-the-sand approach. You may hide your head, but the rest of you is vulnerable. Particularly your heart. And there is a great deal the doctor and cardiologist can do to prevent damage.

When a coronary artery is totally blocked, the blockage is called a *coronary occlusion* or a *coronary thrombosis*. The damage to the heart muscle (myocardium) is called a *myocardial infarction* or a *heart attack*.

We feel that a coronary artery usually has to be narrowed by more than 75 percent before angina occurs. But even though the blood flow is decreased, there may be no symptoms while the person is inactive. Enough nourishment is still getting to the heart muscle.

Stanley R., who is in his mid-40s, has a narrowing in a coronary artery. But the blood supply is adequate when the heart muscle is at rest.

Suppose he goes out for a walk. He walks at a moderate pace for three blocks. Exercise forces the heart to work harder, so it needs more blood.

But if the blood flow isn't forthcoming, Stanley will often develop the symptoms of angina. If he is aware of his coronary problem, he will pause and put a nitroglycerine tablet under his tongue. The work load of the heart will diminish. The blood supply will become adequate. If this condition has persisted for no longer than five or ten minutes, no damage will occur.

But suppose Stanley were to ignore the warning and continue walking, perhaps even increasing his pace?

If the inadequate supply of blood persists for twenty to thirty minutes, actual heart damage will develop. Stanley can actually produce a heart attack in this way. Exertion is not the only triggering factor. It can be an argument, too much excitement, even a large rich meal.

If the person is under stress—in an argument with his boss or playing singles in a competitive tennis match—his heart is suddenly faced with an increased work load. It's got to pump harder and faster to meet the demands of the body. Like a gallant warrior, it responds. Flow through the coronary arteries is stepped up to fuel (with oxygenated blood) the heart's extra effort. The coronaries do this by dilating.

Normal arteries can deliver as much as a three-fold increase in flow, while the heart muscle flexes, beat after beat, under the increased work load.

A narrowed coronary artery also tries to answer the call. But it cannot respond. The flow through the narrowed vessel isn't enough to give the heart muscle what it needs. An imbalance is taking place. A deficit has occurred.

This is *ischemia:* not enough blood flow for the heart's need.

Now the heart is laboring. The heart's limited oxygen stores are quickly exhausted.

Heberdon's original report described angina as a severe seizure. But time and experience have taught us that even mild chest pains may indicate severe and dangerous coronary disease. A narrowing greater than 75 percent causes angina pains when the heart is stressed. A narrowing greater than 90 percent may cause anginal discomfort, even when the patient is at rest.

Anginal episodes, however, are usually brief, lasting a few minutes. They are relieved by placing a nitroglycerine tablet under the tongue or by stopping the activity that prompted the attack.

"What do you mean by stable angina patterns?" a patient with angina wants to know.

"A predictable pattern of symptoms in relation to your activities over a period of time," we tell him. "As long as you are comfortable and can go about your life to your satisfaction, nothing further needs to be done for you."

"And what is unstable angina?"

"It means that there is the appearance of frequent or more severe symptoms over a length of time. If this occurs during a period of several weeks to several months, it is called the *chronic* form of unstable angina. It usually means the coronary circulation is gradually deteriorating."

The patient should see his physician. He may go on to a heart attack.

There is also *acute* unstable angina. In this case, the patient experiences a sudden change over a period of minutes, or hours or a few days. This would lead his doctor to suspect a significant change in the blood flow to his heart. His doctor would apply prompt therapy.

Patients have said: "Doctor, I never had a chest pain before, and this one woke me out of a deep sleep."

Angina often starts in the night. It may be a danger signal and the patient should turn to his doctor for immediate care.

The patient who has been diagnosed as a victim of anginal pattern learns to differentiate between his pains.

He recognizes danger. He knows if there is some change in his anginal pains, or if they are compounded by a feeling of fear or insecurity. If the pains persist, if the patient breaks out in a sweat, has palpitations, or feels sick to his stomach, he should get to a hospital Emergency Room immediately.

These symptoms are often the indication of an impending heart attack. It makes no difference whether the pain is severe or not.

Pain is not the only warning. Anyone with coronary heart disease who has unusual fatigue without a recognizable cause should seek medical help. This kind of fatigue is a common premonitory symptom of myocardial infarction.

Not all people who suffer a heart attack have earlier anginal discomfort. Those who do, can clearly tell the difference.

When it happens, the pain of a heart attack is usually crushing. The chest is gripped by an unrelenting vise. "An elephant sitting on my chest," patients often say. Frequently, there is weakness, sweating, nausea, an urge to move the bowels. The pain may start at the center of the chest and spread from there radiating up to the shoulders, arms (on the left more than the right, but often both), and even up to the jaw, teeth and ears. There may be palpitations (irregular heartbeat). Breathing may be labored, with a feeling of not getting enough air (dyspnea). The patient may pass out.

People never have exactly identical symptoms but most agree that the pain is severe. As important as the pain, is the sense of overall, impending catastrophe that accompanies it: weakness and a profound sense of doom. Yet there are some people who have "silent infarction" without pain. The attack is detected after the fact on a routine electrocardiogram. This is uncommon.

The pain of an infarction is usually felt at the beginning of the attack, and often comes on without exertion. A heart attack can occur at rest while sleeping, as well as while shoveling snow. Most severe heart attacks do *not* develop during strenuous physical exercise.

The pain of a heart attack persists, sometimes for hours. Nitroglycerine doesn't help. It may ease the discomfort momentarily, but the pain quickly returns. A strong narcotic is necessary to relax the patient and ease his agony. Morphine or a related drug is most often used.

False heart pains

But does all chest pain mean angina or a heart attack? Naturally not. We all have occasional twinges, aches, muscle spasms in the chest that are totally unrelated to the heart. An illness in another part of the body may cause chest pains. Gall bladder problems, indigestion, ulcers, pressure on a nerve in the neck or hiatus hernia can all be felt as terrible chest pains. Yet the heart may be perfectly well. A pain in the chest may be due to Tzietze's Syndrome, an inflammation of a part of the breast bone. The list is endless, but these symptoms do require evaluation.

Another frequent misleading symptom is overbreathing. It causes a condition known as hyperventilation syndrome. No lung or heart problems are involved, but the person breathes too rapidly (see page 117, chapter 9). Hyperventilation is very common, and easy to correct.

You've developed chest pains? You fear it may be your heart.

If they began while you were reading the last ten pages, be reassured. The possibility is strong that you've become infected with the "medical student's syndrome." Often medical students "develop" symptoms that match the disease they happen to be studying. You've been in their company for the past several chapters. So your concern is natural.

Causes of coronary heart attack

There are three coronary arteries as described in the last chapter, but four danger spots, where narrowing may lead to a severe heart attack.

1. The most dangerous spot: a narrowing in the left main stem (the left coronary artery) *before* it branches into its two main subdivisions. A patient rarely survives a heart attack if there is total blockage at this point. When coronary arteriograms show a severe narrowing here, the patient is in urgent need of surgery. Fortunately, it is not a frequent finding.

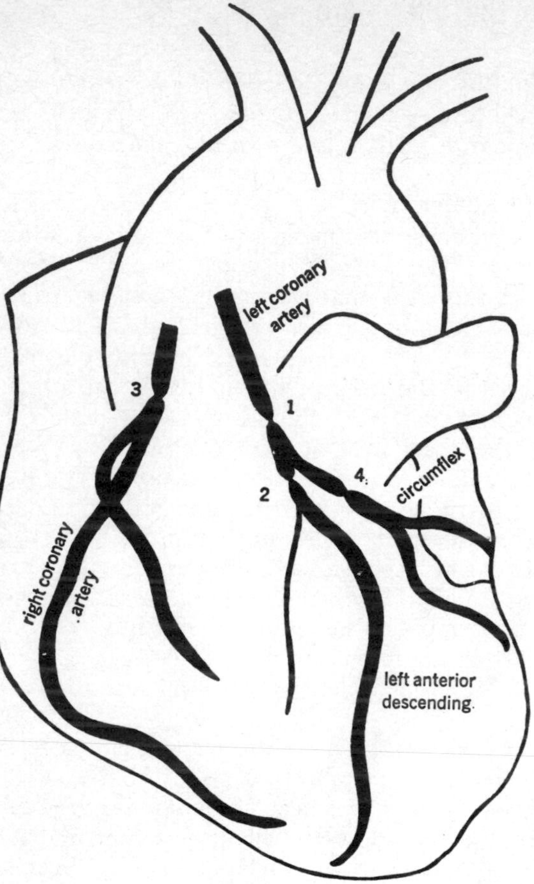

The coronary arteries: four points of narrowing

2. The next most deadly site is the left anterior descending *before* it gives off any branches. It is not uncommon to find serious narrowing here. While not as dangerous as the first site, it is much more common and therefore critical for more people. Dr. Donald Effler, the internationally known heart surgeon at The Cleveland Clinic, has aptly named this narrowing, "The Widow Maker." When we find severe narrowing here without good collaterals to help out the damaged artery we feel an operation is needed.

3. Another site is the right coronary artery which is usually large.

4. The fourth is the circumflex branch of the left coronary, which is often the smallest of the three.

When any of these coronaries close completely with arteriosclerosis (rust in the pipes), the heart muscle may be damaged.

This is a heart attack.

The larger and longer the blood vessel, the greater the amount of heart muscle it supplies. And the greater is the damage to the heart if the vessel is blocked. The greater the damage, the more the danger.

Heart attack damage

A heart attack damages the main pumping chamber, the left ventricle. When the attack occurs, damage doesn't involve the entire ventricle. Just a segment, perhaps at the tip

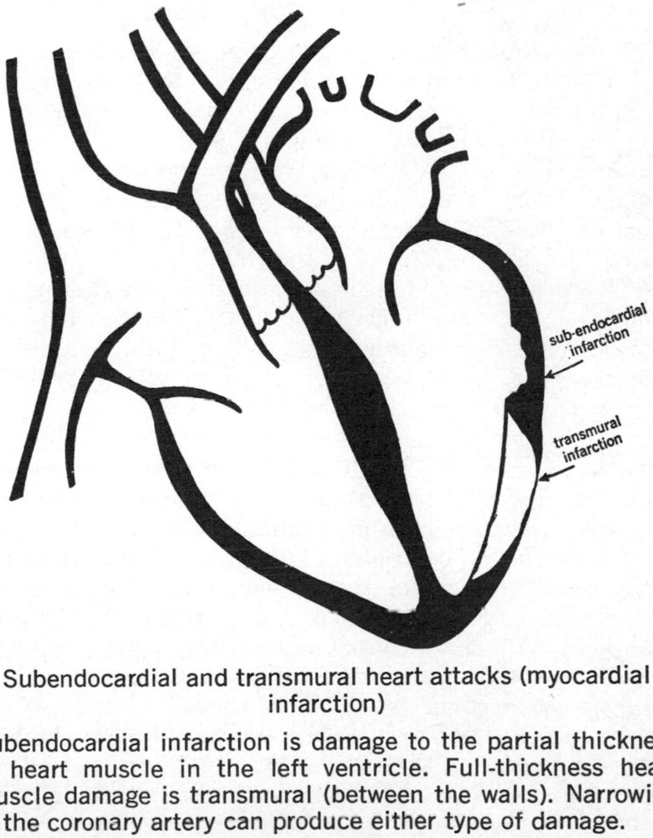

Subendocardial and transmural heart attacks (myocardial infarction)

Subendocardial infarction is damage to the partial thickness of heart muscle in the left ventricle. Full-thickness heart muscle damage is transmural (between the walls). Narrowing of the coronary artery can produce either type of damage.

or along the side. A more severe heart attack might damage more than one area. But usually just one part is involved. So there are infarctions of different size depending on where along the artery the extreme narrowing or closure occurred and how much muscle was dependent on nourishing blood from that coronary artery.

The inner lining of the heart is called the *endocardium.* When only part of the ventricular wall's thickness is damaged, the involved area is usually just next to this inner lining. Therefore, a *sub-endocardial infarction* is partial damage to the ventricle's wall.

In other cases, the damaged segment may go all the way through the wall, from the outer surface of the heart to its inner lining. This is a *transmural infarction.* It is usually larger. It destroys more heart muscle and leaves the heart weaker, especially in the early stages of recovery.

The thickness and size of the damaged area are important factors. The physician will consider them in deciding when his patient is ready to sit up, feed himself, begin to walk and return to work. And when he is ready for sexual relations with his wife again. Size and thickness of the damaged piece of heart muscle aren't the only points evaluated by the doctor, but they are the most important.

After a heart attack, part of the vital left ventricular wall is replaced by scar. The scar becomes tough and strong as it heals. But it is no longer muscle, which means it is stiff and has no give. It cannot contract and relax. As a result, it decreases the heart's ability to pump as well as its ability to accept blood at low pressure from the lungs.

The left ventricle can lose 20 to 25 percent of its muscle and still perform well.

However, if more than 25 percent of the left ventricle is destroyed, heart function may suffer. The heart's ability to relax is the first to deteriorate. Drainage of blood from the lungs to the left ventricle can be hampered. The lungs can become congested. The patient has difficulty in breathing (dyspnea). The more heart muscle lost, the greater the congestion. Since the symptoms of this congestion may build up slowly, it is usually first noticed by the patient during some form of activity. Shortness of breath with exertion. The flight of stairs to the attic seems steeper. Halfway up, it feels good to stop and catch one's breath. Finally, shortness of breath even at rest. This means the person is severely ill, needs hospitalization and intensive medical care.

Sometimes, this form of congestion builds up quickly. It may be triggered by infection. Or by a meal containing too much salt. Or by stopping medication too soon. Or it may be set off by a new heart attack. In this case, fluid collects rapidly in the lungs. The patient has great difficulty breathing. This is *pulmonary edema,* which can be life threatening. Immediate hospitalization is mandatory.

A very large heart attack strains the reserve capacity of the left ventricle. The heart is barely pumping enough blood to keep the body alive. Blood pressure is low. The organs of the body aren't nourished properly. The kidneys cannot clear the blood stream of waste products. The patient may be confused because not enough oxygenated blood is reaching the brain.

This is *shock.* It is extremely serious. Fortunately, it doesn't occur often in heart attack patients.

The patient suffering a heart attack of moderate size will probably experience no congestion or shock. But as he recovers, he may find it difficult to recapture his old vitality. He may fatigue more easily. The supermarket may seem farther from the parking lot. And the packages heavier. The 11:00 P.M. news is less interesting, because the body insists on an earlier bedtime.

The wise patient listens to these messages from within. A damaged heart is no longer normal. Readjustments to a life style are to be expected.

Collaterals and a heart attack

A collateral, as described in the previous chapter, is that bridging vessel between coronary arteries. (They also occur in other parts of the body.) But the collateral vessel is only as good as the arteries it is attached to. It is only as good as its supply, the supply that comes from another of the coronary arteries. If a narrowing developed in the supplying vessel (the one that feeds the collaterals), it decreases the flow through the collaterals as well as to the endangered heart muscle. The collateral is open but the source is closing. This is serious. Because if the donating coronary artery closes, you have in effect, two coronary arteries closing at the same time. The result may be a very large heart attack. Surgery may be needed to prevent it.

Collaterals have puzzled and intrigued physicians for

years. Many doctors have felt that they had to be a protective device to help the heart, that when they did exist, they would save the heart muscle from damage. Yet any number of people with collaterals were felled by heart attacks. Dr. Franklin wanted to know why they weren't protected.

He reviewed hundreds of the "maps" of the heart called coronary arteriograms (see chapter 15, "The Heart in Motion Photography"), trying to form a conclusion about collaterals. He came up with two.

The first was that timing is important.

If the coronary artery closed off in a person who had no collaterals, a heart attack would occur. But sometimes, he discovered, collaterals developed *after* the heart attack. Too late to help. This explained why arteriograms showed collaterals in some patients who had suffered heart damage.

The next logical theory was that collaterals should protect the heart from damage if they were present before the coronary artery closed and the heart attack might have occurred.

Over the next year, Dr. Franklin carefully followed a number of patients who had narrowed coronary arteries and collaterals, but no heart damage. The heart muscle supplied by the narrowed coronary artery was getting a portion of its blood supply from the collaterals. The collaterals seemed to be protecting the heart muscle. But would they continue to do so?

His observations went well into a second year. Patients with collaterals responded well to medical treatment. (This was in the early years of heart surgery for coronary problems.) In spite of severe coronary narrowings, symptoms in these patients lessened. None had heart attacks. The few who had occasional anginal episodes were able to work and live comfortably.

At the end of the second year, one of these patients did have a heart attack. The damaged area of the left ventricle was in the region fed by the collaterals. Dr. Franklin was again puzzled. He reviewed the arteriograms. And then he saw it!

The vessel that gave rise to the collaterals was itself narrowed.

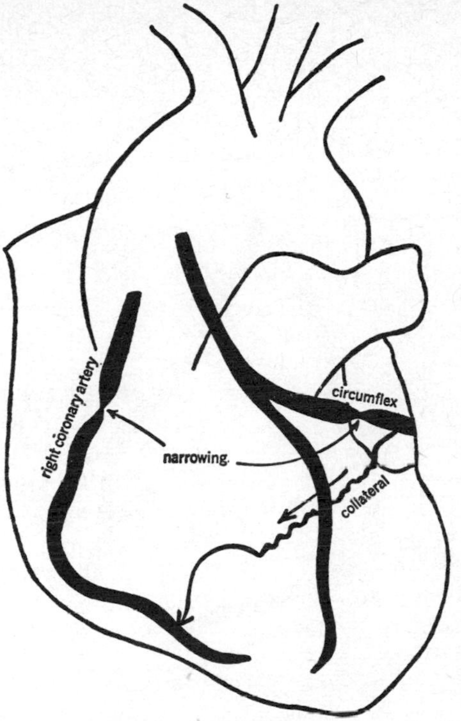

Jeopardized collateral

The right coronary artery is severely narrowed. Complete blockage of this artery would ordinarily produce a major heart attack.

A collateral arises from the severely narrowed circumflex artery—a major branch of the left coronary artery. Because the donor vessel is severely narrowed, it cannot provide full protection to the heart muscle supplied by the severely narrowed right coronary artery.

Blockage of the two severely narrowed vessels would produce massive heart attack.

Patients with this problem are often best treated by surgery with double by-pass operations.

Although the collaterals were there, their source of supply from one of the other coronary arteries was endangered. The collaterals were jeopardized.

This suggested to Dr. Franklin a second concept:

Collaterals had to have a parent vessel that was open and free of any significant narrowing. A life preserver that leaks

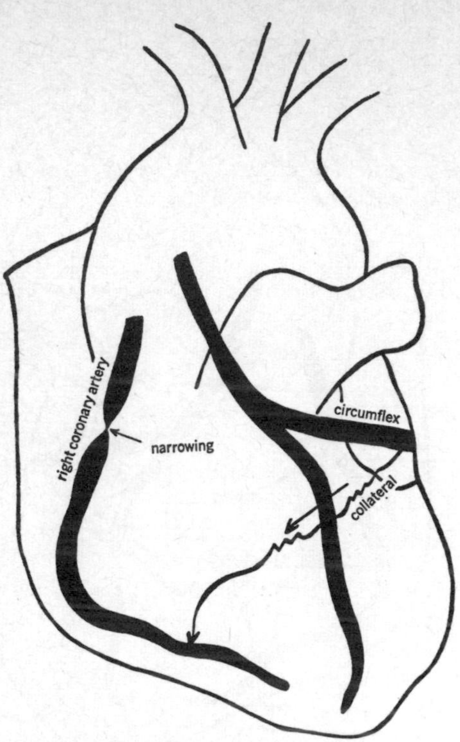

Unjeopardized collateral

The right coronary artery is severely narrowed. Complete blockage of this artery would ordinarily produce a major heart attack.

An extra vessel (collateral) arises from the clean circumflex artery.

Collaterals arising from a source of this kind are called *unjeopardized collaterals.* They protect the heart muscle previously supplied by the now severely narrowed right coronary artery. In this case, occlusions may not cause a heart attack.

The quality of a collateral can help us to decide specific treatment.

or is waterlogged can keep you afloat only for awhile. It postpones the catastrophe, but doesn't avoid it.

These concepts have held up. As a result, we now have many patients, alive, working, and with minimal symptoms. Yet each one has a major coronary artery that is narrowed by 90 percent or even totally blocked. The heart muscle that should be fed by the narrowed or blocked vessel is supplied by the collaterals.

Unjeopardized collaterals are good.

Jeopardized collaterals, those that are supplied from a narrowed source vessel, are risky. We now recommend surgery for most patients with jeopardized collaterals.

So collaterals, like an insurance policy, are good to have. We value their presence, especially if they come early enough and in the right place.

DR. KRAUTHAMER:

You would never associate Karl S. with heart disease. At 58, he was a spare, youthful-looking man, with a quiet, relaxed manner and a gentle philosophy of life seldom seen in our present hectic times. After having survived a siege of tuberculosis in his youth, which gave him plenty of time to meditate in the sanitarium, he taught himself the value of every moment of his day and how to enjoy it.

He has a small law practice in a nearby commuter town, a happy marriage, and children who have given him few of the ordinary problems.

One spring Sunday morning, as he was bicycling on a lonely stretch of beach against a harsh wind, he was suddenly aware of a funny feeling in his chest—heavy, but not really painful. He stopped pedaling and the discomfort disappeared. Two weeks later he went skiing without any trouble. Routine activity presented no problems.

Then it recurred. This time, his wife was bicycling with him, and he told her why he'd asked her to come along. They pedaled home slowly, and he noticed a mild recurrence while wheeling the bicycle up the hill to the garage. A few seconds later, it was gone.

He called me that afternoon. He was feeling well and had no other symptoms. We agreed that there was no need for emergency care but cautioned him to carry nitroglycerine with him until we could do a complete evaluation.

Monday morning, I did his history, physical examination and resting ECG. Everything seemed normal. Wednesday morning, he took the treadmill stress test (see page 170, chapter 14, "Testing, Testing"). This was markedly abnormal and diagnostic of coronary disease. He went for cardiac catheterization on Friday (see chapter 15, "Catheterization, Heart in Motion Photography").

We found the anterior descending artery more than 90

percent narrowed. Fortunately, the right coronary artery had sent connecting branches—collaterals—to this vessel. This secondary supply was enough to preserve the heart muscle, but not enough to prevent symptoms. However, since it did keep the heart muscle alive, there was no need for surgery. We started him on an intensive program of medication, and a specific regimen of diet, exercise and activity.

Six months later, a repeat treadmill test was perfectly normal.

He continues to do well, works actively and enjoys a rich full life. We were obliged to curtail a few activities. He can still bicycle, but not against the wind on a cold day. He continues to enjoy the important things in his life.

The coronary arteriograms were helpful in predicting the outcome of this case of *unjeopardized collaterals.*

DR. TAI:

Jack Z. was an asthmatic child. As he grew older, his health improved somewhat, but by the time he was in his early 50s, the asthma returned, full-blown, and accompanied by emphysema, which was slowly destroying his capacity to function. He visited his family physician regularly for medications to keep him breathing adequately.

"He follows all of the doctor's instructions," his wife, Fay, reported. "Except for cigarettes."

"I'm addicted," Jack admitted morosely.

His doctor and his wife had both given up on him. Jack continued smoking. One winter day, he was conscious of an uneasy feeling in his chest as he climbed the hill to his doctor's office. The symptoms persisted for a month and finally Jack said to his doctor: "Look, this bothers me enough so I want an answer."

His doctor thought it might be a mild heart condition and suggested a cardiac consultation. That's how Jack came to us. After his workup, we told him that coronary arteriography would give us a definite answer about the condition of his heart. Even though his symptoms were mild and certainly atypical, there was always a chance that he might have a severe heart condition. We also told him that if surgery were needed, he might not be able to tolerate an operation because of his lung condition.

This was the appropriate moment to make a bargain with Jack. We agreed to do the coronary arteriograms provided he stopped smoking. He accepted the challenge.

We brought him to the hospital a week later, and did the coronary arteriograms without any problems. They showed a total blockage of one of his coronary arteries—the left anterior descending—that dreaded Widow Maker.

But he hadn't had a heart attack. Nor any severe chest pains. His ECG showed no evidence of heart damage.

The answer was *collaterals*. He had a heavy bridging network of small blood vessels leading from his right coronary artery. They connected to the blocked vessel, thus preserving the muscle of the heart.

However, the right coronary artery, the source that fed the collaterals, had a severe narrowing at its beginning. If this narrowing in the right artery closed, Jack would suffer the effect of two large heart attacks at once.

Now we had a problem. Jack needed an operation if he were to have any chance of survival.

We contacted a heart surgeon who agreed to operate as soon as we could get Jack's lungs in shape for cardiac surgery. This required three weeks of intensive inhalation therapy twice a day. His lungs responded well. Jack was finally ready. He was transferred to a university center that had an excellent department of heart surgery and an outstanding section of respiratory therapy.

He was scheduled for surgery the morning of February 15th. On the 12th he was admitted to the university center. They wanted to double-check on his ability to withstand the operation.

On the evening of February 14th, Jack was walking in the corridor with Fay. Suddenly he collapsed and fell to the floor.

The nurse flashed the cardiac arrest signal. Doctors converged on Jack from all parts of the hospital. All available modern medical technology was put to work right there in the hallway. But it was too late. Blockage of the coronary artery, and the lack of blood supply had caused so much damage to the heart muscle that only a new heart would have allowed him to survive.

It's important to note that Jack never had a severe complaint related to his heart. According to his wife, they had been talking about the surgery, and he was relieved that it was going to be done. He complained of no pain, even as he collapsed.

The post-mortem confirmed the cause of death as occlusion of the threadlike narrowing in the right coronary artery. The blockage affected not only the right coronary artery but the left anterior descending as well because of the collateral connection. The heart's electrical system as well as the muscle got caught short. The heart stopped and couldn't be started again.

Had his lung condition cleared up early enough to permit an operation in two weeks, he might have lived.

Chapter 7

Valves—floodgates of the heart

DR. TAI:
"Doctor, I can't understand it. I don't smoke. I don't drink. But I'm getting more and more attacks of bronchitis. It's been a very bad winter for me."

Her name was Olga. She was 56 years old and looked older, but had the general air of a woman who was comfortable in managing her home and her family.

In going over her past history, I asked if she'd had rheumatic fever or scarlet fever.

"Not that I remember," she said. "I had growing pains in my joints, but I was never confined to bed."

Three years ago, Olga came down with a severe case of flu, with irregularities of the heartbeat. She was admitted to the hospital where her major symptom, shortness of breath, was controlled by medication. Afterwards, she tried to function normally, but her husband, a prominent real estate broker, felt that she had slowed down.

He called me and said, "Olga denies it, but it takes her twice as long to climb the stairs. She spends more time cleaning the house. She used to come out on the golf course with me but she's given it up. She always has some excuse. She isn't normal, not as I've known her for thirty years. I wish you'd give her a complete checkup."

By inspection, palpation, listening to the heart sounds, we estimated that her mitral valve was narrowed and there was back pressure in her left atrium as well as in her lungs. The ECG and special types of chest X-rays confirmed our view. We explained the situation to Olga and her husband and suggested treatment.

She had both a cardiac catheterization and an echocardiogram (see chapter 14, "Testing, Testing") which verified our findings. She did require surgery to open the mitral valve. She came through the operation splendidly, and now leads a normal, active life.

"I didn't realize how sick I was," she said, when I saw her for a followup after surgery. "I feel like a new woman."

"For the love of Mike," Robbie said, "just what is *mitral stenosis?*"

There were four patients sitting in a small room off the plant-filled solarium in the hospital, and each of them had valve problems. It was two o'clock in the afternoon, and the hospital was filling up with visitors, but each of these men had warned his family to skip this afternoon's call. I was going to talk to them about valvular problems in an informal seminar. The men were Robbie L., Hank G., Julian S., and Louis R. They were all to be discharged at the end of the week.

"You have four valves," I said. "The two valves on the left side of your heart are tremendously important. Any disease that affects both the mitral and aortic valves will cause greater disability than if it affects the tricuspid or pulmonic valves, on the right side of your heart."

"What's the reason?" Julian asked.

"On the left side, blood pressure is five times higher than on the right. This means the mitral and aortic valves are under much greater stress than the other two. If disease attacks the mitral or aortic valves, there is greater burden on the heart.

"If there is an inflammation of a valve, the edges of its cusps may thicken and partially fuse. As a result, when the valve opens, blood can't flow through easily. The narrowing of a valve is called *stenosis*. If it affects the mitral valve, it's *mitral stenosis*. If it affects the aortic valve, it's *aortic stenosis*. Both can be caused by rheumatic fever. Once in a while, we come across a case that is due to congenital narrowing of the mitral valve. This is rare and requires attention in early infancy."

"What I can't understand," Robbie said, "is this bit about mitral regurgitation."

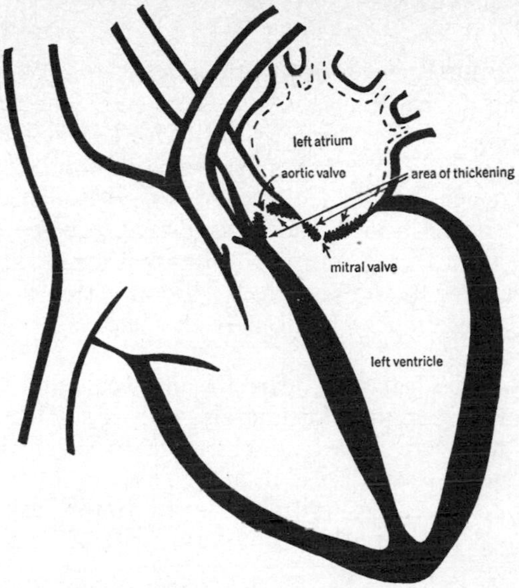

Mitral Stenosis and Aortic Stenosis

Mitral stenosis: Narrowing of the mitral valve blocks blood flow from the lungs. The back pressure dilates the left atrium and raises pressure in the lungs, which become stiff, causing shortness of breath. Too much pressure can cause blood vessels in the lungs to burst and lead to coughing up blood.

Aortic stenosis: Narrowing at the aortic valve blocks outflow from the left ventricle. The left ventricle must then work harder, and it enlarges.

"If the mitral valve cusps are damaged, they can't close properly. They are branded as incompetent valves. The term we use is 'regurgitation' of the valve."

"How does it affect your heart?" Robbie asked. He was a big man, blond and muscular like a Viking, and to an observer, an unlikely candidate for heart disease.

"When the left atrium pours blood into the left ventricle, the mitral valve opens downward into the left ventricle. Once the left ventricle begins to contract, the valve snaps into its closed position. To prevent it from billowing backward into the left atrium, and allowing blood to be squeezed back, nature has provided a kind of support system, of muscles and fibers connecting the valve edges to the heart wall.

"Sometimes, after a heart attack, the muscles and fibers supporting the mitral valve are damaged. The valve loses its tautness and may over-flip into the left atrium leaving a gap that could produce a leakage of blood."

"Is that what happened to me?" asked Louis.

"Yes," I told him. "The leakage is *mitral regurgitation.* If the valve leaks, it means the heart must do extra work with each beat to compensate for blood which is sent backwards in the wrong direction. If the leak is small, it is of no importance.

"But a large leak in a heart already weakened by a heart attack can be serious. Fortunately, only a small number of patients who have heart attacks develop severe leaks. For them, a heart operation is usually necessary."

"What else causes mitral regurgitation?" asked Louis. He was a slight man, too early bald, with a tense, nervous manner.

"There are other factors. A deposit of calcium in the mitral valve apparatus may produce weakness in the function of the mitral valve. The cusps of the mitral valve can be destroyed as a result of rheumatic fever. This usually occurs in children or young people. Some women are born with naturally short support fibers which makes them liable to mitral regurgitation.

"In all these situations, the left ventricle connects freely with the left atrium, when the mitral valve should totally close the space between them, between beats. Instead, some blood goes back into the left atrium, and less blood is pumped into the aorta.

"Fortunately, the heart can tolerate this condition for many years. These patients don't require treatment in the early stages or even later, if the problem remains mild. If it becomes severe and produces enlargement of the heart and incapacity, an artificial valve must be implanted through surgery. You don't need one."

"Well, what precautions should I take?" Louis asked.

"As we told you, Louis, you require no drastic treatment. You can lead a perfectly normal life."

"Are there any risks?" Louis persisted.

"Sometimes if a valve becomes deformed for any reason, it attracts bacteria. They grow on its surface and produce what is called *bacterial* or *infective endocarditis*. The endocardium is the surface covering of the valve as well as the heart. To avoid this complication, a patient with valve disease must take antibiotics before any dental treatment or surgery. This is something you must all remember."

Julian wanted to hear more about the cusps of the mitral valve, where his problem was centered. He was lean, wiry, and looked as though he'd never had a sick day in his life.

"If the mitral valve isn't leaking, but the cusps have thickened and there is decreased movement of the cusps, it means that the opening of the mitral valve will be smaller than it should be. When this happens, the left atrium cannot empty itself normally. Blood coming from the lungs distends the left atrium. As a result, there is distention of the blood vessels that come from the lungs, causing higher pressure in the pulmonary circulation. Some blood can leak into the air passages. This may prevent the proper exchange of oxygen and carbon dioxide, and produce acute pulmonary edema. So the patient has shortness of breath—"

"And a cough," Hank interrupted, "mixed with sputum and blood."

"Right," I said. "A person may be without symptoms for years, then they will show up between the ages of 30 and 50. Once in a while, we see a new patient in his 70s but this is rare. When a patient with mitral stenosis develops shortness of breath, blood-stained sputum, or irregularity of the heartbeat, he requires immediate attention."

"What do you do?" Hank asked sarcastically, "Cut him open?"

"If he needs it, surgery is recommended. The valve is either slit or stretched with the surgeon's finger or a scalpel to enlarge the aperture. Or an artificial valve is put in." (See chapter 18, "Surgery.")

In my discussion with the four men, I had covered only mitral stenosis, not aortic stenosis. In mitral stenosis, the aortic valve is usually alright. But what if it's the aortic valve that is in trouble?

Aortic stenosis is narrowing of the aortic valve.

Normally the left ventricle must exert force to raise its pressure from 10 millimeters to 120 millimeters so it can open the aortic valve and force the blood forward. When the aortic valve is narrowed, the ventricle's work load increases in order to force blood through the tighter valve. The result is that the wall of the left ventricle increases in thickness and also works harder to pump out the same amount of blood. So there is a tremendous waste of energy.

Now as the left ventricle's work load increases, the oxygen supply from its coronary arteries cannot keep up with this demand. There is now a disproportion between supply and demand. The left ventricle isn't functioning normally. The patient is likely to have trouble: shortness of breath, chest pain, even fainting spells. This is not a heart attack but it resembles angina. It needs urgent attention and frequently the patient will require valve replacement. In patients with valve disease, medications aren't used for the condition of the valve itself, but drugs may be used to control the rate and rhythm of the heart (see chapter 16, "Medications").

DR. KRAUTHAMER:

Marcia, 48 years old, and an unusually handsome woman, had become aware of increasing shortness of breath in the last few months. The first time she noticed it was after a Christmas dance. One member of her family was a physician and had treated her for pneumonia. Marcia was admitted to a New York hospital, where her illness was diagnosed as aortic valve regurgitation (leaking) and infective endocarditis.

What had happened was this: Marcia had a dental extraction early in October. Eight weeks later she had chills and fever, and a week later at the dance she was short of breath. Going back over the sequence, she realized that she had been fatigued for several weeks, but had thought it was due to Christmas shopping and the demanding holiday season.

Marcia was treated successfully for infective endocarditis and then referred to us for evaluation.

On examination, I heard a heart murmur which suggested leaking of the aortic valve, but otherwise the heart was only minimally enlarged. Marcia had no acute heart symptoms. She didn't recall having had any manifestations of rheumatic fever or "growing pains" as a child.

After doing a complete catheterization, it was our impression that her aortic valve was leaking but not seriously. This caused mild overloading of the heart. The other valves and heart muscle were normal, the coronary arteries were clean.

We treated Marcia medically. We explained the precautions that would prevent a recurrence of bacterial endocarditis.

She continued to do well, but two years later she was readmitted to the hospital with a history of chills and fever similar to the previous episode. This time, however, her heartbeat was irregular. It was regulated with medication, and the chills and fever were treated as if she had endocarditis.

Her symptoms had now become more progressive. She was fatigued easily. She was beginning to get shortness of breath on less exertion than previously. As a result, we repeated the catheterization and found there was an increase in pressure in the left ventricular chamber.

Marcia underwent surgery and received an artificial aortic valve. She continues to do well and now leads a normal and active life without any symptoms.

The most common cause of valve problems is childhood rheumatic fever. When a child gets rheumatic heart disease brought on by rheumatic fever, it usually involves the valves on the left side of the heart—the mitral or aortic valves. The reason for more frequent involvement of the left-sided valves is probably the high pressure at which the left side of the heart works. With the onset of rheumatic fever, the valve thickens. Later it shrivels. As a result, these cusps do not close properly. A gap is left through which the blood flows back and forth. That means that the one-way traffic pattern, so essential to a healthy heart, is abolished. In rheumatic heart disease, the mobility of the cusps is decreased. They remain slightly open when they should be completely closed. Therefore, the valve opening may be narrowed as well as incompetent.

DR. TAI:
He was christened Michael Daniel, Jr., after his father who had been an outstanding soccer player in England.

When Michael, Sr. visited the United States with his soccer team ten years ago, he was captivated by New England, particularly the Berkshire foothills in Connecticut. He met an American girl at a Tanglewood concert and decided to settle permanently nearby. He had enough money to buy a sizable farm, since land went for $50 an uncultivated acre at the time. The rocky soil proved to be good for nothing but beautiful views and grazing for cattle. It was a trial, but Michael, Sr. wasn't accustomed to luxuries and he worked at his farm with enthusiasm and vitality. Michael's wife was a dreamy, poetic young woman who deeply loved the three children who came in rapid succession.

The children had fresh air, plenty of milk and good food. Mike, Jr. seemed healthy enough the first four years of his life, and his father visualized the boy as a future athlete. That Mike, Jr. was rather delicate and fair like his mother didn't alter Mike, Sr.'s dreams.

Little Mike's first rheumatic episode happened when he was five years old. He'd had a bad sore throat in mid-December. The day before Christmas, the Elks were giving a party for the local children at the Grange Hall. The child was tired, pale and looked wan, but he begged to be allowed to attend, so his mother gave in. He went in a sleigh with the neighbors' kids. A glittering powdery snow softened the landscape, and when Mike returned from the party, he and his playmates had a lively snowball fight. He seemed so happy that his mother didn't worry about the furious color in his cheeks. But on Christmas morning, when he didn't want to leave his bed, she realized he was feverish.

"I feel sick all over," he said, whimpering.

His mother brought him orange juice and helped him get dressed so he could join his younger brothers at the tree. She noticed one knee was swollen, but as he limped around during the morning, she thought it was because he wanted attention. In the evening, when his limp increased, and both knee joints were swollen, she gave him aspirin. Three days later, he was still limping, and she bundled him into the jeep, and drove him into the village to the doctor. The doctor prescribed aspirin, bed rest, and gave his mother a supply of penicillin so the boy could have prolonged antibiotic therapy. She meant well, but her chores and the care of the children overwhelmed her. Besides, Mike, Jr. made a fuss about taking his medication, and he seemed to be quite well again. When she ran out of capsules during a March blizzard, she couldn't get to the village for a fresh supply.

Mike came down with a series of sore throats and several weeks after each, he had aching joints. His mother didn't bother to refill the prescription. It was a case of benign neglect.

After the third episode, Mike, Jr. was hospitalized for more restricted bed rest, continued aspirin therapy, given penicillin and then discharged. His heart was now seriously and permanently damaged.

If he had been kept on penicillin after the first episodes, most likely this could have been prevented.

The third attack of acute rheumatic fever left him with severe insufficiency (improper closure) of his aortic and mitral valves. He is ill now. His heart is twice the normal size, his chest heaves, he can tolerate very little exercise. When he tries to play basketball, he lasts about three minutes.

He is a child with a poor prognosis.

There was a time when the diagnosis of rheumatic fever brought terror to a parent's heart. Rheumatic fever, tuberculosis, polio were the Three Horsemen of the Apocalypse for all children. Modern medicine has brought them under control—sanitariums are closing down, iron lungs and leg braces are nearly obsolete, and the swollen painful joints and enlarged heart of the child with recurring rheumatic fever are seen less often.

It is currently thought that rheumatic fever is a reaction by the body to part of the streptococcus bacteria and that rheumatic heart disease is the result of this reaction on the heart. Recent research suggests that there may be other causes as well, but preventing "strep" infections seems to cut down on the incidence of rheumatic fever.

A recent study in a typical mid-American town of 20,000

people demonstrated how rheumatic fever can be controlled. The school system there decided that whenever a child was absent with a cold and sore throat, he was to have a throat culture before being allowed to return to class. If a strep infection was found, penicillin was prescribed for ten days. The result was startling: not one case of rheumatic fever in the town for over a year.

And even when rheumatic fever does develop, the risk of heart damage can be lessened. If treated with bed rest and medications, only a small percentage of children stricken with rheumatic fever actually develop rheumatic heart disease. The frequency and severity of rheumatic fever and resulting rheumatic heart disease are definitely on the decline. This is due both to proper early treatment of strep infections as well as improved socio-economic conditions.

But there are still serious cases of the disease if children aren't treated promptly and effectively.

Once a child has suffered an attack of rheumatic fever, he is more likely to have a recurrence, and every sore throat should be looked upon as a forerunner of another episode.

How can a parent prevent what happened to Mike?

The child has a sore throat and fever of about 102 degrees. His throat is severely inflamed and there are tiny spots of yellow or whitish pus. It's best to call a doctor and ask about taking a throat culture. Some mothers rely on aspirin, bed rest, plenty of fluids, and often the child recovers uneventfully, and his indisposition is dismissed as a simple cold. But a couple of weeks later, he might be looking pallid, running a fever every afternoon and limping. (Incidentally, a mother should never give her child antibiotics without first checking with her physician.)

We're not trying to make mothers a nationwide group of diagnosticians. We would like to educate and develop awareness about rheumatic fever.

We've never had a call from a mother saying: "Johnny had a sore throat two weeks ago; he was out playing ball today and hurt his knee, but he says it's the other knee that hurts. It's swollen and a bit tender. I've checked him over and he has a little lump on his elbow—"

But this is what we are aiming for.

Often a limp may be dismissed as "growing pains." Then a few years later, a heart murmur might be detected. It is wise for the parents of a child like this to have him checked once a year by the family doctor. What we hope for is not overreaction of the parents but awareness. Fortunately, today many parents are aware of the dangers and the school nurse and physician do check the child who suffers from endless colds and sore throats during the winter.

A single case of rheumatic fever may not damage the heart. But if there are more episodes of fever and pain and what was originally a minimal heart murmur is ignored, the chance of the young patient coming through without permanent cardiac damage is small, even though it may not show up until he is in his mid-40s or 50s.

Therefore, if a child has an attack of acute rheumatic fever, he should be put on continuous pencillin therapy into his adult life, perhaps even longer. If he happens to work in a field that exposes him to children, he should continue taking penicillin for life.

If a young person gets a strep throat, scarlet fever, or even a strep infection of the skin, it can generate an attack of rheumatic fever. But not necessarily rheumatic heart disease. Certain types of streptococcus seem to cause inflammation of the *serosa*, the thin membrane that covers the joints, lungs, heart, intestines. The time span before the patient complains of symptoms from such inflammation is usually three weeks.

The American Heart Association has adopted a group of criteria for making a diagnosis of acute rheumatic fever, since no single test pinpoints it.

The three most important clues are fever, rapid heart rate, fleeting joint pains. When arthritis comes, the joints are red, tender, swollen. The larger joints are usually involved. Not the joints of fingers and toes, but the wrists, ankles, knees and larger joints. The arthritis may clear up, then return, attacking another joint. This is called migratory arthritis and is one of the hallmarks of rheumatic fever.

Inflammation of a valve of the heart (valvulitis) may finally occur, and produce a heart murmur and abnormal function of the valve. Or myocarditis, where the heart muscle itself is inflamed, weakened and damaged.

In addition to fever, arthritis, and valvulitis, there may

be a rash that forms circles on the abdomen and trunk *erythema annulare*. Nodules (lumps) under the skin, which occur over the elbows and feel almost like tumors, are present in some cases of acute rheumatic fever, but fade as it subsides.

Dr. Sydenham was the first physician to fully describe rheumatic fever. He also named Sydenham's *Chorea*, another rarer manifestation of the disease which is popularly called St. Vitus Dance, and is characterized by the patient's nervous gestures. When these "wormlike" motions of the arms and hands, grimacing of the face, are found, involvement of the heart is common. Unfortunately, many parents don't seem to realize what's wrong with the child for too long. If a child has chorea, as one of the signs of rheumatic fever, the chance that he will develop a heart problem is much higher.

Recovery may depend on the severity of the attack. One of the great physicians has said that "rheumatic fever licks the joints and bites the heart." As far as the child's frame is concerned, rheumatic fever leaves no permanent deformity. The damage, if it does occur, is on the inside.

Other diseases causing aortic valve trouble:
The aortic valve can also be damaged by venereal disease, especially syphilis. And another disease called Reiter's Syndrome, which is a venereal disease producing infection of the urethra and inflammation of the heart valves.

The aortic valve can also become incompetent in old age and as a result of high blood pressure. In some very peculiar forms of arthritis, called *ankylosing spondylitis*, it can also become incompetent. Some children are born with a disorder of the tissue supporting the aorta and its valve, which may lead to malfunctioning of the aortic valve. This is called Marfan's Syndrome. Abraham Lincoln had it in a mild form.

The most common cause of aortic stenosis in the older individual is the slow development of a calcium deposit on a valve that may be abnormal at birth.

Chapter 8

Short circuit of the heart

DR. KRAUTHAMER:
Your heart has a natural pacemaker which I described in chapter 6. The sino-atrial (S-A) node, located in the right atrium's upper wall, is in charge of regulating your heartbeat. When it is working properly, it sends an electrical impulse through the upper two chambers of your heart and also reaches the two lower chambers, through the way station, the atrio-ventricular (A-V) node. But sometimes there is a roadblock. The upper chambers receive signals from the pacemaker, the S-A node, but the lower chambers don't receive the electrical signal because of a break in the conduction system. The impulses are not getting through. Where is the block? Sometimes it is in the way station, the A-V node itself. More often the problem is in the conducting pathways beyond the A-V node, that is, in its "fleshy wires."

What happens if no signal reaches the lower chambers? The upper chambers keep on beating. But no blood leaves the heart to go to the rest of the body. If the heart isn't pumping blood, you pass out. This is called heart block.

The lower chambers need a "spark" to get them going. Without an electrical signal, nothing will happen. But the signal cannot get through.

Fortunately, the heart has a "fail-safe" system for just such an emergency, the His-Purkinje system which can be a secondary generator and functions at only 50 beats or less per minute.

This is enough to keep a person alive. So when heart block occurs and the primary pacemaker impulses cannot reach the lower chambers, the secondary generator site takes over and produces the slow but life-saving beat.

The secondary system, however, is unstable. It is subject to fits and starts and occasionally it quits altogether for a few seconds or even a minute. Fortunately, it usually starts right up again. But that is the danger of heart block—the heart can actually stop. No heartbeat for a few seconds.

These episodes are called *Stokes-Adams* attacks in honor of the two physicians who did a detailed analysis of this particular syndrome.

Even if a Stokes-Adams attack doesn't occur, the heart,

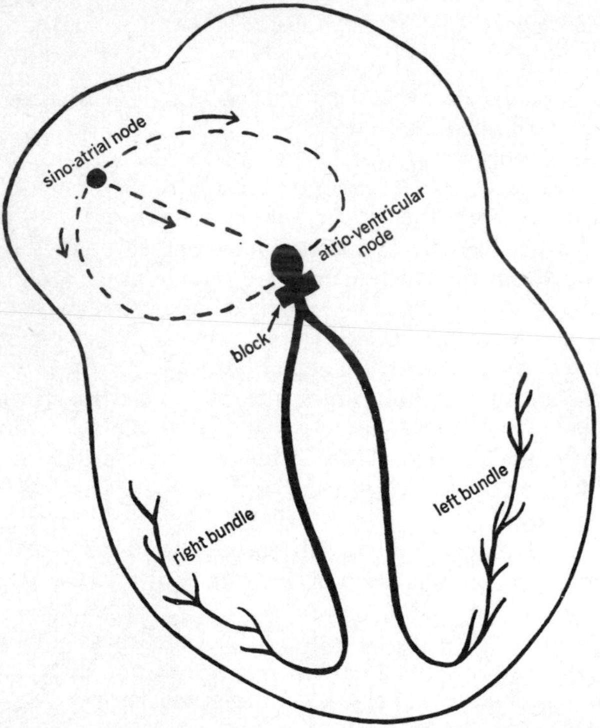

Complete heart block (Stokes-Adams Syndrome)

Impulses are generated normally but do not reach the ventricles.

Disease in part of the electrical system blocks the impulse. A natural secondary pacemaker in the "fleshy wires" usually takes over to keep the heart beating at a slower rate (40–50 beats per minute).

operating on its secondary system, beats at slightly more than half its usual rate. A young person can tolerate this situation without too much difficulty. In an older person, however, this slow heart action can cause fluid to collect in the body. Poor blood flow to the kidneys can affect their function. More insidious is the damage to the brain if there is not enough oxygen. Thinking, reading, even talking, may be impaired, without a stroke or any other neurological problem. In this case, the whole syndrome may be blamed on old age and senility rather than a slow heartbeat. The patient may start to deteriorate and often he is doomed to invalidism.

As cardiologists, we are very much aware of the plight of our elderly patients. Illness often robs them of their dignity and their will to live.

And nothing gives us greater satisfaction than to see a senior citizen rehabilitated. They may come to us withdrawn and moody, but often become delightful when treatment helps them to feel like members of the human race again.

Until recently, this condition was always attributed to hardening of the arteries. It attacked people at the age when arteriosclerosis was to be expected. But modern research proved that this is not so in most cases. The problem for many older patients is not in the heart muscle nor the blood vessels but in the heart's electrical system.

ALTON J.

He was a vigorous man of 62, who took pride in the fact that he had never needed a doctor. He was a success in business, president of a company that manufactured paper bags, and he divided his time between his country home in Connecticut and his condominium in Florida.

He was a guest at a local golf club one July afternoon, when he collapsed on the ninth hole and lost consciousness. The club manager telephoned for a local doctor who rushed to the clubhouse where Mr. J. was now resting, and examined him. Nothing seemed wrong, except for a slightly elevated blood pressure. The doctor reassured Mr. J., gave him a prescription for a mild tranquilizer, and suggested that he see his own doctor for a checkup.

Mr. J. arrived for his appointment with his family physician five days early. "Something peculiar happened to me this morning," he said, rubbing a faint bruise on his tanned forehead. "I had a dizzy spell in the bathroom. I didn't pass out, but I felt my arms going weak, as if they didn't belong to me."

His physician found his heart rate slow, and after taking an electrocardiogram, suggested Mr. J. enter the hospital. "You should be checked by a cardiologist."

"What for?" Mr. J. asked. "Didn't you say my heart was strong?"

"Its beat is strong and steady. But its rate is 40. Normal heart rate is closer to 70."

The doctor picked up his prescription pad and drew a sketch of the heart to illustrate how the heart's pacemaker works.

Mr. J. looked interested. "Where's my trouble? With the pacemaker?"

"Your natural pacemaker is working okay. But the conduction system isn't. The impulse is starting out fine but it doesn't get through to the proper place. The result is a slow heart beat. And fainting spells."

"What do you suggest?"

"It will be up to the cardiologists, but I suspect you will need an artificial pacemaker."

DR. KRAUTHAMER:
The following morning, Mr. J. was in a private room at the hospital. I went in to see him. Mr. J. was remarkably youthful for his age, with a quick way of speaking and a tremendous interest in what was happening to him. He had always been healthy and energetic, and he was irked by the fact that the infirmities of age were present in his system. He had resolved to cooperate fully.

We verified the slow heart rate and also found complete heart block. There was an interruption in the heart's conduction system—a break in one of the fleshy wires.

I explained to Mr. J. that the dizzy spells were due to the unstable nature of the secondary natural pacemaker system which had taken over. It was likely that Mr. J.'s heart had momentarily "stopped" and then started up again.

The brief stops were the fainting spells.

Treatment for heart block is the insertion of a permanent

pacemaker. This would mean a small operation, but the pacemaker would prevent fainting spells and keep Mr. J.'s pulse rate at an appropriate 70 per minute. If this were not done, there was a possibility of sudden death.

He readily agreed to the operation which I performed. He reacted well to it. A man with few emotional hangups, his convalescence was rapid. He knew the operation would make it possible for him to enjoy the future.

He has done extremely well. We recently received a Florida Christmas greeting from his pacemaker. And oranges from Mr. J.

Cases like Mr. J.'s have given us a new slant on the problems of aging and rehabilitation.

At the other end of the spectrum is the child. Sometime we find a newborn infant with congenital heart disease and heart block. The usual heart rate for an infant is 120 to 180 beats per minute. The child with heart block will have a rate of 50 beats per minute at rest. The doctor usually notices the slow heart rate but if there is no murmur, the child may be considered normal. If an electrocardiogram is done, heart block will show up. These children usually do not have any symptoms. When they exercise, their heart rate does rise. As they grow up, many of them are told that their slow heartbeat is no problem, particularly if they are athletic. (When you exercise daily, your pulse tends to become slower.)

Until a few years ago, it was felt that these children had a good prognosis and that their life expectancy would not be affected by a slow rate. Now it has been found that some children with heart block may die suddenly, just as adults do. If a child with heart block has fainting spells (syncope), he too needs a pacemaker. If no fainting spells occur, continued medical observation is suggested.

DR. FRANKLIN:
Burt W., a young man of 21 was referred to us because his electrocardiogram in a pre-employment examination was found to be abnormal. Burt had no previous history of rheumatic fever. He never had a heart murmur nor other form of heart disease. Examination was normal. Electrocardiograms, however, showed a block.

After finishing the evaluation, I talked to him in detail and said I would write a letter to the company. Since Burt was so young, he was rather apprehensive and wanted details.

"Burt, the examination I gave you shows everything to be normal. But your electrocardiogram shows what we call *right bundle branch block,*" I said.

"What do you mean by that, Doctor?"

"When the electrical impulses come from your natural upper pacemaker to the A-V node, they pass normally into two pathways, the left bundle and right bundle. In your case, the right bundle has been blocked. We don't know why—you may have been born with it. The impulses, therefore, come only through the left bundle. First, they activate the left ventricle and then have to cross over to activate the right ventricle. As a result, it takes a long time for the right ventricle to receive the electrical impulse. This shows up on the electrocardiogram."

"Heck," Burt said, "I don't mean to sound sorry for myself, but I'm only 21. What's my future? Will it reduce my life expectancy?"

"From our experience," I said, "and from the experience of other cardiologists, we know that a young healthy person can have a right bundle branch block with no significant effect on the heart. If there is no underlying heart disease, a right bundle branch block by itself will *not* affect your ability to lead a normal life and have a normal life span. You certainly don't require any treatment. Nor do you need any restrictions. You know you have right bundle branch block. Have an ECG done once a year. Otherwise ignore it. Don't ever let it interfere with your life. We'll write a letter to your company recommending that you be employed, and be considered physically fit."

DR. TAI:

Helen C., aged 39, outwardly cheerful and good-natured, was admitted to the hospital by Dr. Sheils, her family physician. Helen has two children. An industrious housewife and mother, she is also an excellent seamstress, never at a loss for work. Her overwhelming ambition is to provide the best of everything for her family. Her house is spotless, her cooking delicious, her daughters are dressed not in jeans and boys' shirts, but in pretty dresses which Helen makes for them. When they complain that they prefer to dress like their friends, Helen is outraged. Helen lost her own mother when she was five, and she tries valiantly to act out her fantasies of what she thinks a good mother should be.

Five years ago, she had a couple of fainting spells. One happened on the street after she had been shopping. When she opened her eyes, she was flat on the pavement, with broken eggs, oranges and dry cereals scattered around, and two elderly ladies trying to help her. She said nothing to the family. There was a recurrence two years afterwards, but she had already forgotten the initial episode. Again she ignored it.

Recently, during the Hong Kong flu epidemic, she caught the virus which left her weak. She was conscious of palpitations of the heart, and near-fainting spells that incapacitated her two or three times a day.

Her ECG showed a *left bundle branch block* with a rather fast heart rate. I attended her and thought she might have *cardiomyopathy* (disease of the heart muscle) with involvement of the conduction system. After our initial workup, she underwent cardiac catheterization. Dr. Sheils was with her in the cath lab while I performed the procedure.

"Dr. Sheils," I said, "I assume the viral infection caused her left bundle branch block and is now responsible for the episodes of complete heart block."

"But she also complained of chest pain," Dr. Sheils said. "I thought it was coronary artery disease."

"No, she's still menstruating, and she doesn't smoke. Nor does she have a family history of coronary artery disease. When we finish the catheterization, we'll know, but I suspect her main problem is that the virus has affected the electrical system of the heart."

I completed the catheterization. The coronary arteries were normal and there was normal function of both the left and right sides of the heart. Indeed, the only problem was in the electrical conduction system.

The following day, Dr. Sheils and I jointly gave her the report. It was likely the viral infection had produced scarring of the heart's electrical system. In order to make sure it was a temporary phenomenon, I suggested a temporary artificial pacemaker at a slow rate, so her own heart could take over. This is called a "demand" pacemaker (see chapter 17).

For the following eight days, we observed her with the temporary pacemaker. Dr. Sheils and I had a consultation.

"There's an interesting feature here," I said. "Whenever her heart rate is rapid, she goes into left bundle branch block. The fast rate causes the left bundle to become fatigued. Even when she goes into complete heart block, and the natural secondary system takes over, her rate is 56 beats per minute."

We decided to remove the temporary pacemaker. Helen remained in the hospital for a continuous ECG monitoring on the tape recorder (dynamic electrocardiography—see chapter 14, "Testing, Testing"). This information verified that her heart rhythm was normal most of the time—72 beats per minute. Intermittently, she showed complete heart block. Yet her heart rate never fell below 56 beats per minute.

Dr. Franklin, Dr. Krauthamer and I discussed the situation with Helen on separate occasions. We discussed it between ourselves. Even if Helen developed a complete heart block again, her own heart rate wasn't likely to go under 56 beats per minute. She wasn't likely to have a catastrophe (cardiac arrest) and sudden death. There would be time to insert an artificial pacemaker. When we talked about time, we meant in terms of days, perhaps even weeks.

"If we can avoid putting in a permanent pacemaker now and hope the initial insult by the viral infection which produced a temporary block will be reversed, then we will have won the game," I said. "If not, if it produces irreversible changes, we can then put in a pacemaker."

Helen was delighted with the news. Particularly since we told her that at present, she needn't limit her activity.

However, if there was another episode of fainting, she was to notify Dr. Sheils immediately. If he wasn't available, she was to call the cardiologists. If her heart rate were to remain permanently at 56 beats per minute, she would be required to have a pacemaker.

Helen agreed to this arrangement, and went home a happy woman. So far, she has been doing well on her own.

DR. TAI:
Maurice was admitted to the Coronary Care Unit of the hospital, the picture-book image of a fat man with a size 46 suit, triple chins, ruddy skin, a small nose, blue eyes nearly lost in the puffy cheeks, and a bluff friendly manner.

No history of heart disease, but some episodes of palpitations, and this time the palpitations were prolonged. He had been playing cards with three friends at the Club, and at first he figured his heart was going crazy because he was on a winning streak. But after he won the jackpot, he didn't feel elated. Instead, he suddenly felt weak. His cronies brought him to the Emergency Room and I was called in.

The electrocardiogram showed an exceedingly fast heart rate. Because his blood pressure had dropped, and his heart was unable to maintain its output, it was necessary to correct the rapid heart rate by electrical shock. He responded nicely and remained in a normal heart rhythm. After he was stabilized, I did a careful examination but the ECG was normal, as were the X-rays. Because Maurice had had similar episodes approximately twice a year for several years, we suspected a condition called *Wolff-Parkinson-White Syndrome.*

I explained the problem to Maurice and placed him on the 24-hour dynamic electrocardiographic monitor (see chapter 14, "Testing, Testing") for two days. During this period, Maurice had an episode. It was recorded by the monitor, and confirmed the diagnosis of Wolff-Parkinson-White Syndrome. By this time, Maurice was able to come to our offices for consultation.

I told him: "Maurice, low blood pressure and weakness are signs that your heart wasn't able to pump enough blood. Instead of beating at 72 times per minute, your heart was racing at 200. At that rate, it does not have enough time to fill properly. As a result, its output of blood to the body decreases, blood pressure falls, and you develop these symptoms."

Maurice listened intently. "Is it something I've done that started this?" he asked.

"No," I answered. "You were born with a condition that is called Wolff-Parkinson-White Syndrome."

In the normal heart, this is what happens: The natural

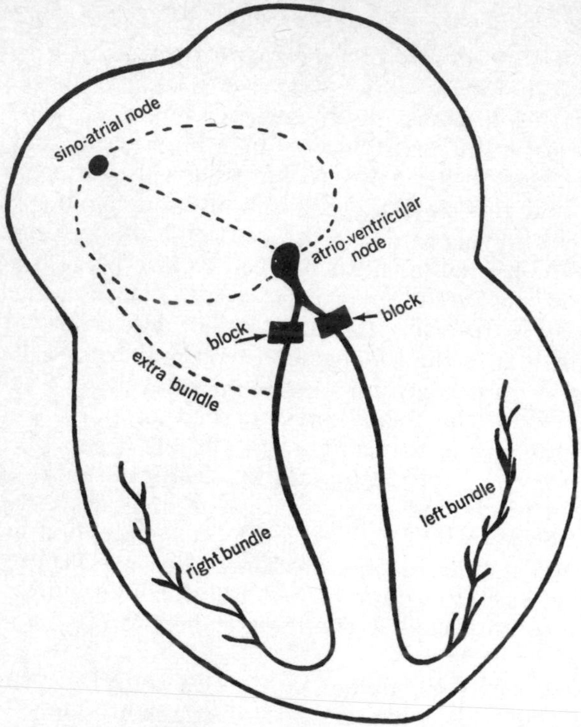

A. Right-and left-branch block
B. Wolff-Parkinson-White Syndrome

A. "Blocks" can also occur in the bundle branches. If both are blocked, complete heart block again occurs.

More commonly, only one bundle is blocked, changing the configuration of the cardiogram because the impulse travels through the normal bundle and reaches the heart muscle of the opposite side a few hundredths of a second later.

B. The "extra bundle," or electrical short circuit, is not usually found with bundle branch block. It is the cause of another cardiac problem: The Wolff-Parkinson-White Syndrome, episodes of rapid heart beating.

An impulse can short-circuit, or by-pass, the A-V node and reach one of the bundles. Then, if circumstances are right, it can go up and down—up to the atria and down to the ventricles. The part of the impulse that goes back up can recycle quickly through the extra bundle.

This recycling also reaches the ventricles and a repeating tachycardia is set. Medication may be needed to prevent this.

pacemaker fires its impulse, which comes down to the traffic station that is called the A-V node. From here the impulse goes into the left bundle to the left ventricle, and into the right bundle and the right ventricle.

In case the main pacemaker grows too active or the upper chambers contract very quickly and irregularly, the A-V node blocks out some of the impulses before they reach the ventricles.

"This is the usual pattern. But some people are born with what we call a bypass or a short circuit. Instead of being screened at the A-V node, the impulse can bypass it and reach the bundles directly. Then it can recycle through the short circuit, causing the fast heart rate. It requires control."

"What kind of control?" Maurice asked.

"Well, in your case, the best drug would be propranolol (see chapter 16, "Medications"). It blocks the bypass route and diverts traffic signals through the A-V node. It also controls the rate of signals reaching the A-V node. As a result, your heart rate slows down. It will minimize the frequency of the palpitations and may even completely abolish them."

Maurice is on the drug, and on a reducing diet, and has remained symptom-free for a year.

Chapter 9

Other heart diseases: serious, benign and masquerade

DR. TAI:
There are a small number of other heart conditions which can cause alarming clinical findings, some of which are serious, others benign.

One of the most serious is cardiomyopathy. It is an abnormality of the heart muscle that cannot be explained on the basis of high blood pressure, rheumatic heart disease, congenital heart disease or coronary artery disease.

It may come from a number of agents, such as alcohol (see chapter 11, "Killer Foods"), virus infections, metabolic disorders, vitamin deficiencies. It can appear after a pregnancy. Sometimes it is hereditary. In more than half the cases we never find the cause.

Gordon L. had no history of rheumatic fever, high blood pressure or chest pain. No physician had ever detected symptoms that might suggest heart disease. But two years ago, he began to feel uncomfortable and his condition had deteriorated. He was referred to us because of increasing fatigue, shortness of breath, swelling of legs and abdomen. He had occasional extra beats in his heart, fluid in his lungs, abdomen and legs. His ability to tolerate physical effort was limited. His ECG showed no evidence of heart attack or coronary artery disease. But his heart was enlarged. He seemed to be happy at his work as a chemist and with his marital life.

My examination confirmed the clinical findings.

After the office evaluation, I sat down to talk to Gordon and his wife.

"I have to confirm your doctor's diagnosis. You do have heart trouble."

They were both silent, not quite believing, yet knowing it was a fact.

"Gordon, our examination has ruled out the chance that you were born with heart disease. There's no evidence of rheumatic heart disease or high blood pressure. Your ECG shows no findings of a heart attack. So we are able to rule out all the major causes of heart disease."

"What is my problem?" Gordon asked. He had a nervous abrupt way of speaking, and a tendency to dominate his wife.

"Well, the only other likely reason the heart might fail is that the pump isn't working as a good pump should. The heart muscle isn't doing its job.

"We don't know why. Many conditions that affect the body can damage the heart. Virus diseases are the best known. They invade the body, often causing fever, upset stomach, cough and the like. They can also invade the heart muscle and cause damage there, which may not show up immediately. After the initial scarring, there may be no symptoms for any time from several days up to fifty years later.

"There are other conditions that can hurt the heart muscle. Alcohol taken in large amounts can also harm the heart. Or other major illness."

Gordon's questions persisted. "You think my condition is the result of a virus?"

"I'm not sure in your case. I'm just giving you the causes that can produce this condition."

"Is there anything else that could have caused this trouble?" Gordon's wife asked timidly.

"Yes, a host of conditions can produce disease of the heart muscle or interfere with its pumping. These include the bacterial infections we used to see before the antibiotic era. Diphtheria, tuberculosis, pneumonia. There are also parasites that abound in under-developed countries. The condition can develop when the thyroid gland isn't functioning properly. Or if there is a severe vitamin deficiency, which is sometimes seen in prisoners of war."

"Why did you ask if I drink?" Gordon wanted to know.

"If you take two bottles of beer, and four to six ounces of whiskey a day, and perhaps a half bottle of wine with your dinner, you are risking damage to your heart. Alcohol affects the liver, everybody knows that. But few people realize it can have a direct effect on the heart muscle and interfere with its function. The end result is similar. The heart muscle is replaced by scar tissue. Alcohol can depress the function of the heart, especially if the heart is already diseased.

"Alcoholics can also suffer from malnutrition which may affect the heart, but that is different and can be corrected with B complex vitamins.

"In people with heart disease, even one cocktail decreases the performance of the heart. (This should debunk the old myth that alcohol is good for the heart.) If there is a latent abnormality of the heart, or a fast pulse, alcohol may precipitate the condition. Magnesium, an ion important to the function of the heart, is lodged inside the heart muscle cell. Alcohol interferes with the storage of magnesium in the heart muscle cell, and can cause damage. Heavy drinkers often harm their heart muscle. The coronaries are clean, there is no sign of valvular disease, but the heart muscle doesn't work.

"The disease is called cardiomyopathy."

"That means if you drink too much and have heart trouble, you can help your heart by giving up alcohol?" Gordon's wife asked, with a triumphant note in her voice.

"Don't nag," Gordon said. "I'll have none of your 'I told you so's.' "

"There is evidence that if the patient gives up liquor entirely, and gets bed rest and proper treatment, the heart is likely to get better, provided the condition is not too far advanced. It will not reverse completely. But there will be a marked improvement and the patient may add many more years to his life."

"Doctor, as a chemist, I'm doubly curious. Why does alcohol cause this reaction?"

"I wish I knew. We see a higher incidence of this kind of heart muscle problem in chronic alcoholics.

"Now, from our clinical examination and X-ray, we're pretty sure you don't have coronary heart disease. But a cardiac catheterization will tell us at what stage your heart is functioning. We need to confirm the findings for future treatment."

Gordon agreed to a cardiac catheterization and the diagnosis was confirmed. He had a severe degree of heart muscle disease—cardiomyopathy.

Gordon took the news stoically. "What's to be done?" he asked.

"There is no surgical treatment for this condition. You'll be put on a form of medical therapy. It's most important to maintain your proper weight and to avoid salt in your diet. You may eat food cooked with salt seasoning, but banish the salt shaker from your table."

"Gordon loves salt. He can eat a bag of potato chips at a time," his wife said.

"Salt retains fluid in your body. When a heart isn't working properly, the fluid accumulates and the heart has to work harder. But the diuretic pills we are giving you, Gordon, will flush the sodium out of your system."

"Give me the rest of the bad news," Gordon said.

"Your job—"

"You mean I should quit?"

"It puts you under too much tension and aggravation. You've got to take it easy. A nap after lunch or before dinner. You can be active around the house. You can even do the marketing for your wife, just as long as you don't overdo it.

"Cigarettes are out. Coffee is out, but you may have decaffeinated coffee. Alcohol is out. And a strict program of medication."

Gordon has been followed over a period of 18 months. He is making slow but encouraging progress.

Men like Gordon can die of cardiomyopathy—failure of the heart muscle.

Yet if the problem is detected early enough and alcohol is given up permanently, this sickness of the heart muscle is reversible.

DR. FRANKLIN:
We don't often see women patients at as early an age as our men patients. Women's hormones seem to protect them from heart attacks during their child-bearing years. Those who come to us for cardiac evaluation are usually beyond their menopause.

But once in a while, we treat a young girl who has heart disease and her family rightly cries out, "Why did it have to happen to her?"

I first saw Joanna B. in 1966. She was a girl "for all seasons." She had an IQ near genius level, a healthy interest in sports and a good-natured contempt for her family's social life. The only girl in the family, she was an outstanding badminton player and trounced her three older brothers regularly. She played to win with a passionate driving intensity. She lived in Philadelphia, but competed in tournaments throughout the Northeast.

A few months earlier she had noticed that a fast game brought discomfort to her chest. She was bothered by palpitations and angina-like pains, but she ignored them.

One humid afternoon, while she was playing a particularly strenuous game at a club in Connecticut, she was stricken with a crushing chest pain. Her friends rushed her to the nearest hospital, and we were called.

During the examination, I heard a heart murmur. I took an ECG which showed an overgrowth of the muscle of the left ventricle.

I was disturbed by her symptoms, because she was so young and full of life. You don't like to associate heart problems with the young.

Cardiac catheterization was recommended. The results showed no coronary artery disease but the marked overgrowth of the left ventricle. This is not cancer. The muscle tissue was growing *inside* the heart chamber and crowding it, which made it difficult for the blood to flow in and out.

This is *hypertrophic cardiomyopathy*, an overgrowth of heart muscle. It is a well-known condition that occurs in many forms, with or without obstruction of blood flow. Joanna's case was the more uncommon type, without obstruction. Since no cause could be found, it was called *idiopathic* (of unknown origin).

The excess size of the heart muscle led to a greater need for nourishing blood. The coronary blood flow was normal, but unable to cope with this extra need. As a result, the heart was starved for adequate blood containing vital oxygen.

After the diagnosis was made, Joanna was given propranolol, which was a new drug at that time. It decreases the heart muscle's need for oxygen. There's a chance it may also decrease the rate of overgrowth of the heart muscle.

I still see her for a checkup every two years. At the last examination, she was feeling well. She is taking a fairly high dose of propranolol and is tolerating it. But she has given up badminton and any other sports that involve running. She swims, she has a busy social life, she travels to Europe each summer and she works in the winter with a group of ghetto children in remedial reading.

No one can foretell what her life span will be. The new drug has prolonged her life without turning her into an invalid. Without propranolol, she might not have made it up to the present time.

We bring up Joanna as an example whenever one of our heart patients grows depressed. None of us knows what new drugs are coming along that will restore many lives (see chapter 16, "Medications").

Being human, we dare to be optimistic.

DR. KRAUTHAMER:
Chris A. is 34 years old, and an executive vice-president of an airline company. He had been under the care of his family physician for episodes of sudden weakness and near fainting spells. A neurologist who checked him suspected an epileptic possibility and put him on the drug Dilantin, without any positive results. During one of Chris' frequent admissions to the hospital, I was asked to see him for a cardiac evaluation, since Chris was apprehensive about the danger of a heart attack. He was in an important, well-paid job, and he didn't want his future ruined by office gossip about his physical problem.

His ECG and chest X-rays were normal. I suggested a treadmill stress test to which Chris agreed. He passed the test at maximum rate. No abnormality was noted. Because I suspected *arrhythmia,* an irregularity of the heartbeat, was responsible for his symptoms, I placed Chris on the 24-hour portable ECG monitoring system. During the first 24 hours, the tape showed no abnormality. During the second 24 hours, Chris did complain of his recurring symptoms. When the tape was scanned, it showed that his heartbeat suddenly sped from 75 beats per minute to 150, and up to 200 beats. When the heart rate slowed down, his symptoms disappeared and he felt fine. At this stage, I had a talk with Chris and his wife.

"Your near fainting spells have nothing to do with epilepsy," I explained. "The tape gave us the clue. You feel symptoms when your heart suddenly races at twice or more the normal pace. This condition is known as *paroxysmal atrial tachycardia*."

"Can you tell me a little more about it?" Chris asked.

"Yes. Your heart normally pumps 72 times a minute. The time interval between one beat and the next is about 0.8 seconds. Now the heart can't keep pumping without a rest. It pumps, then during its rest, it collects blood to start the cycle all over again. When your heart speeds up, each cycle is 0.3 seconds instead of 0.8, because your heart muscle must complete 200 beats in 60 seconds. So in one second, your heart must beat more than three times the normal rate."

"You've lost me," Chris said.

"All right. If the cycle takes 0.3 seconds instead of 0.8, your heart will have 0.2 seconds to beat but only 0.1 second to rest and accumulate blood in order to be ready to pump again. It can't do the job satisfactorily. So the pumping ability of the heart is decreased. Even though the heart muscle is contracting, it isn't putting out enough blood. The brain doesn't get enough blood and you have marked weakness or a fainting spell."

"Why did this happen to Chris," his wife asked. "What's the cause of it?"

"It happens in people who have had rheumatic heart disease, or overactive thyroids, or who take excessive amounts of coffee, or alcohol, or who smoke too many cigarettes. But sometimes, we can't find the cause. This is true in Chris' case."

"What is he supposed to do?" his wife asked anxiously.

"The usual precautions. He must lose weight, he must avoid alcohol and all caffeine beverages. He must avoid overexcitement and fatigue. He should exercise judiciously and try to lead a normal life. He may have to be placed on a drug to slow the heart rate and prevent recurrences of this rhythm."

"How does it work?"

"There is a good chance it will prevent recurrences of the tachycardia. It will keep your heart slow and normal. There should be no problem since there is no underlying heart disease. As long as your heart rate remains normal, you will have no symptoms."

Chris has followed the schedule we laid out for him. In the past six months, he's had no recurrences.

DR. TAI:

The world was astonished when the space program grounded the astronaut, Donald Slayton, for an irregularity of the heart. Many patients spontaneously develop such irregular heart rhythms. In *atrial fibrillation,* the heart's beat is not only irregular but very rapid. It can happen as an abnormal response to exercise. When you exercise moderately, your heart normally goes from 80 to 120 beats per minute. But these people may go suddenly from 80 to 180 beats. Even with a small work load, their heartbeat becomes irregular. So they cannot function normally.

Atrial fibrillation most commonly has its roots in rheumatic heart disease, overactive thyroid, blood clots in the lungs, hypertension, coronary artery disease, or some kind of heart muscle disease. But in some, no cause is found. They check out normally. William Evans of the National Heart Institute has called it, "lone atrial fibrillation" when there is no heart disease.

When Donald Slayton developed this condition, he was grounded on the basis of the old concept that it had to indicate some other problem. He was determined to find out if he actually had heart disease. If not, he couldn't understand why he should be grounded. Physicians who were not aware of Evans' concept had tried different drugs on Slayton. Finally, he went to Mayo Clinic for catheterization. They reported that he did not have coronary artery disease. Or any other heart disease. He was readmitted into the space program.

Slayton's courageous fight and its results were widely reported in the press. It's reassuring to a patient when you can quote an astronaut's experience.

DR. FRANKLIN:

Suppose a heart patient must have non-cardiac surgery, such as an operation to remove an appendix, gall bladder, or to repair a hernia.

Families of heart patients often are deeply concerned

over this prospect. We will do a pre-operative evaluation of the patient and make recommendations to the anesthesiologist. We make two major points:

1. The patient must be kept well oxygenated during anesthesia.
2. His blood pressure must be maintained.

These are both necessary. Even if the patient is adequately oxygenated, he can have a heart attack if his blood pressure falls too low.

Sometimes a patient on the operating table will go into a hypotensive episode, with shock and low blood pressure. He may get a heart attack at the tip of the heart—*apical myocardial infarction*. This part of the heart is more poorly supplied as far as coronary arteries are concerned. Even though the patient is getting enough oxygen, circulation is inadequate. And the most distant parts of the heart from the point of circulation suffer.

The longer the blood pressure is kept low, the larger the area of the heart that will be involved. If a patient has a history of high blood pressure, he will require a bit higher pressure during surgery than a patient who has normal blood pressure.

I saw a case like this when I was at Cleveland Clinic. A 17-year-od boy was brought in after an accident. He had injured an artery behind his knee. He was prepared for surgery to have this corrected. He bled profusely during the operation. His blood pressure dropped and couldn't be brought back quickly to normal. It was nearly thirty minutes before the staff could get the bleeding under control, give him enough blood to replace the loss, and elevate his blood pressure.

Once he was out of anesthesia, an electrocardiogram was taken. He showed a classic electrocardiogram pattern with apical myocardial infarction. Several weeks later he was catheterized and his coronary arteriography showed perfectly normal coronary arteries—the only damage was the infarct at the apex of his heart.

In a routine appendectomy, there is stress on the heart but it is tolerable. In minor surgery, such as hernia repair, a hemorrhoidectomy, a D and C (dilation and curettage), a local anesthesia is preferable to a general one.

The more serious procedures involve organs that have reflex arcs with the autonomic nervous system. (You hit the knee and it jerks; this is an example of a reflex arc.) These are the gastro-intestinal tract, including the stomach, gall bladder, pancreas, where pulling or pushing these organs aside sends impulses through the vagus nerve into the central nervous system. This has a tendency to change the heartbeat; to slow it down.

Part of the routine pre-operative medication which the anesthesiologist gives is medication to block this reflex arc. The medicine is usually atropine.

Major surgery, such as kidney removal, an amputation, a colon resection, a lung removal, all place fairly high stress on the patient. They carry the hazard of bleeding. This is particularly true in vascular surgery, such as the removal of an abdominal aortic aneurysm (ballooning of the vessel) or major vascular surgery to improve blood flow in the legs. If the bleeding becomes uncontrolled, low blood pressure can occur. If there is enough stress, an individual without heart disease can have a heart attack. It is rare, but this is what happened to the young boy in the Cleveland Clinic. In his case, it was a combination of general anesthesia, massive hemorrhage, and low blood pressure.

DR. KRAUTHAMER:
Overexposure to sun is particularly bad for heart patients. They should take the sun in small doses. If your skin is reddened or inflamed, it means that the small vessels in the dermis (the lower portions of the skin) have an increased blood flow through them. There is subsequently dilation of the pre-capillary arterioles. Although this may have a tendency to lower the blood pressure, it also calls for a greater cardiac output. The heart beats faster to put out more blood. The reddened skin makes the heart work harder.

If you're out in the sun too much, you're also bound to sweat profusely and become dehydrated. Consequently, the amount of fluid (plasma) in the blood stream decreases, lost through the skin. The result is a relative increase in the red blood cells or in the concentration of red blood cells. It is called *hemoconcentration*, and since the red cells take up a greater percentage of blood space, they are more likely to clump and clot. Which can then dispose the patient to coronary thrombosis.

Our recommendation to patients who are golfers or beach addicts: If you sweat, drink plenty of liquids.

Father Xavier, a patient of ours, was a football player during his Notre Dame college days. Two decades later, he played golf at the city course near his parish house with such competitive drive and skill that even his most recalcitrant parishioners attended church Sunday morning in order to have him for a partner in the Saturday afternoon foursomes. At fifty-two, Father Xavier, still a big powerful man, had suffered three heart attacks at different times on the golf links.

"Doctor, let's get this straight, I'm not giving up the game," he announced. Since he was then in Emergency, I was not going to argue with him.

His coronary arteriograms showed that the damage done to his heart was confined. His left anterior descending artery was occluded near its middle and a scar was now present on the heart. He had only one other danger area in the coronary tree and that was small.

"When you go back to the game, Father," I suggested, "carry a jug of water with you."

We gave Father Xavier the instructions for taking care of himself. Each spring, he took a month off to play golf in Florida. We received cheery letters from him. His partners couldn't keep up with him. "I've challenged Jackie Gleason to a match." He added, "I'm drinking plenty of H_2O as you advised."

Those four weeks of fresh air and exercise gave him the strength to cope with the demands of his parish for the rest of the year.

He played golf until his death, seven years later, which was due to arteriosclerosis, but in another part of his body. To the end, he didn't have another heart attack.

Sweating and fatigue are not specific symptoms. If you have no diagnosed heart disease, you'd be foolish to ascribe these symptoms to your heart. However, if coronary heart disease is strongly suspected and you find your normal exercise tolerance waning, it may be a warning of a possible heart attack. Today, the physician is alert for his patient's complaint of unusual fatigue.

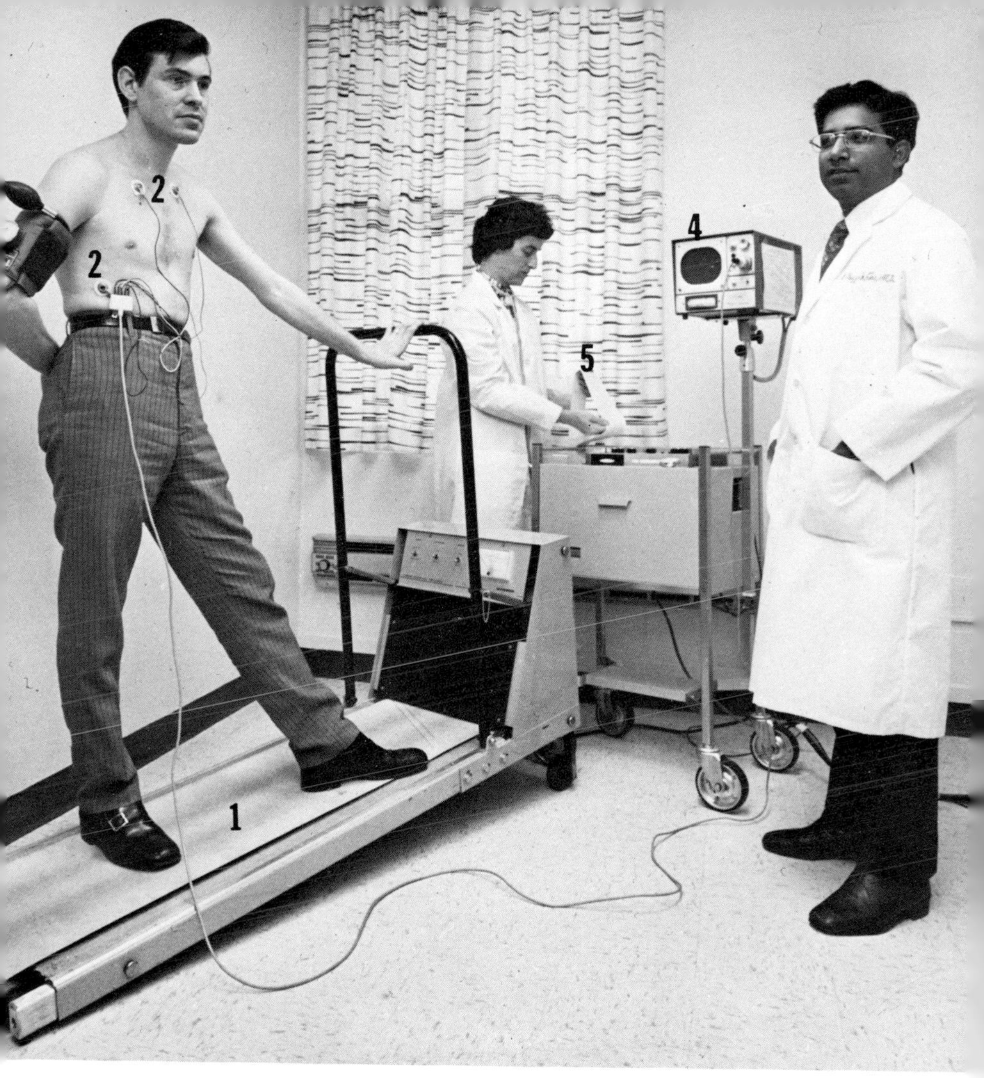

1. *Treadmill electrocardiogram: stress test*
By walking, then running on the treadmill (1), the patient is tested for blood pressure and heartbeat in action. By this means the physician can determine whether the patient has a heart condition and his degree of tolerance of activity, which cannot always be determined by the usual electrocardiogram taken while the patient is still. Here Dr. A. Razzak Tai monitors a patient while the nurse records the stress electrocardiogram.

1. treadmill 2. electrodes 3. blood pressure cuff
4. oscilloscope (ECG monitor) 5. electrocardiogram tracing

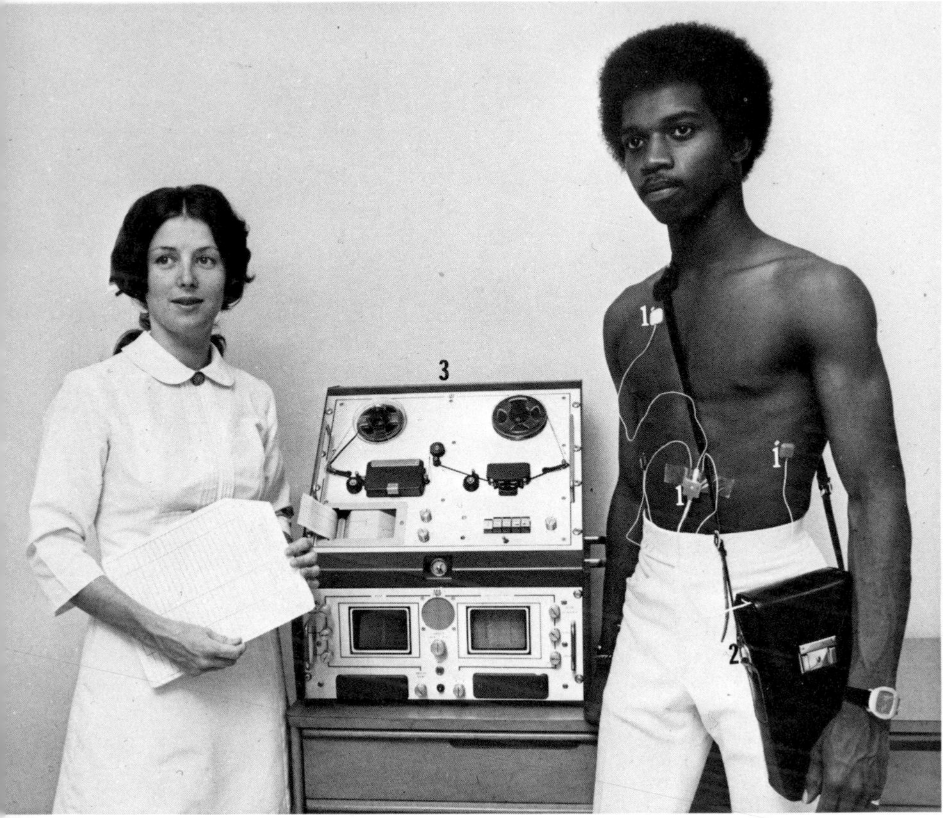

2. *Dynamic electrocardiogram*
The nurse attaches the electrocardiogram electrodes (1) on the patient's chest to the electrocardiogram tape recorder carried in the carrying case (2). The patient's heartbeat is recorded for 24 hours while he is outside the hospital, and the tape can then be replayed on the scanner (3) to detect any irregularities.

1. electrodes 2. tape recorder carrying case 3. scanner

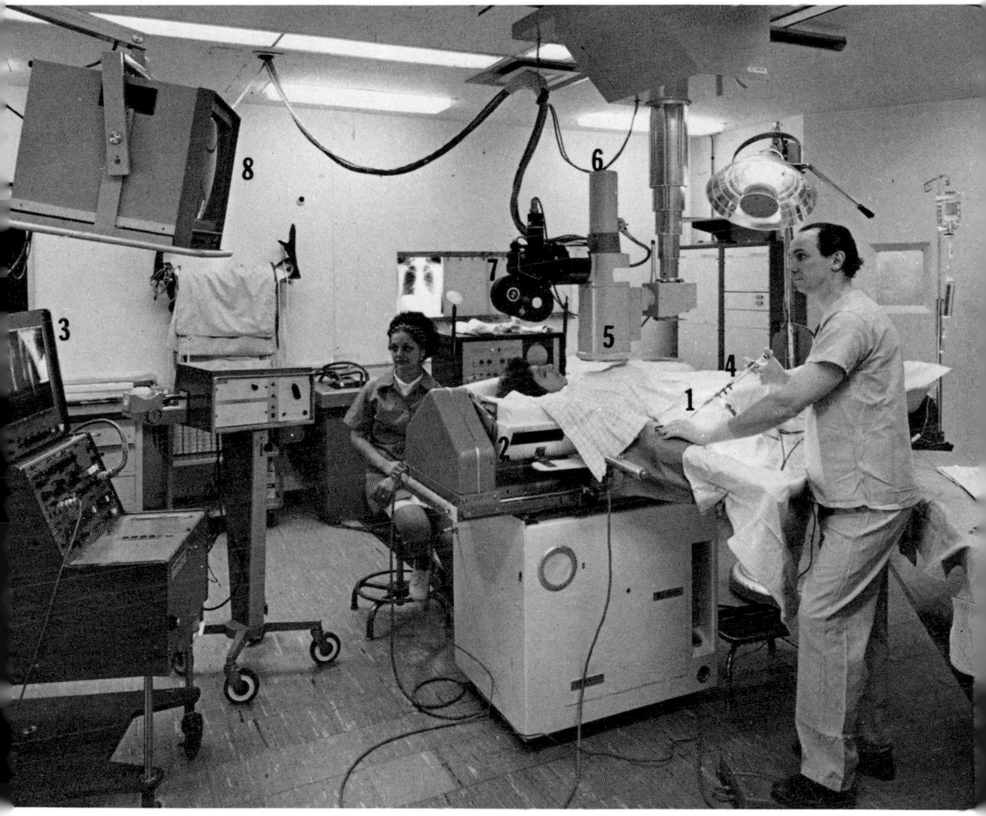

3. *Cardiac catheterization*

In this special procedures laboratory, the cardiologist photographs the arteries of the heart. Here Dr. Marshall Franklin inserts the catheter (1) through a vein in the arm to the patient's heart while she lies in the movable cradle (2) so photos may be taken at different angles. On the biomedical monitor (3) he can observe the patient's blood pressure and electrocardiograph, as he (4) injects dye through the catheter to outline the arteries, and the X-rays are taken by means of the fluoroscope (5), recorded in action by the TV camera (6) and the movie camera (7), which projects the interior of the heart, with arteries clearly shown, on (8) the TV screen. The precise condition of the heart is determined and the photos used by a heart surgeon if surgery is indicated.

1. catheter 2. cradle 3. biomedical monitor 4. dye
5. fluoroscope 6. TV camera 7. movie camera 8. TV monitor

4

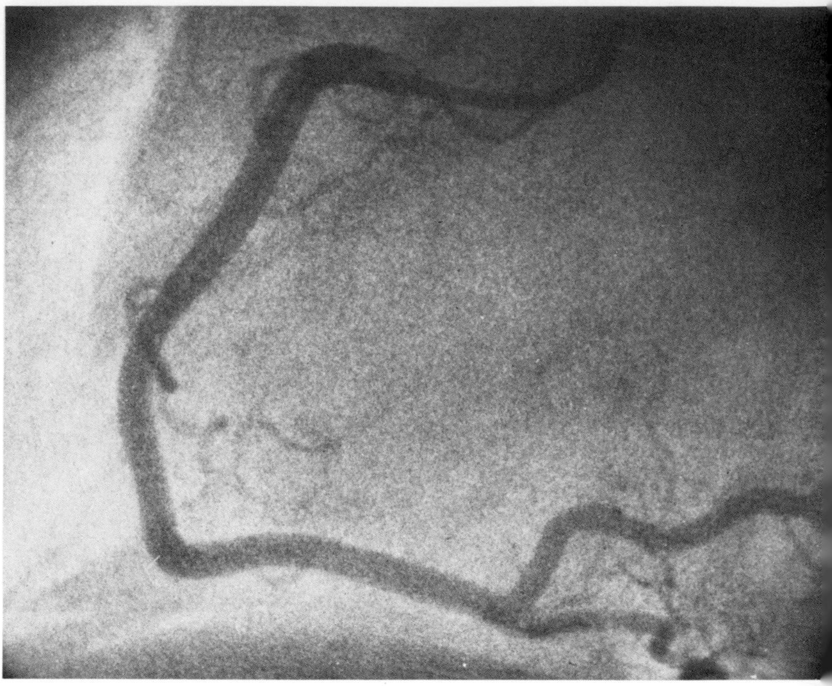

These pictures, taken of coronary arteries in living patients, show three stages of arteriosclerosis and the surgical by-pass.

4. A normal coronary artery with little to no arteriosclerosis.

5. A coronary artery narrowed significantly and causing angina in this patient.

6. A totally blocked coronary artery that has caused a heart attack (myocardial infarction).

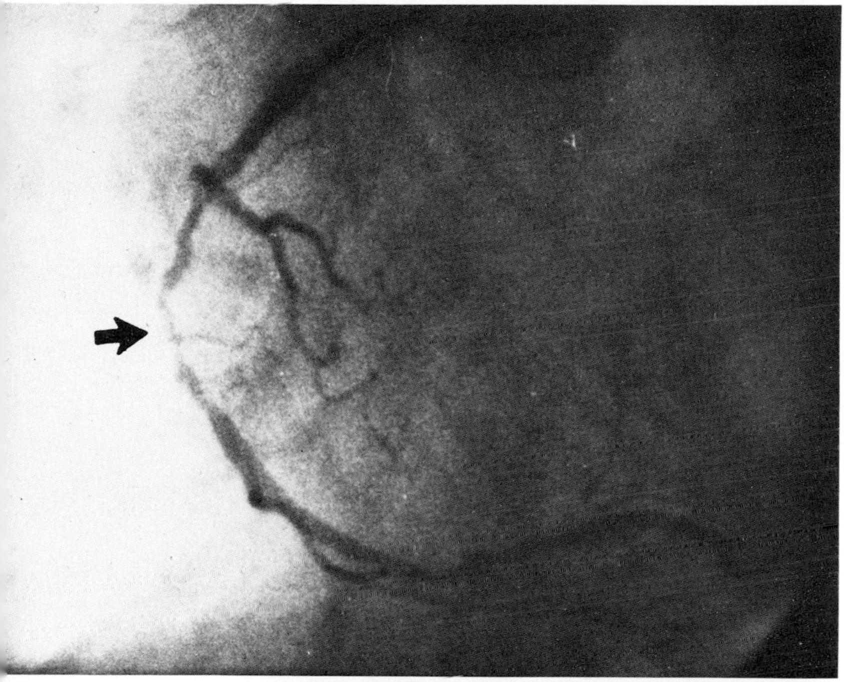
5

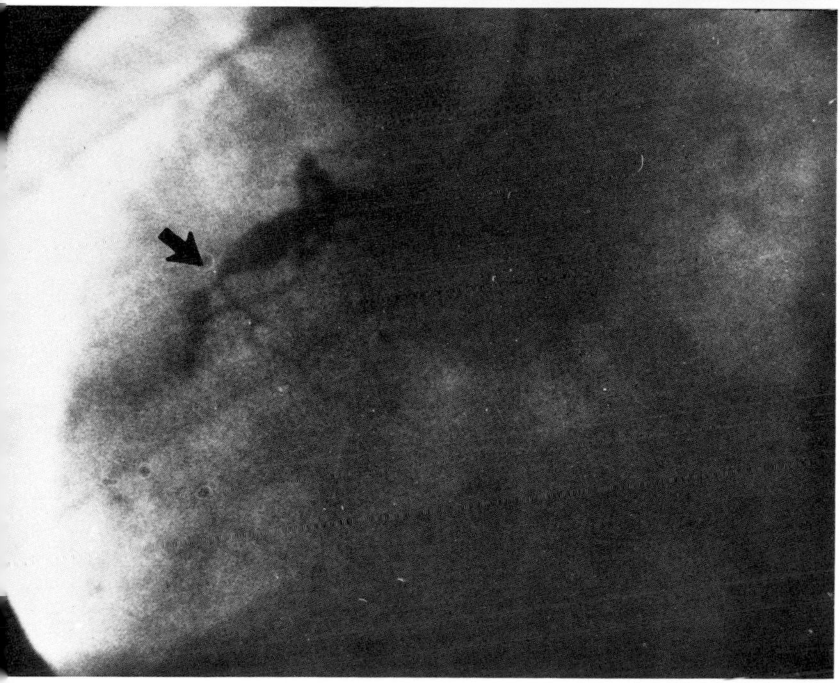
6

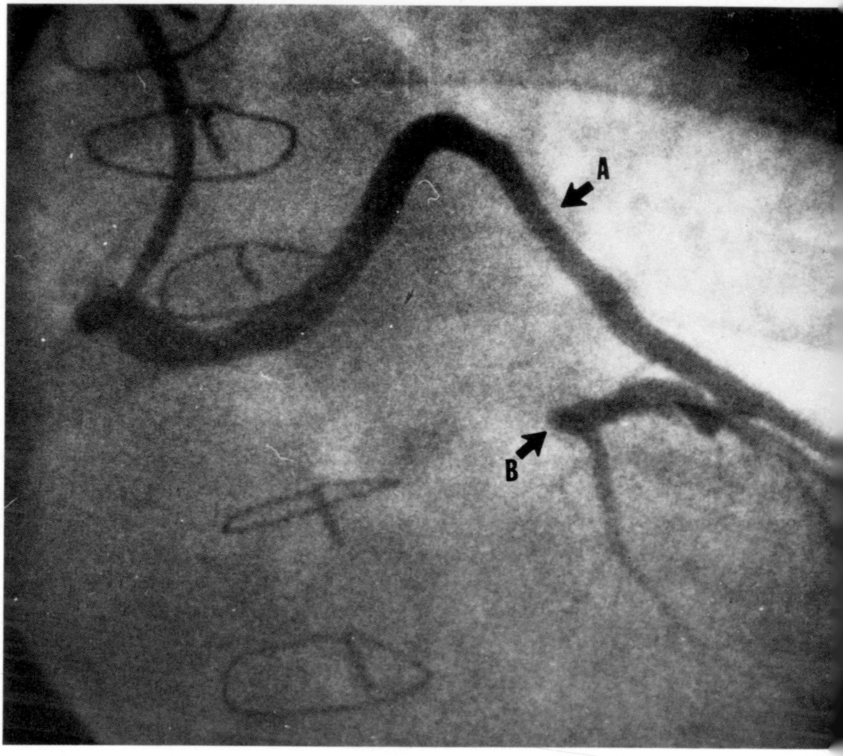

7. Angiogram of a saphenous vein by-pass graft. The coronary artery branching from the end of the by-pass is clearly filled by a good blood supply from the graft. The circles are stitches from the incision in the chest.

A. by-pass B. closed artery

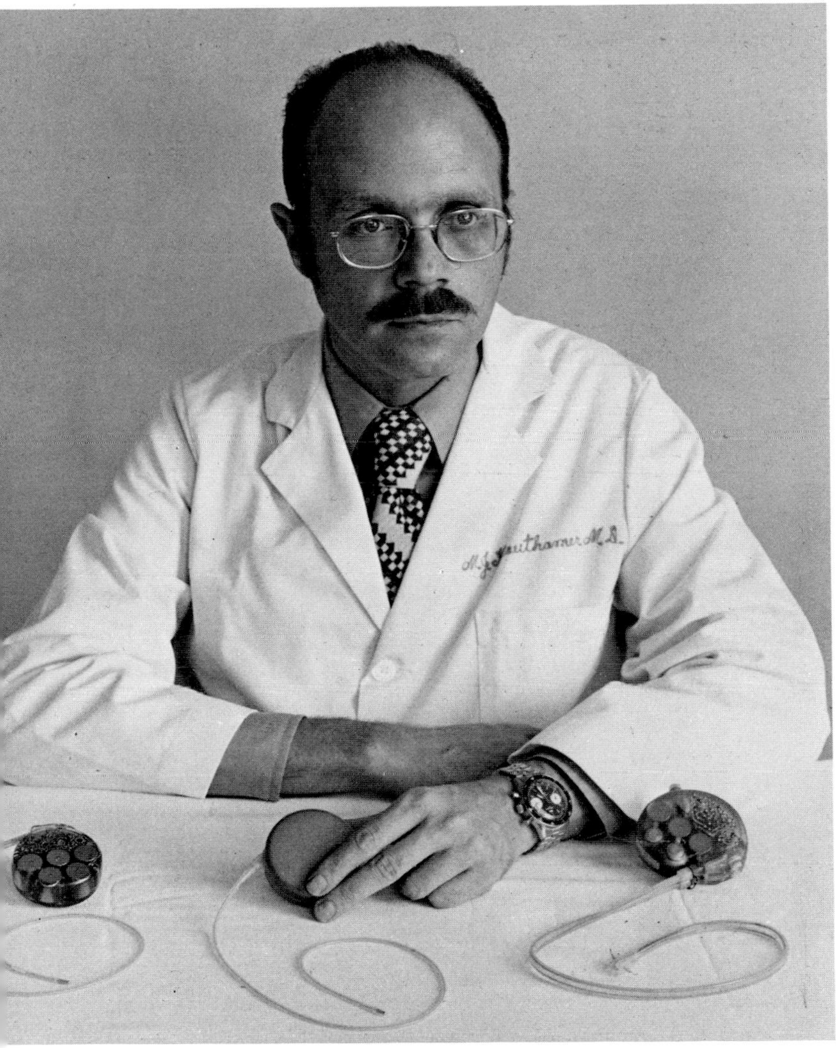

8. Pacemakers demonstrated by Dr. Martin J. Krauthamer. Three units are shown. Each has the battery and electric components sealed into a complete unit. The middle one is metal-encased as well. The electrode (the wire protruding from the powerpack) will be placed within the heart. The unit on the right has a catheter different from the other two. It is meant to be inserted by a chest operation and actually sewn to the heart's surface rather than put through a vein (see Chapter 17).

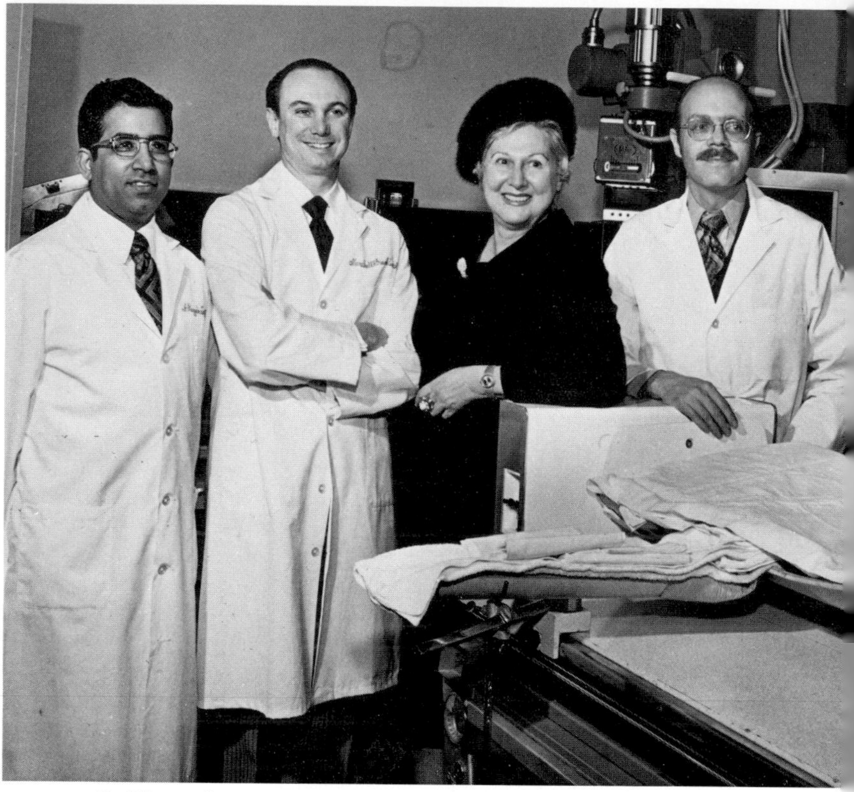

9. The authors in the Special Procedures Laboratory, Stamford, Connecticut. Left to right: Dr. A. Razzak Tai, Dr. Marshall Franklin, Ann Pinchot, Dr. Martin J. Krauthamer.

In our practice, we have discovered that many heart attack victims had been running a fatiguing schedule for months, even years. Several weeks before the attack, they have found themselves bushed, totally depleted, unable to cope physically with a schedule that never before drained them.

"It's as though my strength deserted me the past weeks," a patient who is an executive in the soybean industry confessed. "I could hardly make it through the day." Though hindsight suggested he was developing coronary insufficiency, there was no basis for his family doctor to suspect an impending heart attack until it actually happened.

Of course, in a patient who's already known to have a heart condition, the doctor becomes alert at any complaint. The fatigue should be treated as serious until proven otherwise.

This may be true also of sweating.

A patient usually has a pattern to his angina. For instance, he walks three or four blocks, feels mild discomfort, pauses. It goes away. But then the pattern changes slightly —pain is accompanied by shortness of breath or perspiration. These symptoms suggest a greater degree of severity to his condition. They should never be ignored or passed off lightly, as "Oh, I was a little nervous at the time."

He should telephone his doctor for an appointment, making it clear that he has new symptoms. We cannot blame him for wanting to ignore them. But if the new symptoms test out positively, they are indicative of what we call *unstable angina*. This usually indicates a decreasing coronary blood flow. *It is a danger signal.*

DR. KRAUTHAMER:
"Doctor, I have pains in my legs." This is a familiar complaint. We hear it often from our patients.

There are two distinct causes of pains in the legs that involve the vascular system: Leg pains may be the result of a) vein disease, or b) arterial disease.

The pain due to arterial disease is very much like the pain of coronary disease. In coronary disease, you remember, the heart is calling for added blood supply, and doesn't get it. So the heart starts hurting.

The same thing happens in the legs. The obstruction is

in the arteries that carry blood to the legs. When the person walks, his legs begin to hurt. If he stops, the pain goes away. Once he starts walking again, the pain may return. It is usually a cramping in the calf, and is called *intermittent claudication.* Or window shoppers' disease. Or store-front syndrome.

"Doctor," one middle-aged woman confided to me, "I like to walk midtown where the shops are. When my legs start hurting, I stop and stand in front of a window as if I was interested in buying something. I can walk only so far before my legs cramp, and I just have to stop and rest. Sometimes I go into a coffee shop and have a snack, even if I'm not hungry, just to rest my feet. When the cramping stops, I walk a little more—until it starts up again."

When cramping occurs in the calf, the arterial blockage is usually in the thigh area.

When the cramping shows up in the thigh, the blockage is usually in the pelvic area.

When the cramping is in the buttocks, the blockage is usually above the pelvic area.

If the blockage shows up above the bifurcation (dividing) of the aorta into the iliac arteries, this combination of symptoms is called the *Leriche Syndrome* and it includes impotence. Patients sometimes come to us with a complaint of leg and hip pain, but they never mention impotence until the information is extracted from them.

If the discomfort is due to vascular disease, we do an arteriogram and pinpoint the location and extent of the blockages. Then corrective surgery can be done. It is possible that surgery will improve a man's sexual performance, but sometimes the loss of sexual potency is permanent. No doctor can guarantee that potency will be restored. One can only wait to see what happens after the operation. The legs, however, return to good condition in nearly every case.

A patient of ours, Dell W., a busy dynamic lawyer who is known to the public for his dramatics in the courtroom, had both coronary arteriosclerosis and arteriosclerosis of the blood vessels in his legs. The condition was so bad that he couldn't walk a block. Surgeons did bypass grafts from the *femoral* artery (in the groin) to the *popliteal* artery (behind the knee). He is now able to walk twenty blocks without discomfort.

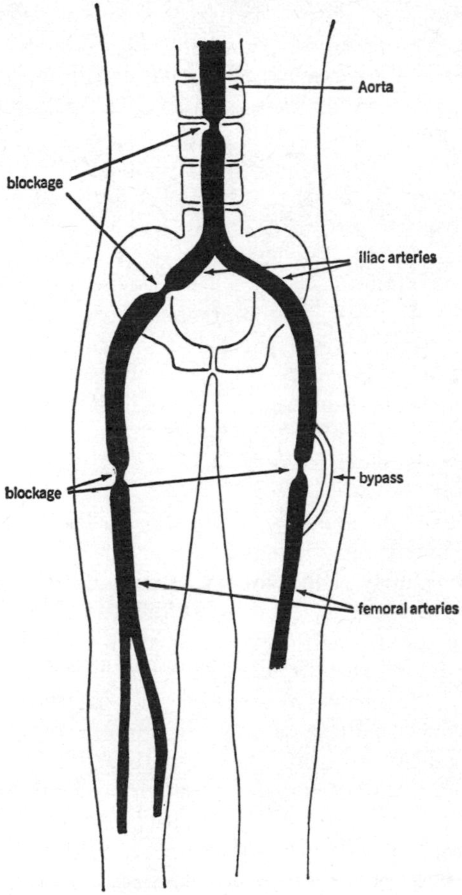

Arteriosclerosis of the aorta and the femoral arteries

The aorta, after it exits from the heart, passes down through the chest and abdomen. A severe narrowing in the aorta within the abdomen can cause a Leriche Syndrome.

Blockages below the bifurcation of the aorta causes symptoms in the leg being supplied. The narrowed right iliac artery might cause intermittent claudication (cramping pain) in the buttocks region on that side. The partially blocked femoral arteries would cause claudication in the calves. The left femoral artery shows a by-pass graft across the narrowing.

For the patient with beginning symptoms of claudication, the main exercise is walking. The more he uses his legs, the greater is the chance that he will develop collaterals that will take over the job which his regular vessels can no longer service. This may make it possible to avoid surgery. But the obstruction in the vessel must be located in a place where the collaterals can help out.

DR. TAI:

Cardiac masquerade

Some non-cardiac conditions present alarming symptoms of heart disease even when there is no proven heart disease. These include pulmonary embolism; hyperventilation syndrome; gastro-intestinal problems such as peptic ulcer, gall bladder disease, hiatal hernia; heart murmur in the absence of heart disease; and some ECG changes in the absence of heart disease.

Pulmonary embolism (a blood clot to the lung) is often mistaken for coronary disease.

Most frequently, this clot will form in the veins of the pelvis or the lower extremities. It breaks off and travels in the blood stream to the right side of the heart, and then lodges in a pulmonary artery. This condition can cause an acute rise of blood pressure in the pulmonary artery, which in turn, can cause chest pains and simulate angina with one additional feature—shortness of breath.

If the blood clot is large enough, infarction, or death of tissue in the lung can take place. Just as myocardial infarction can occur from a blocked coronary artery, a pulmonary infarction can occur from a blocked pulmonary artery. Some form of lung disease is usually present beforehand. Pulmonary embolism can cause changes in the ECG that suggest coronary insufficiency and an anginal attack.

It can be diagnosed in its early stages by the use of a test called a *lung scan:* Radioactive material is injected into a vein in the arm and is carried to the lungs. On a screen, the radioactive material is seen and photographed as it outlines those portions of the lung it can reach. It will not reach portions blocked by blood clots. This causes a "blank spot" or "defect" in the scan.

Coronary disease and pulmonary embolism can mimic one another, but treatment and outlook are quite different.

Patients with pulmonary embolism are treated with anti-coagulant therapy to diminish the possibility of additional blood clots coming to the lungs. If anti-coagulants are not effective, surgery may be needed (see chapter 23, "Pregnancy, the Pill, and Children").

DR. TAI:
Some middle-aged women with chronic anxiety or emotional problems often develop symptoms even when circumstances do not warrant it. They are victims of *hyperventilation syndrome*, which is characterized by over-breathing. Too much carbon dioxide is exhaled, decreasing acid content in the blood and leading to what is called

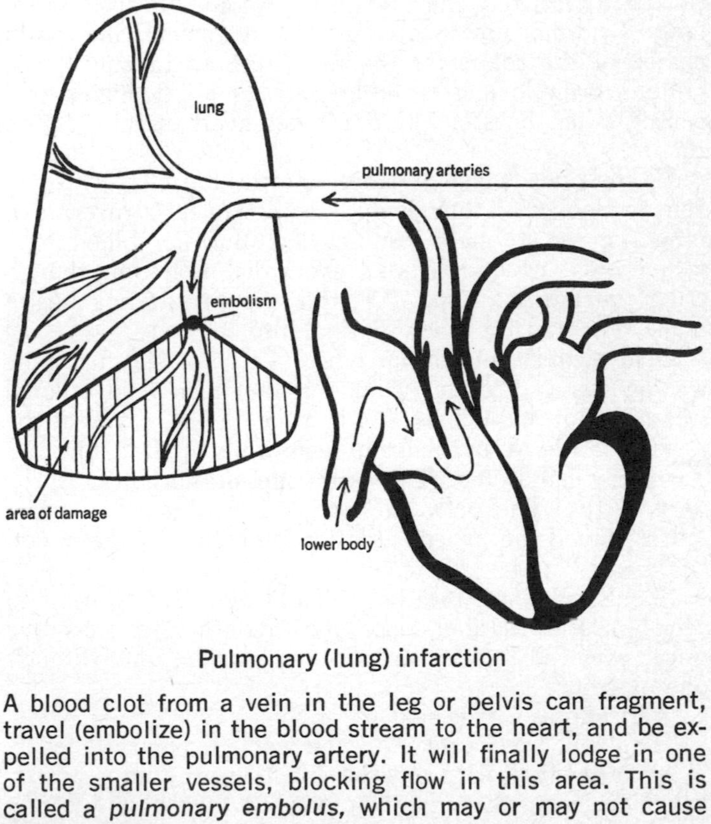

Pulmonary (lung) infarction

A blood clot from a vein in the leg or pelvis can fragment, travel (embolize) in the blood stream to the heart, and be expelled into the pulmonary artery. It will finally lodge in one of the smaller vessels, blocking flow in this area. This is called a *pulmonary embolus*, which may or may not cause lung damage.

respiratory alkalosis. The chemical changes cause numbness and tingling in the fingertips and toes, a flush on the face and a sense of lightheadedness. In extreme cases, it can lead to fainting and convulsions. The fingers of the hand may become stiff just before the victim faints.

A good many of these people, in addition (and frequently during their hyperventilation) experience chest discomfort in one form or another, sometimes palpitations and tachycardia.

The strange thing is that respiratory alkalosis may cause the electrocardiogram to change in a manner suggestive of coronary insufficiency.

Gladys R., a tense, nervous career woman in her late thirties, appeared at the Emergency Room with hyperventilation syndrome and an attack of severe anxiety. She was in charge of the colors for the new lipsticks in one of the famous cosmetic houses, and her boss, an erratic high-strung genius, often boasted: "I don't get heart attacks. I give them."

He had already given Gladys an ulcer, but now, in Emergency it looked as though she was also in for a myocardial infarction or coronary insufficiency. But her blood tests were normal, which ruled out myocardial infarction, though not coronary insufficiency. We did coronary arteriograms to make sure, and they were normal also.

Gladys later came to our office. This was the first time we saw her as a career woman in her glen-plaid tailored suit and white silk blouse, her hair combed in a knot at the nape of her head, her makeup beautifully applied. She was startlingly handsome. The only sign of tension was the deep vertical line between her glossy eyebrows.

I explained the hyperventilation problem and she understood.

"You're a mouth breather," I told her. "If you want to avert hyperventilation, close your mouth and press one finger over the right nostril, so you breathe only through one nostril."

"I'll suffocate," she said.

"You won't suffocate. And you won't hyperventilate.

"Another trick is to breathe and rebreathe into a paper bag. This means that when you blow off the carbon dioxide, you'll end up rebreathing it. Because of the concentration of carbon dioxide in the bag, you'll get some back in your system. And you'll save yourself a case of alkalosis and all its symptoms."

"If you say so," she agreed but uncertainly. Perhaps it seemed too easy. Blowing into a paper bag to spare yourself chest pains.

"That's one tip I won't give my boss," she said, with a wry smile. She went back to her color charts, her forecasts of fashion lipsticks and her irascible boss. The next time we saw her she was visiting the Cosmetics Czar, who was himself in CCU, recovering from a heart attack.

A recent patient of ours is Bernard G., a pianist who plays with one of the smaller symphony orchestras. One day as he was rushing from lunch to rehearsal, Bernard found himself climbing the steep steps up to the rehearsal hall two at a time. Midway, he paused on the landing, feeling breathless and aware of a sharp pain in his breastbone.

"It was the corned beef on rye," he said to the first violinist.

But when the conductor strode in with his quick walk and piercing glance, which seemed to search out someone to humiliate during this rehearsal, Bernard felt the pains increase, and he agreed with the violinist that he should leave the rehearsal and check with a doctor. (They were rehearsing Ravel's *Bolero*, a piece that he loathed.)

His physician found nothing wrong with his heart, but discovered he did have a *hiatal hernia.* Anger and frustration can cause the stomach acid to rise up to the hernia in the lower esophagus. The fierce pain is like a heart attack. Nevertheless, the doctor sent Bernard to us for a workup. The pianist did have some cardiac manifestations. However, all of them could be caused by anxiety. Palpitations, extra systoles (heartbeats), increased perspiration, tachycardia, cold hands or feet, a feeling of faintness are all common anxiety symptoms.

We found nothing wrong with Bernard and he returned to his piano and his hatred of the tyrannical conductor.

Other diseases masquerading as cardiac conditions such as peptic ulcer and gall bladder do not fall within the province of this book.

PART III

THE BIG RISKS

Chapter 10

High blood pressure: the silent foe

DR. FRANKLIN:
It was 1942, and Morton Franklin was happily married, the father of two girls and a young son, and a partner in a successful hardware business in Baltimore. He seemed to have everything going for him. Except for one thing that turned his face a little puffy, his skin a little pale, and made it difficult for him to get life insurance in order to protect his family. He consulted a number of physicians and their verdict was unanimous.

"You have high blood pressure, Mr. Franklin, and there is nothing we can do about it."

One morning in January, the mother, daughters, and son were seated at the oval breakfast table, waiting for the father to appear. Finally, the son was sent to fetch him. The bedroom door was closed. The boy knocked. No answer.

"Dad, breakfast is ready."

Still no answer. The boy opened the door cautiously. His father, still in pajamas, was lying motionless on the floor.

The doctor's office was three houses away. Fortunately, the doctor was in. His expression was grim as he spoke to the mother in the hallway, "Your husband has had a stroke." The boy was sent to stay at a relative's, and two days later, he was brought back home. The boy had seen two of his grandparents die, but they were very old. People said it was their time to go. But his father wasn't that old.

His mother took him by the hand and led him into the

room. His father lay in his bed, covered by a large cellophane tent. A tank with OXYGEN printed on it was being moved by a nurse.

The son was led to a chair near the bedside and sat there, looking at his father. The father's eyes turned briefly toward his son. Their eyes met. It was the last time.

Morton Franklin died in January 1942 at the age of 49 years. The cause of death was malignant hypertension. There was no treatment for it then. People who had it rarely lived longer than two years. The man made it for a year and a half and died of a stroke.

He was my father, and I am his son.

My mother and older sisters couldn't have been more understanding and helpful. But I don't enjoy remembering what it was like to be a growing boy without a father.

My partners and I feel fortunate in being in a profession which helps keep families together. Death is never a welcome visitor.

We take our responsibilities very seriously. Sometimes, we've been accused of taking them too seriously. But never by our patients.

High blood pressure, hypertension, is today the most common ailment to affect the heart and blood vessels.

It is a risk factor in nearly one-half the men and three-fourths of the women suffering from coronary heart disease.

Life expectancy of the person with untreated high blood pressure averages fifty-two years, depending on the elevation of pressure.

Twenty million Americans—10 percent of the population—probably suffer from high blood pressure. Possibly more. Symptoms come from the complications of high blood presssure, not the high blood pressure itself. Headache, dizziness, ringing in the ears are no more frequent in someone with hypertension than in someone with normal blood pressure, which is why it goes on so many years undetected, though detection is easy at the earliest stage.

The complications of high blood pressure

The left ventricle of the heart carries the burden of high blood pressure. At first, it grows stronger under the extra pressure, and like the muscles of a weight lifter, the heart muscle enlarges. Carrying the burden for many years, however exacts its toll. The left ventricle eventually weakens and dilates. Congestion of the lungs follows. The patient feels fatigued or short of breath. At first, this is only with exertion. Mowing the lawn becomes tiring, the work day seems longer, that game of catch with the kids leaves one panting, and any incline feels like a mountain. In later stages, the patient may find breathing easier if he sleeps on two or three pillows. He may awaken during the night feeling short of breath, he finds sitting up brings temporary relief. His ankles begin to swell. Every day is filled with misery.

Chronic high blood pressure damages blood vessels in many parts of the body, particularly in the heart, aorta, brain and kidneys. It does so in two ways, by arteriosclerosis causing blockages. Or by an aneurysm, a ballooning of a vessel which carries the danger of a blowout.

Complications resulting from untreated elevated blood pressure are:

1. Coronary insufficiency and myocardial infarction, due to somewhat premature arteriosclerosis.

2. Heart failure. This happens when the heart muscle becomes weakened after years of overwork from high blood pressure.

3. Stroke, due to blockage of blood vessels to the brain or hemorrhage through weak points in the blood vessel wall.

4. Aneurysm of the aorta, which is a bulging in the aorta due to weakness of its wall.

5. Aortic dissection, a tearing of the inner lining of the aorta.

6. Loss of kidney function due to damage of blood vessels that filter waste products as well as those that nourish kidney tissue. If this damage is extensive, kidney failure will result.

If organ damage to the heart, brain or kidney is present, the condition is known as *complicated hypertension*. This condition suggests a poorer outcome than *uncomplicated hypertension,* where there is no demonstrable organ damage.

In the complicated form, high blood pressure has already damaged body tissues to a measurable degree. This means the body has less "reserve" to draw on in the future.

DR. TAI:

Caroline G. walked into the Emergency Room of the hospital with her husband at two A.M. on a hot summer's night. Caroline G. was 58 years old, a pleasant, motherly woman, overweight and with graying hair, a worried expression on her lined face, and a manner of holding her hands together, palm to palm, as though in prayer.

As I was on call that evening, her family doctor asked me to see her.

"I started to feel uncomfortable about nine o'clock tonight," she said in a low breathless voice. "I figured it was due to the humidity. I just can't stand that kind of heat. But even with the air conditioning in the kitchen, I felt worse. Our son and daughter-in-law were over for dinner and I didn't want to scare them. So I lay down for a while. But I didn't feel any better, so Ed called our doctor and he said, 'Take Carrie over to the hospital.' "

She was in acute congestive heart failure. Her blood pressure was 220/130.

We put her on blood pressure therapy, and she gradually improved, but her blood pressure remained high. As I went over her physician's records, I found she'd had an episode of dangerously high blood pressure some eight years previously. Her family doctor confided the news to her husband, but both of them took it on themselves not to tell her or give her treatment, which might frighten her, but to watch her carefully. With this new dangerous flareup, Ed and her doctor decided to put her in our hands. She underwent a complete investigation for high blood pressure and is now on treatment with good control of her condition. She is leading a normal and active life.

What high blood pressure is

You go to your doctor's office for a checkup. The doctor wraps the blood pressure cuff on your bare upper arm, pumping it up until it's tight. He listens with the stethoscope placed carefully against the inside crook of your elbow, then releases the cuff pressure a bit at a time. A gauge attached to the cuff by a tube tells him what your blood pressure is. This is the simple and accurate method of measuring the pressure under which blood is circulating in your body.

Blood pressure is the tension (or pressure) built up by

the blood against the inside walls of the arteries. It results from a delicate balance of the pumping action of the heart (cardiac output), the "tightness" of the pre-capillary arterioles (see chapter 6) and the amount of blood in the vascular system (blood volume).

There are two pressures in your circulation, known as *systolic* and *diastolic*. When the left ventricle pumps blood into the arteries, the strong pumping action causes the higher, *systolic* pressure.

When the left ventricle relaxes, the aortic valve closes and the blood flows into the capillaries. This causes the lower *diastolic* pressure.

When the doctor takes your blood pressure, he looks for two readings on the blood pressure gauge: the upper, systolic, which is usually 120 millimeters of mercury; and the lower, diastolic, which is usually 80 millimeters of mercury. (This has nothing to do with your heart rate).

The normal upper range is 120 to 160.

The normal lower range is 70 to 90.

Blood pressure is reported as a fraction: Systolic/Diastolic. So when the doctor says your blood pressure is 120/80 you're in a normal range.

High blood pressure is an increase in blood pressure above the accepted normal.

It is thought that diastolic high blood pressure is more dangerous than systolic high blood pressure, but both are dangerous.

Nervousness can cause temporary high blood pressure, which is usually not serious. Temporary hypertension due to nervousness does not seem to be a forerunner of permanent high blood pressure and its dangers. The physician is usually aware of his patient's nervous state. He knows that the sight of the blood pressure cuff is enough to create anxiety that makes a patient's pressure rise. He may therefore take the blood pressure reading several times, so the patient grows accustomed to the cuff and he can get a valid reading.

Occasionally, the patient is so nervous that the doctor cannot get a reading to his satisfaction. He may want to take the blood pressure while the patient is on his job or at home.

There is another temporary form called *labile hypertension* which is the prelude to a permanent condition.

When he finds a high reading, the doctor will carefully examine eyes, heart, and the neurologic reflexes to uncover any complications. Sometimes the blood pressure is taken in both arms and the legs to detect certain disorders. When there is a difference in blood pressure between the arm and the leg, it means a blockage in the aorta. When our patients ask for more details, we tell them: High blood pressure is divided into categories according to the cause.

Primary high blood pressure is essential hypertension. Secondary high blood pressure is due to some other illness. In primary, the cause is unknown; in secondary, the cause is known.

Today, more than 90 percent of high blood pressure is primary, and three-fourths of those who have it, have inherited the tendency.

Secondary high blood pressure is most often due to diseases of the kidney or a hormone abnormality.

There is a direct relationship between the level of your blood and your life expectancy.

LIFE EXPECTANCY (Average Years to Live)
Related to Blood Pressure—(Males/Females)

	Age at measurement (years) f (female), m (male)		
Blood Pressure	35	45	55
120/80	41.5	32m–37f	23.5m–27.5f
130/90	37.5	29m–35.5f	22.5m–27f
140/95	32.5	26m–32f	19.5m–24.5f
150/100	25	20.5m–28.5f	17.5m–23.5f

Example: At age 35, a blood pressure reading of 140/95 indicates a life expectancy of 32.5 more years. With pressure of 120/80 at the same age, there is an added nine years of life expectancy.

DR. KRAUTHAMER:
At the age of 45, Luke was told by his family doctor that he had high blood pressure, but it was mild and needed no treatment at that time. He had a strong family history of hypertension and stroke. Over the years, he was examined but at irregular intervals. When his blood pressure began to climb, he reluctantly took medication prescribed by the doctor, but as soon as his blood pressure returned to normal and remained stable for several months, he discontinued the medication.

"It's ridiculous to take medicine when I feel okay," he told his doctor.

He also ignored the warning to stay away from salt. He liked plenty of seasoning in his food.

When he was finally referred to us, he was 52 and his blood pressure was 190/115. My physical examination indicated definite changes in the blood vessels of the eyes compatible with chronic hypertension. The examination also suggested some enlargement of the heart which was confirmed by chest X-ray. Auscultation of the abdomen revealed no murmur, and the pulses in the legs were well preserved. Blood tests showed kidney damage was present. Luke still felt well at this time, and gave me a little argument when I prescribed medication for control of his blood pressure. He agreed finally to give it a try and embarked on a treatment program.

He returned to the office for followup visits. His blood pressure did not respond to the initial group of drugs. I prescribed more potent medicine and Luke began to experience some side effects—if he stood up quickly after getting out of bed, he would feel light-headed for a brief period. Once he fell down.

He said irritably, "The medicine is worse than the disease."

I tried to convince him it was important to reduce his blood pressure, but he refused to follow the medical program.

We did not see him again for several years. Then, one night, I was summoned because Luke had appeared in the hospital emergency room with severe chest pains. All the tests I gave him strongly suggested coronary insufficiency. His blood pressure was now 200/120, and now he was more amenable to treatment.

We got along well over the next year as Luke took his medication and his blood pressure returned to near normal level. But once again, as he began to feel better, he started complaining about the side effects. After all, his blood pressure hadn't been very high for over a year. Again, he refused to continue his regular medical treatment again.

The next time I saw him was in the Emergency Room when he was brought in with a stroke. His right side was paralyzed, he was unable to speak coherently, and in his frustration, he muttered over and over again, "Damn, damn, damn." (It's always a curse word with stroke patients.)

We asked a neurologist to evaluate him while we attempted to bring his blood pressure under control again. Finally with the help of the neurologist and physical therapist, Luke started on a long rehabilitation program. After fourteen months of therapy, he walked with only a slight dragging of his right leg. His speech was quite good. The right side of his face showed only a slight droop, and he was able to return to work at a desk job.

He is very cooperative now, takes his medication regularly and follows instructions explicitly. It's been two years since his stroke and we are hopeful he will have many good years ahead of him as long as he takes care of himself. There is no question that permanent damage has been done to the brain and the kidneys but we hope these organs will hold out.

DR. KRAUTHAMER and DR. TAI: One afternoon during office hours, we had a call from a local general practitioner, who asked us to see a young patient with high blood pressure.

Shirley was 18 years old, had graduated from high school and was now working in the public library. She had no idea that she was having a problem with high blood pressure until she applied for an insurance policy to protect her elderly infirm parents.

As a child, Shirley had what was then suspected to be glomerular nephritis, an involvement of the kidneys because of a streptococcal infection—the same kind of infection which produces rheumatic fever. She was treated medically. The physician felt there had been minimal damage to the kidney tissue.

Her blood pressure was now 165/90, clearly abnormal for

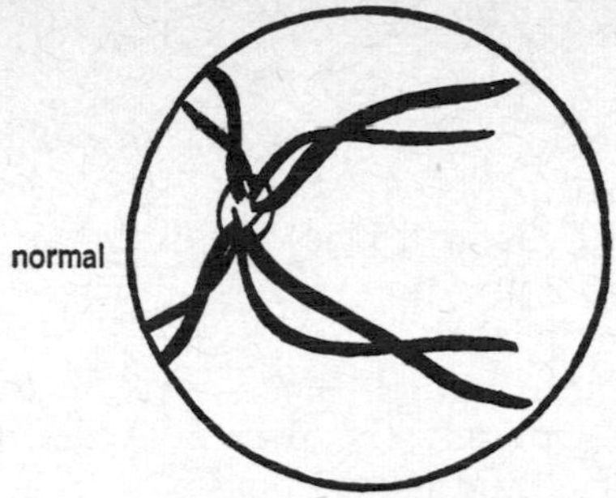

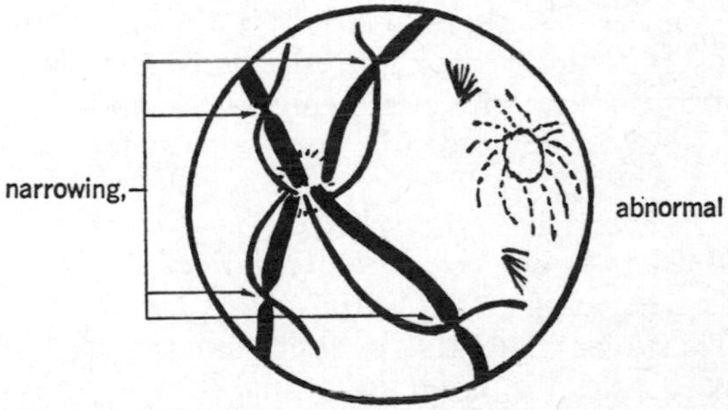

Normal and abnormal blood vessels in the eye

The top figure shows normal arteries (narrower vessels) and veins (thicker vessels) as they look to the doctor when he uses an ophthalmoscope.

When high blood pressure damages blood vessels (bottom figure), narrowings appear where the vessels cross each other. The eye nerve is also affected. An "exudate," an area of damage to the eye lining where a small vessel has ruptured and then healed over, is also seen.

a thin young woman. During the time she was under our care, each of us followed her case, but Dr. Krauthamer did the original workup. Whichever doctor she saw, Shirley bombarded him with questions.

One day in the office, Shirley asked, "Dr. Krauthamer, why do you look into my eyes with that gadget?"

The gadget was an ophthalmoscope, which is used to inspect the blood vessels on the retina at the back of the eyes. Those blood vessels are arterioles, the smaller branches of the arteries. We may find a spasm of the blood vessels or an increase in the thickness of the blood vessel wall, which gives us a clue to the duration and severity of the high blood pressure.

"By the time the blood reaches the arterioles, there has been a decrease in its pressure," Dr. Krauthamer explained. "But these vessels in back of the eyes are more delicate than other arterioles, so high blood pressure can destroy some of them. I can tell the degree of destruction by looking through the ophthalmoscope."

"Another thing I'm curious about, Doctor. You were comparing the vessels in my groin with the vessels in my arm."

"Normally, the pulse in the blood vessel of the groin, the femoral artery, should be felt at the same time as the pulse of the blood vessel in the wrist. If there is any delay, it is because of a narrowing in the aorta. This delay is brief—only micro-seconds—but with practice, it can be felt."

"Do I have that?" she asked.

"We don't know yet. We'll need to make some tests. But the narrowing of an aorta, called *coarctation*, can be cured by surgery and the patient, relieved of high blood pressure, can lead a perfectly normal life."

While Shirley was in the hospital for her tests, Dr. Krauthamer was away and Dr. Tai came to see her on rounds.

"Dr. Tai, maybe I'm too nosy," she said with an apologetic smile, "but I'd like to know what's going on. After all, it's my body."

"There are three conditions you could have," Dr. Tai told her.

"Dr. Krauthamer mentioned narrowing of the aorta."

"Possibly. Another is narrowing of an artery to the kidney. To keep the blood vessels at the right tension in the body, we have what's called the Renin-Angiotensin System. The renin enzyme is produced by the kidneys. Whenever there is a decrease in blood pressure to the kidneys, more of this enzyme will be produced and discharged into the blood. It works on another substance and creates a product called *angiotensin*, which constricts the small blood vessels (arterioles). The result is that blood pressure rises. Narrowing of a main artery to the kidney—and it need not be arteriosclerosis—is one of the causes of high blood pressure."

"What happens if I have that?"

"If you have a narrowing of a large artery to the kidney, we might hear a murmur over it. If so, there is a good chance of curing your hypertension." She didn't ask about the third condition until the next day.

The following morning, Dr. Tai visited Shirley and brought the news that her heart and lungs were normal, as well as her electrocardiogram. "We've scheduled you for kidney X-rays."

"Why a kidney X-ray? And still more tests?" Her relief at the good news was negated by this announcement.

"As I told you, if there is a narrowing in the aorta or the kidney artery, the condition is curable. Another cause of your high pressure could be a benign growth in your adrenal gland. That's why we are testing your urine."

"You've lost me, Doctor."

"The adrenal gland is small and sits on top of the kidney. A part of this gland puts out a substance called *aldosterone*. If there is a tumor, more aldosterone is produced than is necessary, and we can detect it in the urine. This triggers a rise in blood pressure."

Shirley had the IVP (kidney X-rays). The radiologist felt there was a strong possibility that the artery to one kidney was narrowed. Additional tests were needed.

She went through many special kidney tests. X-rays of the blood vessels to the kidneys (renal arteriograms) confirmed the final diagnosis of a narrowing in a renal artery. That was why she had hypertension.

We recommended surgery and Shirley agreed. Before she was discharged from the hospital, her blood pressure was down to normal.

Other kidney disorders, such as cysts and obstructions that cause hypertension can also be corrected.

Prostaglandins are receiving considerable attention now. These are substances manufactured by the body and affect blood pressure. One type of prostaglandin is produced by the kidneys and lowers blood pressure. This research gives us hope for the future.

DR. FRANKLIN:
It was late afternoon when Dr. Kulick asked us for a rush consultation on Zack, a seemingly healthy 23-year old who

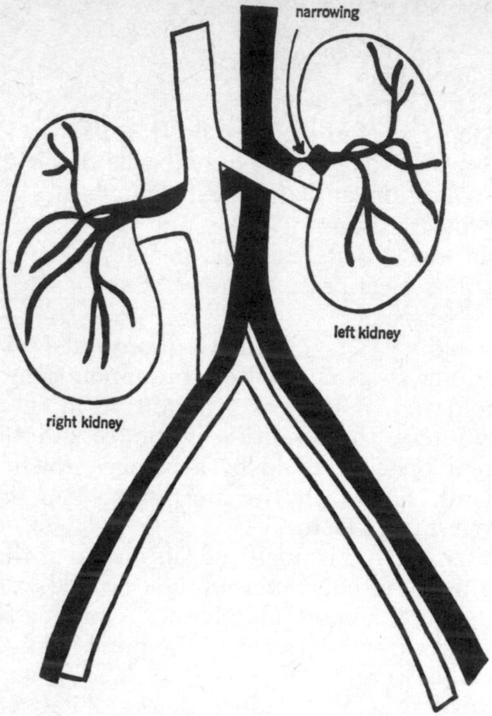

Narrowing of kidney artery

A rare cause of hypertension is a narrowing in the renal artery—the blood vessel that feeds the kidney.

The left renal artery in the diagram is severely narrowed. The kidney, which is not getting enough blood, manufactures a hormone that in turn elevates blood pressure.

had recently been turned down for insurance because of high blood pressure. He was hospitalized for evaluation. Tests suggested a narrowed renal artery, but were inconclusive.

"I need a favor," Dr. Kulick said. "Zack needs renal arteriograms (X-rays of the arteries to the kidneys), but he won't stay in the hospital. Can you do it today?"

Although it was close to quitting time, the nurses agreed to stay. Zack was rushed to the Cath Lab and prepped before I got a chance to say "hello." I quickly examined him.

Zack said he had been told about a heart murmur at age 10, but had not needed any medical attention until this insurance exam. I noticed that the murmur was heard better over his upper back and also in the abdomen. His blood pressure was 180/95 in both arms, but only 80 in his legs, with weak femoral pulses.

I called Dr. Kulick, "I think Zack has a coarctation (narrowing) of the aorta."

Dr. Kulick was in the lab within five minutes examining Zack himself. His dismay and embarrassment were obvious. "How could I have missed it," and when I tried to make excuses for him, he wouldn't accept them. Dr. Kulick is an excellent physician. He knows that all of us at some time in our practice make a mistake. He realizes that making unnecessary excuses for a mistake is the end of intellectual honesty and the beginning of accepting second best instead of excellence. We respect that kind of honesty and feel patients get better care from physicians like Dr. Kulick because of that attitude.

We explained the situation to Zack. He agreed to stay in the hospital. The next day we did a "combined procedure" —cardiac catheterization, arteriograms of the aorta and the renal arteries.

The coarctation was confirmed as his only abnormality and surgically corrected without complication. He is now able to get insurance without any qualifications, and is living a full life.

Mollie was a case of accelerated, or malignant, high blood pressure. On the surface, she was bluff, caustic and loudmouthed. She reminded one of our secretaries, a devoted fan of late movies, of a young but no less hefty Marie Dressler.

When we saw her, she was already confined to the hospital and was eligible for an award as the most difficult patient of the year.

"I hope you can persuade her to stay," her physician said. "She insists on checking out—and her blood pressure is 220/130."

I stopped by her room. It was eleven in the morning when most patients have been bathed, changed, their rooms tidied. Mollie's side of a semi-private room was a tangle of clothes and shopping bags, and Mollie herself, sitting on the stripped bed, fully dressed and boiling mad. When a person is sick, he is not always in control of his temper. I was prepared to be tolerant with Mollie.

"I'm Doctor Franklin."

"And I'm the Queen of Sheba," she roared. "Get on with what you want to do so I can get the hell outa here."

"You sound angry," I said. Her plump cheeks were raspberry red, her eyes nearly lost in the fat, gleamed wickedly.

"Angry," she mimicked. "I'm so mad I'll bust a gut."

This was no time for a full cardiovascular evaluation. I compromised. "What seems to be the trouble?"

"Sit down, dammit, and I'll spill it. But if you're smart, you'll just sign me out of here."

I sat down on a chair opposite her and showed I was ready to listen.

"While I'm here and you doctors are messing around with my blood pressure, my brother is at my house, messing around with my 17-year-old daughter. I don't trust the S.O.B. She'll be a mother before she's a wife."

The ten-day stay in the hospital had caused her nothing but grief, Mollie reported. And while she was being evaluated, no treatment was given for her hypertension. This is a routine procedure because treatment can mislead the diagnostic testing.

"I haven't peed in the bathroom for ten days," Mollie complained. "You've got a bunch of urine freaks around here. They treasure every drop, like gold. What's going on anyway?"

I explained that she was only thirty-four years old and the physicians were doing everything to find the cause of her high blood pressure, so that it could be cured.

"These urine tests are a search for certain hormones that can cause high blood pressure."

"Well, did you find them?" she demanded.

"Unfortunately, no."

"Oh, hell, what's the use!" She was growing angry again. She held her right hand spread out and started to count off with the fingers of her left—"X-rays, chest X-rays, ECGs, blood tests. And then—" she wiggled her finger as she spoke, "eat this, don't eat that. Don't smoke. Stay in bed. Get up. Walk around. I'm going home and throw my brother out of the house."

"At least let me examine you first," I suggested.

She dropped her 240 pounds on the bed. She ripped open the fasteners on her blouse. "Close the damn curtain," she ordered, although the other bed was vacant. I complied and quickly examined her, while she was willing to cooperate even in a grudging way. There was evidence of damage in the retinas of her eyes, and of course, there was her excess weight, and her blood pressure, which had been as high as 240/140. According to her chart, her X-rays were normal, but her ECG was abnormal. There was evidence of kidney damage in the blood tests, and an elevated blood sugar suggested early diabetes.

"Don't go home, Mollie," I said. "We can help you. Your life is in danger."

"My daughter's in danger," she said grimly. And signed herself out of the hospital at noon.

The next time I saw Mollie was a year later. I was checking on a patient in the hospital and saw her name on a chart heading at the nurse's station. I dropped in to say hello and ask how things were going for her.

No questions were necessary. Mollie was unconscious and on a respirator. I called her family doctor to find out what had happened. Mollie had ignored her high blood pressure. She refused to go to her physician's office, so he made frequent housecalls. She wasn't taking her medication. She hadn't lost weight.

Several days earlier, he got a call from her daughter. Mollie was having severe and frequent headaches. He couldn't go to see Mollie but he telephoned and asked her to come into the hospital. She refused. Yesterday, the ambulance brought her to the Emergency Room, after she had collapsed at home. She'd had a stroke. She looked terminal. None of the emergency measures helped. She never woke up. She died two days later from kidney failure.

It happens all too frequently, if not so dramatically. If Mollie had accepted treatment, she would have prolonged her life. She felt sick only after her hypertension was complicated by severe organ damage. We couldn't help after that.

No illness ever seems to come at a convenient time—plans are disrupted, and work has to be left undone. But some illnesses are more difficult to treat if they have been neglected. It's obviously better to treat a potentially serious illness while there is still time.

Chapter 11

Killer foods: cholesterol and triglycerides

DR. KRAUTHAMER:
"The world's turned into a giant computer," said an elderly general practitioner, who goes back to the horse-and-buggy era of medicine.

"Social security, credit cards, zip codes—everything's broken down in ciphers, even the patient. In my day, I knew the patient from the time he came into the world until he left it. I knew him, and I knew his folks. Now, he's not a patient. He's a number. Heart patients are classified in groups. And hyperlipoproteinemia has five groups —" He shrugged his frail shoulders in a kind of Sam Levenson humor, "Enough already!"

The volunteer fire company ambulance braked before the doors of the Emergency Room. The men hopped off their stations and the door of the ambulance flew open. They lifted the stretcher out and carried it inside.

The patient was a small boy wrapped in blankets, an oxygen mask over his face. Dr. Tai, awaiting his own patient, stepped forward to help. The boy looked no more than seven. His sandy hair fell over his forehead, and on the stretcher beside him was a small baseball mitt.

Efforts to revive him were futile. The dreaded phrase was written on the medical report. D.O.A. Dead on Arrival.

Dr. Tai spoke to the parents, seeking to comfort them. They said the child was thought to have had pneumonia.

A week later, the pathologist's report came in.

The report spoke of the extensive hardening of the boy's arteries.

Arteriosclerosis in a child? How could they explain this to parents, particularly his mother? Isn't it a condition of aging blood vessels? She had tried so hard to take care of her boy, feeding him the "Basic Seven" foods, seeing to it that he was well nourished, that he took his vitamins and wore his boots in bad weather. He was a Little Leaguer and soon to be a choir boy at St. Brigit's.

What comfort could we give her except an explanation of what arteriosclerosis is and what is being done to conquer it.

Arteriosclerosis is related to fatty substances in the blood.

The two most important fatty substances in the blood are cholesterol and triglycerides. Cholesterol can be manufactured by the body, or obtained from animal fat and other saturated fats in food.

Triglycerides come predominantly from the breakdown of starches (grains), carbohydrates (sweets), and some fatty substances.

When cholesterol and triglycerides are incorporated into the wall of a blood vessel, they associate with other substances to form what is known as *atheromatous plaque.* The buildup of the plaque is arteriosclerosis.

It is your cholesterol and triglyceride levels that give your physician an index of your risk in developing coronary artery disease.

The average normal American male has a cholesterol level of about 250 mgm.

If a person's cholesterol is higher, the danger of coronary heart disease increases. But that doesn't entirely rule out people with less than 200 mgm. as future victims. Cholesterol is only one of the contributing factors, and there are many, some still unknown. However, a low cholesterol level does reduce the risk.

In our Western culture, we enjoy a diet that is easy to prepare and pleasant to eat. Unfortunately, many tasty foods are high in cholesterol, fat and carbohydrates. We indulge our craving for sweets in large amounts, as much as 100 pounds of sugar per individual a year. The coffee break with a donut or Danish, both rich in carbohydrates, is a part of the office ritual. We enjoy our liquor, as the cocktail business lunches and bar cars on commuter trains will attest.

When you've had a fatty dinner of Kansas City beef, well marbleized, with crisp French fries, and well-buttered garlic bread, or roast duckling or a loin of pork, the fat you eat is broken down into succeedingly smaller particles by the intestines. Their fats do not dissolve in water. So nature has devised a system of combining these fats (lipids) with protein to create a soluble substance.

Since it is soluble, it dissolves in the blood and contributes to the blood fat level. The fat (lipid) part of the lipoprotein can be cholesterol, triglyceride, or both in varying proportions.

If the level of fat in the blood goes too high, it is called *hyperlipoproteinemia.*

It is a major risk factor.

The key question for the cardiologist is: How much is present in the patient's blood stream? And in what proportions?

Scientists have discovered five varieties of hyperlipoproteinemia. These have been classified by special blood tests which separate the various fatty substances (Appendix D).

The most common and those which will concern us the most are Type II and Type IV.

Type I

Butter, beef drippings, fatty lamb chops, peanut butter, even vegetable oils are digested into smaller molecules and then absorbed through the intestinal wall into your circulation. These tiny molecules are called *chylomicrons.* Since they are tiny, they circulate in the blood stream without actually dissolving.

After a rich meal, the chylomicrons in your blood are increased because your food is being actively absorbed. This is normal. When your physician wants an accurate reading, he'll ask you to fast for fourteen to sixteen hours and then he will draw a blood sample. By this time, all those fat globules in your circulation should have cleared.

If not, your system may be missing an enzyme.

Your body can't get rid of the chylomicrons even after fourteen hours, and it will show up in your blood test. The physician has put a sample tube of your blood in the refrigerator overnight. In the morning, he'll find a layer of fat in the tube. The fat rises, just like cream rises to the top of a bottle of milk.

There's your Type I.

Life can be uncomfortable for the Type I person. Aches and pains in the abdomen may lead the physician to treat his patient for stomach or pancreatic problems. Sometimes the pain is so severe that an operation is performed. Unnecessarily.

But the problem is essentially in the blood. Keeping a person with Type I away from alcohol and fats and feeding him from a special menu can relieve him of all his symptoms.

Type I is always genetic. You cannot possibly convert yourself to Type I. Your are either born with it or not.

But you can turn yourself into a Type II or Type IV if you aren't disciplined in your eating habits.

Type II

In Type II, the cholesterol level is high and the incidence of coronary artery disease is directly related to the level of cholesterol in the patient's blood. Type II people may have fatty spots of cholesterol on their eyelids and under their skin.

Some patients cannot understand (nor can the medical profession) why, even when they cut down on cholesterol in food, their cholesterol levels remain elevated.

Cholesterol comes from two sources:

1. Extrinsic: Foods that contain cholesterol.
2. Intrinsic: Cholesterol manufactured by the body.

When you eat animal fat (saturated fat) a large portion may be converted to cholesterol in your blood.

However, if you eat some vegetable fat (polyunsaturated) you get double benefits. It will not be converted to cholesterol and it is likely to reduce the cholesterol level already in your body. This is why you should be using polyunsaturated fats.

All of us make cholesterol, but some manufacture more than others. If you have inherited the gene that mass produces cholesterol, your body may produce it in greater quantities over the years. This may increase your risk of coronary arteriosclerosis. If your cholesterol count is high, it is possible you are Type II.

Some people are born with perfectly normal levels of cholesterol and triglycerides. But if they eat cholesterol to excess or are under persistent strain, they may become Type II by default.

If the physician is treating a patient in the Type II category, he must convince the patient to reduce his weight and cholesterol consumption. The normal cholesterol intake in the American diet is about 800 milligrams daily. The doctor may suggest reducing it to 300 milligrams, which means that these foods are limited: eggs, butter, artificial whipped cream, shell fish, animal fats. Coconut oil must be avoided, since it is a saturated fat. It is used in many cream substitutes. (See Appendix E, for a more detailed list.)

This cuts down on the rich goodies in the patient's menu but it leaves him plenty of good nourishing foods.

If diet alone doesn't work, the physician can give the patient a drug which will bind the cholesterol in the intestine so it is not absorbed in the circulation but is excreted.

The person who has inherited the Type II gene from mother as well as father has an 80 percent chance of dying from coronary artery disease before the age of twenty years, because of the excessive cholesterol.

When this occurs, treatment must begin as soon as the child is born. When the infant emerges from the womb, the blood from the placenta or umbilical cord can be examined in order to discover whether the child's cholesterol is high. If it is, preventive measures must be started in the hope of improving the long-term outlook.

The infant son of a friend of Dr. Franklin's died of coronary disease two days after his birth. Dr. Franklin knew the family's history of coronary heart disease. But this happened in 1960, when the lipoprotein groups hadn't yet been discovered. Fortunately, this is very rare. *Most of those with Type II either inherit it from one parent only or it is due to an acquired condition.*

George W. was a prime example of Type II. He had just turned 39, an age that is an emotional milestone in a man's life. He should be reaching the peak of his life's work, backed by a solid marriage, and a couple of growing children. But he's aware of the fact that time is fleeting, particularly when he sees some of the senior officers in the plant, no longer bucking for promotion, just treading water until retirement.

George's ethnic background was Irish, Slavic and German. He was a big fellow, over six feet tall and beginning to spread in the middle, so he was always pulling up his pants and tightening his belt. He had a square face with a blunt nose, the result of an old hockey injury, and his eyes looked at you directly.

"I've got no complaints," George often said, over a can of beer and the evening paper. "The world's treated me real well."

He, his wife Marge, and their sons lived in a pleasant community. His neighbors gathered around the big barbecue he built and the above-ground redwood swimming pool was a magnet for the local kids. They were all welcome.

George and his two brothers were all expert handymen. George's brothers gave up evenings and weekends to line the kitchen with cabinets and they built a cabinet for the stereo and TV set. George was working in the basement one night, cutting boards for bookshelves, when it happened. He couldn't explain it, he didn't believe he'd blacked out. But suddenly he was holding his left hand to his chest, and the blood was dripping on his T-shirt.

His wife drove him to the hospital. Their family doctor met them in the Emergency Room. George's hand was wrapped in a bloodstained towel. His forefinger was nearly severed. He was pale and clammy.

"Doc, I've got this funny feeling—" he began.

"The sight of blood always makes George sick," Marge interrupted.

The doctor asked more questions. "Where is this feeling?" he asked.

"In my chest, sort of. It's like my heart is going in high." After George's hand was sewn and bandaged, he was not allowed to leave. Instead, he was taken to the Coronary Care Unit. His physician called us for a consultation.

Dr. Krauthamer examined him.

"Have you had chest pains before?" he asked.

"Well, yes, I had a little trouble five years ago. My brothers were helping me with an addition to my house. It was August, the dog days. I took a shower, and as I was drying myself, my heart kicked up. I could feel it in my chest. Some pain, too, like a burning sensation."

"Were you checked?" Dr. Krauthamer asked.

"Yes, the doctor found nothing wrong. He said I got overheated and sweated too much. Maybe it was dehydration."

We performed coronary arteriography. His arteries were very bad, and he was sent for open heart surgery. The first surgery for his widespread disease wasn't entirely successful.

"I'm afraid he'll need another operation," the surgeon told his wife.

During the second operation, he didn't come out of anesthesia.

We offered our comfort, for what it was worth, to Marge and the boys. When the first shock of George's death had eased, we had a consultation with her, and explained that George had had a Type II hyperlipoproteinemia.

Then we learned that three of George's brothers had died between the ages of 35 and 37. We did blood tests on his two remaining brothers. They were both Type II. Even more worrisome was the fact that George's younger son, Roger, aged ten, was also Type II.

We've had the boy on the Type II diet for about twenty months, but it is too soon to form any conclusion.

We use no medication on Type II children. They are put on a diet that emphasizes fish, poultry, lean meat, skim milk. This isn't easy for the parents, since too many of our children today live on hamburgers, hot dogs, French fries, malted milks, ice cream, chocolate bars. It means re-educating the child's taste buds and an explanation of why he must confine himself to specific foods. Doctors are watching the progress of these Type II children. A new drug is being tested over a ten year span on children of Type II parents. In ten or fifteen years, we are hopeful that we will be able to control their high cholesterol.

At present, we have only a few weapons against the build-up of cholesterol: maintenance of normal weight, diet, exercise, avoiding stress. Whenever we see a patient with heart disease, we try to investigate his family background to discover whether there is a family tendency to heart disease, and then we suggest a program of prevention for the children in the family.

To combat risk, to diminish the toll of the killer factors, we must start prevention early.

Type III

Type III is a mixture of Types II and IV and seems to combine the elevation of both cholesterol and triglycerides. Like Type I, it is quite rare, and also is a familial trait. Those who have inherited the gene tend to have coronary vessel disease, often before the age of forty.

Treatment of Type III is simple. Lose weight. Reduce the intake of cholesterol and triglycerides. If the levels fail to come down, the physician may prescribe a drug called *clofibrate* (see chapter 16, "Medications"). We hope that the chances of heart disease are reduced by this treatment.

Type IV

This type of individual is usually obese. He eats a lot of carbohydrates (bread, pastries, pastas) and sugar, and has a high intake of alcohol. When sugar is absorbed into the body, some of it is converted into fat particles called triglycerides. In Type IV people, these triglycerides levels can be very high. Fifty percent of these people have an abnormal glucose tolerance curve, indicating a tendency to diabetes. Blood analysis of Type IV shows that while triglyceride level is high, the cholesterol level will be normal or only slightly elevated. Evidence suggests that triglycerides have as much to do with arteriosclerosis as cholesterol.

Those who drink alcohol frequently fall into Type IV. Yet alcohol is accepted as part of our Western culture, and does not have the opprobrium of taking drugs. Often, a person's alcohol consumption increases with his professional success, and its attendant tensions.

A person born with the gene that increases the level of triglycerides can be helped with clofibrate. If this drug doesn't help, there are still others which the doctor can prescribe. But even with the use of medication, he must avoid sweets and liquor.

DR. TAI:
One of our patients, Mike F., is a construction worker. He is a big-boned man of 39, an athlete from his teens. On weekends, he played softball with his friends. One afternoon, he felt a burning sensation in his chest. He broke off early, went home and took a cold shower.

The pain recurred while he was showering. He called his doctor who ordered him to go to the Emergency Room of a nearby hospital. There the doctor on duty did an electrocardiogram and told Mike that nothing showed up.

The pain didn't subside. I was called in consultation. The ECG was still normal and his pain was still intense. We suggested that he be admitted to the Coronary Care Unit. His tests showed a myocardial infarction. He recovered uneventfully.

Twelve weeks later, the blood tests showed that he was a Type IV hyperlipoproteinemia, with a high triglyceride level from excess sweets and pastry. He was then smoking about twenty cigarettes a day. His weight was still high. His father had died at age 33 of a heart attack.

I did a cardiac catheterization. Coronary angiograms showed two of his three coronary arteries severely narrowed. The heart muscle was good.

He had coronary by-pass surgery and came out of it splendidly. I told Mike that even though he had a saphenous vein by-pass (see chapter 19, "Surgery") and no severe heart damage, it was essential that he stay on his diet. Mike also receives drugs because I did not want to take a chance on diet alone controlling the triglycerides.

Time alone will tell us the answer to Mike's future. Initial data suggests that it should be hopeful.

Type V

Type V is a combination of Type I, with elevated chylomicrons, and Type IV with elevated triglycerides. Like Types I and III, it is rare.

In Type V, weight reduction works miracles. If the rare patient needs more help, the doctor will prescribe medication.

Reduction to normal weight is the most important prescription in all types of hyperlipoproteinemia.

Types II, III, or IV have a greater risk of early arteriosclerosis, unless it is caused by other illnesses. Obstruction to the liver's bile flow can cause Type II. Low thyroid function and a certain kidney disorder can cause Types II or IV. Type IV can also be caused by an inflamed pancreas (pancreatitis), a certain blood disorder, pregnancy or contraceptive pills. Diabetes mellitus (sugar diabetes) can cause Types III or IV, and is also itself a risk factor for coronary arteriosclerosis.

Often correction of such causative conditions will relieve the hyperlipoproteinemia, and early arteriosclerosis need not occur.

Obesity

Obese is an unattractive word and our overweight patients cringe when they hear it used to describe them. But the adage that you can dig your grave with your teeth is still painfully true.

"The longer the belt, the shorter the life," we tell our overweight patients.

Yet unless high blood pressure or diabetes is present, obesity has little to do with arteriosclerosis. It's the increased work load of the heart, caused by all those extra pounds, that may trigger coronary heart disease. Overweight contributes to high blood pressure, diabetes and high cholesterol. If there's a tire of fat around the waistline, your diaphragm cannot work properly for the proper exchange of air in the lungs. There's a greater danger of blood clotting in the veins. An overworked heart is exceedingly vulnerable. No rapid loss diet will melt weight and *keep it off*. There are no miracle shortcuts (see chapter 21, "Diet for Survival").

If you go on any sensible reducing diet and stabilize your weight, there is a chance of outsmarting your arteries.

Chapter 12

Killer habits and heart-prone diseases

We all know people who are compulsive in their habits, given to excesses that are self-destructive. Too many cigarettes, too much rich food, alcohol for a pick-up until it becomes habitual. The busy man who smokes his way through the tense world of deadlines and business luncheons, with too little exercise and not enough sleep, is asking for trouble.

Those who pursue this behavior are apt to become hostile, objectionable or upset when we physicians call their attention to the reality: Their life style encourages coronary risk. We recommend denying themselves foods that are pleasurable, we suggest exercise that involves discomfort, inconvenience and tired muscles, or we may prescribe medications that they do not want to take. In our society, a man often considers taking pills a reflection on his masculinity.

"You mean I'm dependent on this for life?" he will exclaim, holding a pill that can reduce cholesterol. "That's not my idea of living."

What he doesn't realize is that the end result of this belligerent attitude is not always sudden death. It could also be a gradual and progressive disability that leads to an uncomfortable, even a horrible end.

If high blood pressure invites so many disasters, and cholesterol and triglycerides boost arteriosclerosis, what's left that could be worse? There's a list of familiar risks that are all too easy to disregard if you happen to enjoy them—they are all killer habits.

Smoking

Smoking is a crime against the heart as well as the lungs.

Among the victims of fatal heart attacks, cigarette smokers rank high. A smoker inhales nicotine plus other toxic substances, which produce changes in the blood and raise blood pressure. Tobacco addicts have a tendency to develop irregular heartbeats, which means danger of sudden death. Smoking may cause changes in the electrocardiogram. We ask our patients not to smoke for at least 12 hours before they come in for an exercise ECG (see chapter 14, "Testing, Testing").

If a person is a heavy smoker, or lives in an environment where there is considerable air pollution, he can accumulate a good deal of carbon monoxide in his blood. The hemoglobin has an affiinity for carbon monoxide, and mixes with it, resulting in a combination called *carboxyhemoglobin.* Hemoglobin's affiinity to combine with carbon monoxide is 200 times greater than combining with oxygen. So only a minimal amount of carbon monoxide is needed to displace oxygen from the hemoglobin.

This can predispose you to angina, even at a low level of activity. People who have switched to non-nicotine cigarettes still have this problem. A West Coast doctor tested his patients with nicotine, and with non-nicotine cigarettes, and found no difference in the effect on the smoker's electrocardiogram, stress tests and level of aerobic capacity (see chapter 14). Although cigar and pipe smokers have less of a tendency to inhale, they also run risks.

With the recent epidemic of hysterectomies, younger women seem to be more cardiac prone. Heart attacks are rare in a normally menstruating woman. After menopause (whether natural or artificial) the heart attack rate does increase in women, and it may be compounded by their addiction to cigarettes.

Sudden death among American women under the age of 45 has risen fourfold since 1949. Oddly enough, women find it harder than men to abstain from cigarettes. As women compete in the business world, they are more subject to stress and anxiety. And as in men, the incidence of sudden cardiac death is greater in the woman smoker than in the non-smoker.

"I realize that no fully sane individual smokes because he

thinks it's healthy," admitted a recent patient with a two-pack-a-day habit. "I'd like to stop if I could, but there's a fire at both ends of every cigarette. The fire in me forces me to light the match to the other end of that cigarette."

The American Heart Association has booklets on how to stop smoking, which many of our patients have found helpful.

Behavioral scientists believe smoking is a habit, not an addiction, and that the smoker who is motivated to quit can. It's not easy but it can be done.

Coffee

The routine "waker-upper" for many of us is a cigarette and a cup of coffee.

And we may use the coffee break, at eleven in the morning and three in the afternoon, to tide us over the low points of our day, when energy is flagging. It is an effective stimulant.

Most diets encourage the reducer to drink as much black coffee as he wants. Young children are allowed to have numerous cola drinks, which are laced with caffeine.

But like other stimulants, coffee should be used with discretion. It should be self-rationed. At the tag end of a party, you would be wise to take coffee rather than alcohol as "one for the road." But the late Dr. Paul Dudley White was one of many doctors who believed that coffee is apt to make a person nervous and weary. "It stimulates the adrenal glands and nerve endings, and releases catecholamines, which speed up the heart!"

A recent study has indicated that coffee, *either regular or decaffeinated*, taken in large amounts—more than five cups per day—may contribute toward a higher incidence of heart attacks. The hazard may stem from a substance in the skin of the coffee bean. Even though tea contains a similar amount of this substance, it does not seem to lead to an increase in the saturated fats in the blood, and therefore, it doesn't add to the higher incidence of heart attacks. Other studies fail to confirm this.

Gout

Gout is one of the metabolic disorders that predisposes a person to coronary artery disease. It is often associated with premature arteriosclerosis. Recent studies have shown that people with high uric acid in the blood are in greater danger of a heart attack.

The classic victim of gout is the middle-aged male, sometimes overweight, who drinks too much and eats rich food. The initial attack usually occurs during the night, often lodging in the big toe of either foot.

Sometimes a larger joint is involved, such as the knee. It may be so tender and swollen that it hurts the patient to walk. Gout can also affect the hands and fingers. Often the skin over the inflamed joint will scale or flake.

In some cases, gout can be permanently crippling because of uric acid deposits in the joints and surrounding tissues. An attack of gout, usually very painful, lasts several hours or a day or more and with rest, it gradually subsides.

"What causes gout?" a patient asks Dr. Franklin.

"It is a hereditary disorder," the physician answers.

"How can you help me?"

An attack of gout responds to a drug called colchicine. It doesn't relieve pain in any condition other than gout, and is therefore a diagnostic test as well as a treatment. Equally effective are phenylbutazone and cortisone. We prescribe allopurinol, a drug that lowers uric acid, to decrease frequency of attacks.

High uric acid seems to be a part of an affluent society. When the physician discovers a high uric acid level in a high-powered executive, it may clue him in on future trouble.

Diabetes

Diabetes mellitus is a disorder of sugar metabolism, and is an important risk factor.

Sugar, or starch that has been converted to sugar, must be metabolized into energy by insulin. Insulin is produced by the pancreas. When insulin isn't doing its job, the body cannot burn sugar properly. Sugar accumulates in the blood and spills over into the urine.

Fatty substances also increase in the blood. These may be deposited in the blood vessel walls, and the result is often a narrowing. For this reason, diabetics are often prone to multiple heart attacks in early to mid-adulthood.

A blood sugar test is part of our routine evaluation for coronary heart disease. Two hours after he has taken a sugar meal, the patient's blood is checked for sugar. If it is abnormal, the patient is then checked with more refined tests for diabetes.

Drugs

Tranquilizers are prescribed very frequently nowadays. Taken over a long period, some of these drugs may produce changes in the electrocardiogram without actually damaging the heart. These changes usually go away if the drug is stopped.

Among stimulants, amphetamines are favorites. A close relative of adrenalin, amphetamine was first synthesized in 1927, and was acclaimed as a cure for asthma, nasal stuffiness, depression, epilepsy—and obesity.

MARIA G.:

A family physician was treating Maria G., a middle-aged Italian woman, who was grossly overweight—she was five feet tall and weighed 198 pounds. The thyroid he prescribed had no effect on her weight. In six weeks, she lost only 2½ pounds. And there were side effects: She was anxious, her hands shook, she dropped things, and she was suddenly quite high-strung. She couldn't tolerate warm weather. She had to take barbiturates to counteract her insomnia.

Since the thyroid hadn't helped in weight reduction, she went to another doctor who gave her Dexedrine spansules, which are long-acting amphetamines. The first result was excellent. She felt active and her appetite was under control. But gradually, the initial effect wore off. She needed more Dexedrine to function, until she was finally up to three spansules a day. But her appetite returned, and there was no weight loss. Her heart rate was rapid and her breath was short.

Her physician asked us to check her. Dr. Krauthamer found her pulse rate at 138 per minute and her blood pressure elevated. The electrocardiogram showed some abnormal changes. She was admitted to the hospital, where a complete workup demonstrated that the cause was amphetamines. The drug was discontinued and after several months, her blood pressure gradually returned to normal and her tachycardia was controlled.

She now weighs 208 pounds and enjoys overeating. Her physician has written her off as a lost cause until the time when she again has medical problems.

Used simply for kicks, or sometimes to increase performance, illegal amphetamines are widely used by teenagers. "Speed" has been mixed with marijuana, alcohol, or sleeping pills. Amphetamines are used by some people who must stay awake for long periods of time. In World War II, various armies permitted their soldiers to use them to overcome fatigue. Athletes have been known to take them before meets, and race horses have received illegal injections of the drug prior to important races.

The use of amphetamines is controversial in medicine today. Researchers discount its long-range value in fighting obesity. Students who take the drug may produce more work, but their efficiency is always reduced. Depression is common, even though it may be taken to overcome depression.

One percent of the amount of amphetamines produced today is sufficient to satisfy medical requirements. The rest goes to the pep-happy populace.

Amphetamine addiction is rampant throughout the United States, and many physicians are only now becoming aware of the serious side effects of this drug.

Cardiac complications develop, especially changes in blood pressure and irregularities of heart rhythm. Taken intravenously, speed is a fast stimulant. It can also produce sudden death. "Speed kills" is no exaggeration.

Recently Billy R., a 25-year-old amphetamine addict, was brought to the hospital's Emergency Room with severe chest pains. He was in the habit of taking from 120 to 150 mgs. of amphetamines daily by injection into his veins. He couldn't function without his dose.

His electrocardiogram showed changes that indicated either a myocardial infarction or coronary heart disease. Yet after he went through cardiac catheterization and arteriography, his heart was pronounced normal. He stayed in the hospital for two weeks and during this time, he had no pain. His tests were all normal. He was discharged, but reappeared a fortnight later with recurrence of his original symptoms. This time, even minimal exercise stimulated pain, showing increased heart rate and irregular rhythm.

"Speed" finally killed him. His body, paced high with the drug, wore out prematurely.

Barbiturates

Barbiturates (sleeping pills) are particularly popular with nervous women who use them to get a good night's sleep and often a permanent one. They are used by those bent on suicide. The chronic use of barbiturates often causes mental derangement, confusion and depression. These pills disturb the natural rhythm of sleep. Taken in large doses, they depress the area of the brain that controls the heart and respiration, and can cause death.

Most of us at some time in our lives have taken sedatives, tranquilizers or even psychic energizers. They are a part of our way of life. If used in small amounts, as prescribed bv a responsible physician, they can be enormously helpful. But in the hands of fun seekers, they are lethal weapons.

Glue

Youngsters have discovered that they can get a charge out of sniffing airplane glue. Unfortunately, this product has a chemical which has an immediate effect on the heart. By reducing the rate of the heart, it can cause a sudden collapse and death. It is not a diversion to be recommended.

Heroin

We are interested in heroin because of its effect on the heart and what we have recently observed among young addicts.

The heroin that reaches the street by the pusher is no longer pure. It has been cut many times and diluted with quinine and milk sugar. If an addict is accustomed to "shooting" anywhere from 10 to 30 bags of heroin daily, he is also injecting between 1.5 and 7 grams of quinine at the same time.

Quinine in that dosage can produce irregularity of the heart and instant death. It is a poison that can affect the brain, heart, muscles, gastro-intestinal tract, ears and eyes. Recently, there have been reports of young addicts who have become completely blind following an injection.

If an addict happens to buy a bag of undiluted heroin (much stronger than the stuff he's accustomed to using) the shot can result in respiratory arrest. The brain center that stimulates breathing falters. No air enters the lungs. The heart perishes for want of oxygen. This kills quickly. It may be the reason some addicts are found, collapsed in the bathroom, with the needle still stabbing the vein.

Now, pure heroin in sterile ampules will cause no direct damage to the heart. But heroin in large doses will produce side effects because it depresses the brain centers which control breathing and heart action. It also lowers blood pressure. However, once the effect of the drug has worn off, the bodily functions usually return to normal.

Many addicts become infected by unsterile needles. Their veins are in bad shape. The whole vein is often clotted. If a clot breaks off and flows through the right side of the heart and lodges in the lung, it is a pulmonary embolus. Fortunately, it does not happen often. More frequently, the unsterile needle can produce an infection which travels to the heart and settles on the valves, causing damage (endocarditis).

It is possible for heroin addicts to get endocarditis even when their valves are normal. They acquire a fulminating or an acute malignant type of infection which is usually fatal. Since they are generous in sharing their unsterile needles and syringes, they also share fungus infections and hepatitis. When a fungus infection settles on the valves, there is little hope for the victim. Eighty to ninety percent die in the immediate phase. This is fungal endocarditis.

Anthony, 25 years old, arrived at the Emergency Room of the local hospital, looking pale and undernourished. He complained of feeling ill, and had chills and fever. His appetite was poor and he had lost considerable weight. Eight years ago, he had been examined routinely, after an arrest for drug addiction, but he was then organically sound. Now he had a heart murmur and valvular damage. Dr. Krauthamer diagnosed his condition. Endocarditis was present. His blood culture grew yeast, which had settled like a mold on his valves.

He was willing to go for valve replacement, but the

surgeon decided not to operate as he was already too weak. Even after the valve is replaced, fungus can settle on the new artificial valve. He was going to die, so we took a calculated risk. He was given a potent drug to kill the fungus. His kidneys reacted to it. He developed kidney failure and died. We found a green mold on his heart valves at the autopsy. It was like something out of science fiction.

Stress

Stress is another great culprit. But it's hard to think of it as a killer habit, like drinking, drugs, or eating the killer foods—all of which are attempts to *avoid* stress.

Dr. Meyer Friedman and Dr. Ray H. Rosenman of Mount Sinai Hospital in San Francisco checked 3,500 men over a 4-year span. They found that the Type A man had 2½ times as many heart attacks as Type B.

The Type A person is aggressive, ambitious, success oriented. He talks too fast, he is always on the run trying to meet deadlines, and he is always competing against himself. The rags-to-millionaire is Type A. He not only is a genius in business, but is a success in any field—government, education, whatever.

Type B is placid. He is a quiet man who works at his own pace and doesn't respond in a hyperthyroid way to environmental change. He is not a victim of mental stress.

Whether stress is physical or mental, there is an outpouring of adrenalin into the body. Adrenalin increases the heart rate and raises the blood pressure, thus creating a greater demand of the heart for oxygen.

The heart of a Type A person may need oxygen in greater amounts. He is not only compulsive, in his work and play, but also careless in his eating habits, which may add to his problems. Characteristically, he indulges in high cholesterol foods, which increase the level of fatty acids or fat substance in his blood.

Cool it!

This advice should be imprinted on everyone's mind. "Cool it!" should dominate your life style.

The person prone to heart attack needs a built-in self-regulator for his emotions and state of mind. He is at the mercy of those around him, whose behavior can often trigger a gut reaction in his system. A great surgeon, John Hunter, himself a cardiac patient, once admitted wryly, "My life is at the mercy of any scoundrel who chooses to put me in a passion."

If it isn't the boss or the traffic snarls, or the inflated economy, it's the family. A person is most sensitive and vulnerable to his family. In this area, he usually tries for self-control.

One of our patients, David R., was the newly elected head of an old woolen mill in New Hampshire, with offices in New York, which made it possible for him to live in our county. A Boston boy with a degree from the Harvard School of Business Administration, David had come from Dorchester, where his father ran a small candy and newspaper stand. As he became successful, the chasm between him and his family had widened to total separation. His wife, Allis, was a Vassar girl and like many of her group, she had a deep sense of responsibility for those who were called the underprivileged a decade ago. They had everything, including a 16-year-old daughter, Barbara, whom they adored.

Whether David's drive stemmed from a genetic strain, or fierce anger against his own childhood deprivation, or an unflagging ambition to be admired, was never clear to Allis or his associates. His enthusiasm for forging ahead was so contagious that his staff often overlooked the fact that it was an insatiable compulsive drive. He offered generous bonuses and few sharp words. He goaded the staff but they found it hard to complain because he was always there beside them.

David was a classic Type A personality. He was always keyed up, running behind time, and setting schedules that he couldn't possibly meet.

Nobody ever said of him, " 'What makes Sammy run?' " But then nobody was surprised when he suffered his first heart attack at the age of 42.

David's heart attack, though precipitated by his life style, was not "caused" by it. His coronary arteriosclerosis, the narrowing in his blood vessels that nourish the heart, took many years to develop.

Fortunately, the attack happened on a mild autumn

Sunday morning. He was on the court, playing a tough game of singles with one of his junior executives. He collapsed near the net. Quietly efficient, Allis immediately called the local volunteer fire department, which had an ambulance and firemen trained and equipped for cardio-pulmonary resuscitation. They responded quickly.

David's recovery was uneventful as far as the healing of his heart was concerned. He did experience the depression that is characteristic during this time.

The highlight of his convalescence was his daughter. He looked forward to Barbara's visits even more than his wife's. She was an extension of himself, bright, inquisitive, a good athlete. He had to play a sharp game of tennis to beat her.

He counted on seeing a good deal of his daughter when he convalesced at home. She'd just received her driver's license and she could ferry him around until he got permission to take the wheel again.

But oddly enough, once he came home again, he saw less of Barbara than during his hospital stay. She came home from school in time for dinner and then dashed out again. David soon discovered her new interests were focused on a group of kids he didn't cotton to. He didn't take well to kids who showed their contempt of parental affluence by raveled, dirty jeans, unwashed bare feet and hairstyle of a guru.

What bothered him even more was the break in their communications. She had become a stranger, absent-minded but polite. When he tried to persuade her to drop her new friends, he was greeted with hostility and anger.

David usually went to bed at ten, and didn't need to be coaxed. One night, after midnight, the telephone woke him. Barbara and three of her friends were at police headquarters. They had been picked up in an empty house, whose owners were on vacation: pot and group sex.

It took two tranquilizers to quiet David until they reached headquarters. By then, he needed another.

"Dammit, I tried to help you," he shouted at Barbara. "I told you to stay away from these bums!"

Barbara was cool, remote and singularly unrepentant.

When they got her home and locked her into her bedroom, David was too excited to relax. He felt the first twinge of a chest pain, a flutter, a shortness of breath. He tried to be quiet, although inwardly he was raging. By morning, he was in serious trouble, and Allis drove him to the Emergency Room.

After his second heart attack, David definitely needed a psychiatrist. Barbara was living away from home and made it plain that she had no intention of following her family's middle-class life style.

"She's in the drug scene," the counselor said. "I'm afraid there's nothing that you can do until she wants to turn to you."

David found it impossible to accept such advice. Constant aggravation, anger, reconciliations that were pleas on his part and rejection on hers, created a mounting tension. He lived in a state of such rage that his circulatory system threatened to explode.

No one could help David now except perhaps his wife. And his deep fundamental will to live.

He spent a year in analysis and in the process discovered truths about himself and his relationship with his daughter. He finally realized that he had to accept the current situation. Barbara might come back. Or not. It was out of his hands.

We have had a good many cases similar to David's, with an initial heart attack or a second one triggered by explosive confrontrations. Confrontations may mean a series of cardiac incidents—or a fatal one.

"All that keeps me going," a patient told us recently, "is the fact that change need not be negative."

PART IV

WHAT THE DOCTOR TEAM DOES

Chapter 13

Your annual physical exam is a safety belt

DR. TAI:
Whenever the family practitioner or internist calls us for a consultation, we continue to regard the patient as his, and we report our findings to him. If the patient proves to have a heart condition, we keep in touch with his family physician either by in-person conversation, telephone or notes on the patient's chart, and letters. We carefully discuss the details of treatment, and when we can put him back in the care of his family doctor.

The family practitioner is the main support of the specialists, and everybody gains when he gives his patient expert care. This is of critical importance today as the complexity of medicine is increasing. Many family practitioners continue to read countless medical articles and take courses in various fields to keep them up to the minute on medical developments. They are in an improved position to take care of their patients. This is vital in the field of cardiology because so many advances are being made.

What happens to a patient when his doctor gives him a general examination? What is he doing? What does he discover? Why does he sometimes make an appointment for his patient, presumably healthy, to see a specialist?

Often the most important step any person can take is to have an annual physical examination by his family doctor or internist. You don't wait for a toothache before you go to your dentist. If there *is* something wrong, it will be spotted. And it could be serious even without any symptoms you are aware of. An annual physical can be done in one or more office visits. Further tests or the attention of a specialist will be requested if indicated. Over 20 million Americans have that silent killer, high blood pressure, and this can be detected only if blood pressure is taken. Has yours been checked recently?

EUGENE BABCOCK, M.D.:

I am Eugene Babcock, M.D., a physician in family practice, which includes pediatrics, gynecology and obstetrics. I have been in practice fifteen years. Most of my patients are as familiar to me as my own kin. I know their backgrounds, their personalities. I try to assess each one in relation to his family, his social environment, and his work.

Even though my practice is in a large town, my role as a family doctor retains the small-town community flavor. I realize that many city doctors may not be in such a favorable position because they have so many patients, but their methods will be the same as mine. A physician is above all a diagnostician, catching any sign of trouble. We are lucky because we have at our fingertips resources that the family physician lacked even a decade ago. When one of my patients needs specialized diagnosis and treatment, there are any number of specialists I can call on whether it is a persistent stomach ache or a heart attack.

If there is reason to suspect a serious cardiac problem, I can be on the telephone with a cardiologist at any time. If needed, he will see the patient immediately at the Emergency Room of the hospital. I am acutely conscious of the need for speed in a heart attack.

Once my heart patient is stabilized, I can follow up his care with recommendations outlined by the cardiologist. I never feel I am losing a patient but rather that I am gaining specialized assistance.

As a family physician, I follow my patient regularly, so I am in the position to spot any deterioration in his health. The cardiologists and I are a team, safeguarding his future.

My secretary received a call one morning from Bill S., who wanted to make an appointment for a general physical examination, and mentioned one of my patients who had told him about me. The secretary made an appointment for Friday of the next week and reminded him not to eat for fourteen hours before his appointment and to have an enema to prepare for some tests.

I reached my office at nine that morning, having already made hospital rounds. While Bill S., my first patient, was completing a health questionnaire, I made some telephone calls to sick patients and dictated reports from yesterday.

The nurse brought Bill into my office. As we shook hands and chatted briefly, I was observing my new patient. At such times, I frequently recalled what a greatly admired professor had told my class. "Don't be afraid. Let your heart be like a lion's, your eyes like an eagle's, your hands like flowers, your ears like a leopard's. Watch. Feel. Percuss. Auscultate." After talking with Bill briefly, I felt that although he was a reluctant patient, he was genuinely interested in protecting his health and would cooperate fully. He had had his last physical ten years before when he took out a new insurance policy.

What brought Bill to my office was a friend's death the previous week. Bill, Harold and a group of their friends—all men in their late 30s and 40s—belonged to the auxiliary police and once a week, they went out to Stone Ridge for target practice. Harold had just fired his first shot when Bill saw him hunch over, holding on to himself, his ruddy face turning pale. He was gasping for breath and he crumpled up before Bill could catch him.

After Harold's funeral, Bill's wife, Dottie said, "Bill, I want you to get a checkup. I'm tired of telling you. I don't want to nag, but you're in a dangerous age."

At the next opportunity, Bill talked with some of his friends who'd known Harold too, and came up with my name as a physician.

With the relationship established, I turned Bill over to my nurse for his ECG and chest X-rays, asking for two views of the chest—front and side. Some physicians, of course, have all X-rays taken by a radiologist, not in their own offices. My nurse had also taken blood and urine specimens, and had given him the health questionnaire to fill out. Bill was undoubtedly astonished at the long list of questions he was expected to answer. By scanning the data sheets later, I could pinpoint areas of importance and follow up these points with a more thorough personal review.

Bill S. was nearing his 44th birthday. In the 1950s, he

had started an oil delivery business with one truck. The business had prospered and grown, and now, was not only in fuel supplies and furnace repairs, but Bill had bid on the installation of heating units in the condominium that was going to be built next to the new state highway.

In his health questionnaire I looked for specific problems. Bill was overweight and a heavy smoker. He reported a morning cough and some vague chest pains several months before. His family history was good, no premature deaths from heart disease, no diabetes, nor unusually high blood pressure.

My nurse brought Bill into the examining room, where she recorded his height and weight, and gave him a disposable paper dressing gown. I asked him to sit down on the examining table and talked a bit, trying to be reassuring. I referred to the reason for his coming—the death of his friend, Harold. "It happens whenever somebody loses a friend from a heart attack. And when national figures like Gil Hodges or Jackie Robinson die, the doctors' offices fill with people who want heart examinations."

To get the most out of a general physical, it is most helpful if you prepare yourself before seeing your family physician. Bill hadn't thought about it, so I had to ask him a good many questions as I went along. If you have chest pain, be prepared to tell your doctor *when* it first started, *what* seems to cause or relieve it and *where* you feel it. Wrong information may mislead him. Just tell him what you know—his examination and tests given later if needed, will detect any trouble.

I proceeded with a physical examination that is routine for most physicians—an invariable series of medical checks that include examining the chest, front and back, listening to the lungs, and for the heart sounds. While listening to the heart sounds, I heard a murmur.

"Bill, are you sure you never had rheumatic fever?"

"Never. I was the healthiest kid in my class."

I listened again at different positions on Bill's chest.

During the course of the examination, I checked the rest of his body in addition to his heart. After a rectal examination, Bill had a sigmoidoscopy and I explained that over half of all cancers in men are in the colon. In a woman I would check her breasts for any slight suspicion of a growth that would indicate an early cancer. In fact I would instruct her in how to check this herself. She would also have a Pap smear to detect any sign of cancer of the uterus.

Though I gave Bill a thorough examination and would do various blood tests, I will describe only the heart examination, because I did discover a heart condition and later referred my new patient to the cardiologists in Darien, Connecticut.

To check your heart, the physician does a number of different things during the examination. When you are on the examination table, he takes your pulse. It may be fast, because of nervousness. But he can tell whether your heartbeat is regular or irregular. He can detect a bounding pulse or a weak one. Both may turn out to be normal, but each acts as a medical clue. He will check the pulse in both wrists and compare the wrist pulse with the groin pulse to rule out coarctation.

He may take your blood pressure in both arms. If he finds any abnormality, suspects certain conditions, he may take it again later to confirm the reading. (See chapter 10, "High Blood Pressure," page 124.) He taps your chest with his fingers (percusses) and listens intently for the sound it makes. Lungs are hollow and contain air, so the sound should be drum-like. If fluid is collecting at the bottom of the lungs, the sound is solid. He feels the chest as you breathe to discover if the lungs are expanding fully. He can outline the heart by percussion (tapping). The X-ray is more exact but it cannot duplicate the information from palpating (feeling) over the heart. The doctor can actually feel your heart beat. So can you, if you lie on your left side, and put your palm under your left breast, take a deep breath and let it out. Slowly. Now, feel carefully. With the lungs partly empty of air and therefore smaller, the heart is closer to the chest and can be felt easier. While palpating your abdomen, he will ask you to breathe deeply in and out. If your liver is enlarged, he can feel it ever so gently against his fingertips.

Next the stethoscope, the doctor's symbol. You are now sitting up and he presses the flat part of the stethoscope over your back, asking you to breathe with your mouth open. He listens to the air going in and out of your lungs. It is much like the sighing of the wind in the trees on a summer night. If you smoke heavily and have bronchitis with some mucus in the air tubes, there is a rattle as the air passes over. The doctor hears this rattle. If fluid collects in the small air sacs of the lungs at the ends of the breathing tubes, the walls of these tiny air sacs become sticky. As you breathe in, the walls of the air sacs separate to allow the air in. Because they are sticky, a tiny crackle is heard as the walls separate. When the heart muscle weakens, and fluid collects in thousands of such sacs, moist crackles are easily heard. These are râles, which indicate something is wrong, not necessarily with the heart. Infection in the lungs (pneumonia) also makes the walls of the air sacs sticky but without much fluid. The experienced doctor can tell whether these crackles are "wet" and due to fluid or "dry" and due to an infection. Naturally, a patient with pneumonia has other symptoms which help reveal his illness.

While you are lying on the table, the doctor asks you to turn your head and he inspects your neck. He is checking the pulsations in the neck veins. This tells him whether or not your heart is able to accept blood returning from the body in a normal manner. Abnormalities often show up in the pulse of the jugular vein. If the heart is weak, and cannot carry the normal work load, the veins may become distended. The physician can actually see this distention.

He places the stethoscope over your heart, first one place, then another. He hears "lub-dup," the two heart sounds.

When I had completed the general examination, I asked Bill further questions. After the examination, I knew he might recall some things that he did not remember earlier when he was more tense. I assured him that his next visit the following year would be shorter, since the background material would be on file. If he moved to another location, I would, of course, send his records to the new physician, though most doctors prefer to do their own workup on a new patient.

Then I asked him to come into my office.

"Bill," I said, "most of the preliminaries were negative. But you have a heart murmur."

"A heart murmur? What does that mean?"

"I think you have a narrowing of the mitral valve. It isn't opening properly. You have no significant symptoms, so it's probably mild to moderate. But I'd like to send you to a cardiologist."

When I called the cardiologists' office to set up the appointment, they reminded me that another patient of mine, Ollie T. would be seen this week. I made a note to expect a report, so I could discuss Ollie's heart condition during his next visit to my office.

Chapter 14

Testing, testing

DR. TAI:

The visit to a consultant can be alarming to some apprehensive patients. But when the family physician explains the situation to him as Dr. Babcock did for Bill S., the patient feels more comfortable and his fears are allayed. The fact that his doctor has arranged for a specialist should be reassuring if the patient knows what he's going for.

When Bill arrived at our offices, he already knew he had a mitral valve condition, and Dr. Babcock left it to us to give him details. We told this large, heavy set man that we would be checking his heart thoroughly in the general course of examination. We asked him all the pertinent questions relating to heart murmur. We put him through an even more detailed cardiac examination than Dr. Babcock had done, and would report to him when our examination was complete.

We believe in making a "clinical judgment," or diagnosis, based on the patient's story. Even with all our technical cardiac resources, we find that it pays to spend time with each patient. We learn from listening to them.

Some sixth sense, some unrecognized apprehension may bring the patient into the office. The clinical judgment of the doctor, is, therefore, most important. Dr. Babcock pinpointed the problem, and left it to us to verify it and determine Bill's condition with modern cardiology techniques.

Even though Dr. Babcock had provided complete information, including chest X-rays and ECG, we repeated the questioning with added emphasis on questions regarding the heart.

The examination is similar to the one conducted by your physician. We do not include a sigmoidoscopy or Pap smear in our routine. We are cardiologists and look at the cardiovascular system in minute detail.

After checking his pulse, blood vessels, and blood pressure, I began a systematic examination of the heart. While listening to his murmur, I turned him on his left side and listened with the bell of the stethoscope. I had him sit up and bend forward. While he exhaled fully, I listened to the heart searching for the murmur of aortic valve disease. It was not present. We sometimes exercise the patient and listen to his heart again. The heart sounds are analyzed while the patient is straining and changes position, such as squatting or standing up. This helps us pinpoint heart disease accurately and tell the difference between innocent and serious murmurs.

After completing the examination and reviewing the chest X-rays and ECG, I concurred with Dr. Babcock's diagnosis. I explained the situation to Bill.

"You have a narrowing of the mitral valve," I told Bill. "It seems only mild to moderate by my examination."

"What caused it?"

"Most likely rheumatic fever, possibly some virus. There may be no history of either."

"But I was never told about the murmur and I have no symptoms."

"It can be missed if the examination is hurried and the narrowing is mild," I answered. "Since you have no symptoms, we don't have to do anything but keep you under observation—check you once a year." I explained to him the precautions for preventing endocarditis (chapter 12, "Killer Habits")—taking antibiotics prior to and after any operation or dental treatment.

"Do I need other tests to confirm your findings? Now that Dr. Babcock brought my attention to the heart condition, I have become aware of extra beats on occasion."

"Yes, we do have many sophisticated pieces of equipment to confirm the clinical diagnosis—both qualitatively and quantitatively."

I did a series of tests on Bill in addition to the X-ray, ECG, and stress ECG. This included phonocardiogram, vectorcardiogram, echocardiogram, and dynamic cardiogram screening for irregular heartbeats. These confirmed my findings: mild mitral stenosis. Cardiac catheterization was not indicated at the present time. Bill was encouraged to lead a normal and active life.

These are non-invasive tests. They do not invade the body. All information is gathered externally. They are extremely helpful in evaluating all heart patients. In our opinion, they are the most important and valuable weapons the cardiologist has, next to his clinical examination.

Cardiac series

Bill S. had his X-rays taken at Dr. Babcock's offices. The plain chest X-ray, routine in nature, outlines the heart against the thinner lung fields so the doctor can see its overall size and shape. Looking at the ribs is an important part of the evaluation of congenital heart disease. (Children born with a certain form of congenital heart disease will have a "notching" deformity of the ribs.) But the single X-ray of the chest performed for the detection of tuberculosis, for instance, is not sufficient for cardiac evaluation, because portions of the heart may not be seen in just one picture.

"We need a cardiac series," I requested, indicating four chest X-rays. The heart is near the center of the chest, in close proximity to the gullet (esophagus) and the windpipe (trachea). Enlargement of certain chambers of the heart is likely to produce distortions of the gullet as well as the windpipe. The physician may even outline your gullet by having you swallow barium, so he can see whether the heart is displacing or deforming it. Bill had a slight enlargement of the left atrium because of the narrowing of the mitral valve and the resultant backlogging of blood.

In the cardiac series, one X-ray is taken from the front, and the others are taken facing from the side and obliquely. The purpose of these is to show the shape of the heart and its relation to the areas around it.

X-rays of the lungs outline arteries carrying blood to the lungs as well as veins that return it to the heart. When the heart is overloaded, these vessels become enlarged, giving the doctor a clue to a problem. In some forms of congenital heart disease, the vessels are smaller. Determining the blood vessel pattern of the lung helps the physician decide what kind of heart disease the patient has and how severe it may be.

It is not the whole answer, but leads to the answer.

DR. TAI:

Electrocardiogram

The most common electrical instrument used to test the heart is the electrocardiogram (ECG or EKG). It is done at rest, or while exercising. We did both with another of Dr. Babcock's patients, Ollie T., 53 years old, and a carpenter. For the last several months he had noticed pressure in his chest when working outdoors. It was getting harder to climb steps in the tall buildings in which he worked. He now had to stop at every landing for a minute or two to let the ache in his chest ease. Two months ago it was every other flight.

His blood pressure had been high for several years. Now it was 160/98. The blood vessels in his eyes showed the effects of the elevated pressure and he had a fourth heart sound (see page 176). The remainder of his examination was normal.

The electrocardiograph machine was wheeled in by the nurse. It is about the size of a portable television set, and can work on batteries or an AC outlet.

"What can that thing tell you?" Ollie asked.

"It will only record the electrical activity of the heart." I told him. "Sometimes it helps tell us if the muscle cells of the heart are normal or not. Or if the heart's electrical system is misbehaving."

Later, I would show Ollie his cardiogram and explain how the tall pointed squiggles in certain portions of the tracing suggested a thickened heart muscle, probably due to his high blood pressure.

"Is that why I get chest pains?" He wanted to know.

"No, your pains are probably due to a narrowing in one of your coronary arteries." I explained as I showed him a picture of the heart and its blood vessels.

"Can you see that on the piece of paper from that machine?"

"I wish I could. But your resting ECG does not tell us if the heart is getting a good oxygen supply."

"How do we find out?" Ollie wanted to know.

"First a stress test. A cardiogram done while you are exercising. It can tell us a lot more about your heart and its blood vessels." And I made the appointment for him.

Stress cardiogram

After fasting overnight, Ollie went to the hospital as an outpatient, changed to walking shorts and was connected to an oscilloscope and ECG machine. Electrodes were attached to each arm and leg, as well as to his chest, just as they were for a resting ECG. But now they were taped on so they wouldn't move as he walked.

In front of him stood a machine the size of a doctor's upright scale. But instead of the stand to weigh yourself there was a treadmill with a four-foot long conveyor belt on which the patient walks, then runs.

Like most active people, he was fascinated by this device.

After routine questions by the nurse about shortness of breath, chest pains, and any medications he was taking, he was given instructions on how to walk on the moving belt. Slowly at first, maintaining balance by lightly holding the stabilizing bar in front of him. Too tight a grip caused interference in the cardiogram. Now the machine was going faster. He had been cautioned to alert us at the first sign of chest pains. The treadmill could be tilted gradually to simulate a hill and add an extra work load. The elevation could be raised to a 20 percent grade and the speed increased to four miles per hour or more.

The oscilloscope displaying his heartbeat was watched by Dr. Tai who noted its rate and shape. He asked occasionally if there was any pain in the chest or shortness of breath. He was testing the level at which Ollie's heart could work without distress or change in his ECG. It would continue until his heart rate came to a pre-determined level or Dr. Tai saw a reason to stop the test.

The age of the patient determines the level at which the treadmill will be stopped. Researchers have come up with an index for maximal stress of the heart—a maximal heart rate to be achieved while exercising. The formula is an arbitrary figure—220 heartbeats per minute minus the age of the patient. If the patient can meet this work load with no symptoms or changes in the ECG it is assumed that the heart is getting adequate oxygen supply under maximum stress. And adequate oxygen supply means adequate blood flow through the coronary arteries and probably no significant coronary narrowing.

The stress test can be classified as "maximal" if the rate described above (220-age) is achieved. Some physicians prefer a "submaximal" stress test and then the rate aimed for is 80 percent or 90 percent of the maximum.

Ollie was perspiring freely as he walked faster and faster. After minutes of exercise he began to feel the first hint of the ache in the breastbone that he was so familiar with. He motioned to Dr. Tai, but the doctor had already signaled the nurse to slow the treadmill and decrease the grade. Within twenty to thirty seconds he was walking at a slow pace, with no upgrade. He felt the doctor guide him by the elbow from the still slowly moving treadmill to the waiting cot. As this was happening the nurse was busy recording the cardiogram on the ECG machine. His blood pressure was checked and almost simultaneously he was asked by Dr. Tai how his chest was feeling.

"Much better," he answered, as Dr. Tai put away the nitroglycerine tablet he had gotten ready.

"It always goes away as soon as I stop," he added. "How did you know when I was going to get the pain? You started to slow the gadget even before I signaled."

"Your cardiogram gave you away. This part here—the ST segment it's called, becomes depressed in a particular way when the heart isn't getting enough oxygen. That's why we watch carefully. We want to slow things down at the right time, whether you tell us or not."

Ollie turned to the doctor.

"Why didn't that show up on the cardiogram you did in the office yesterday?"

"Even though a coronary artery is severely narrowed the heart may still get enough oxygen while you are at rest. So the cardiogram done with you quietly lying on the table remains normal. With stress, like during the treadmill test, the heart needs more oxygen. The narrowed coronary artery cannot meet this extra demand. The heart muscle is not getting enough oxygen, your cardiogram changes and your chest hurts," Dr. Tai said.

"Now what?" Ollie asked as the tape adhesive and electrodes were removed.

"Medications—nitroglycerine and some others. A full report will be sent to Dr. Babcock, of course. Another test—coronary arteriograms will be needed but we will talk about that some more after I speak with Dr. Babcock," Dr. Tai said.

Ollie had catheterization and angiograms done two weeks later. We found a severe narrowing in one of the major coronary arteries. A large area of the heart muscle was endangered by this. Surgery was recommended and performed successfully (see chapter 18). Ollie is back at work, but limited to working on buildings less than five stories tall. He is also on medication and on a low cholesterol diet (see Appendix E).

There are two other commonly used methods of testing the heart's blood supply by exercise. The bicycle ergometer and the Master's two-step test.

The bicycle ergometer is a stationary bicycle fitted with weights or a clutch so that an increasing load can be applied. In the same manner as with the treadmill the ECG is monitored with increasing work loads until a heart rate limit or a certain work load is reached.

In the Master's two-step test, named after the late Dr. Arthur Master, the patient walks up and down a specially constructed set of steps. Two steps up, two down, turn, repeat. The number of trips to be done in three minutes is determined by age, sex and weight. There is now a double Master's and an augmented double Master's, each with a greater number of trips to be done in three minutes.

Of the three we prefer the treadmill. It is the closest thing to a natural activity, walking. The stress is easy to decrease or increase. Bicycling is trying on the thighs, which is not what we are testing.

"How accurate is the stress test?" we are often asked.

When it demonstrates classic changes in the ST segment (as in Ollie's) the chances are high that the patient has a severely narrowed coronary artery.

If thc tcst is normal and the stress is maximal the coronary arteries probably have no serious narrowings, but false negatives do occur.

Handgrip

Another simple method being evaluated as a test for detection of coronary artery disease is the grip test. A special, calibrated spring handgrip is used. The patient rolls up his sleeve and squeezes as instructed. A continuous ECG is recorded. The exercise is isometric. It puts a stress on the heart by increasing the work load through an increase in the blood pressure. Abnormalities may be detected on the cardiogram, as during the treadmill test. It takes approximately thirty to forty *seconds*, compared to twenty to forty minutes for the treadmill.

It is still very new, and standardization in comparison to known methods of stress testing is now underway. If it should prove valid it may add a valuable and simple procedure to those available for detection of coronary artery disease.

Vectorcardiogram

The heart is a three-dimensional muscular organ. The electrocardiogram records its electrical activity in only two dimensions. This presents certain limitations. An abnormality from the back surface (posterior wall) will sometimes be missed on the standard ECG.

This is one of the reasons patients admitted to a Coronary Care Unit with chest pains and myocardial infarction have sometimes been reported to have a normal ECG. Yet other tests, such as blood tests, will confirm the illness. Research has demonstrated that some of these patients suffered a heart attack at the back of the heart. The vectorcardiogram (VCG) will pinpoint the problem.

Wilkes A., a 54-year-old janitor, complained to his physician of pain in the chest. The physician could find nothing wrong and conferred with us. "As long as he complains of chest pain," I said, "we have to act as though he has heart disease, until we prove otherwise."

With the vectorcardiogram, the electrodes are placed not only on the side and front of the chest, but also on the back. Sure enough the vectorcardiogram showed a heart attack affecting the back of his heart. The regular ECG was normal because the attack was in the area that it couldn't pick up.

Wilkes underwent a heart catheterization which confirmed exactly what the vectorcardiogram had shown.

The vectorcardiogram has been available for about forty years, but is not yet standardized. As it is more complicated and more time-consuming than the ECG, it is used less frequently. The VCG is recorded photographically, often using a Polaroid system for a permanent record. It detects other conditions as well, such as enlargement of heart muscle or abnormal conduction of the heart's electrical impulse.

Donald J. was the owner of a big hardware store and an athlete who was participating with enthusiasm in the Y.M.C.A.'s aerobic program. He checked in for his annual executive physical examination routine, arranged by the medical director whom he had hired to check on the health of his sales staff.

During the routine electrocardiogram exercise, Donald's ECG suddenly showed a very rapid heartbeat. He refused to be flustered by this incident, but the medical director was upset. He called Dr. Krauthamer to evaluate his boss.

The vectorcardiogram showed his problem:

Wolff-Parkinson-White Syndrome (see page 100, chapter 9).

This is abnormal electrical conduction in the heart, which may or may not be detected on the ECG. Patients afflicted with this condition usually have episodes of tachycardia which may be a problem. The physician, who is unaware of this condition or doesn't detect it, is apt to be overly concerned and may create a good deal of anxiety for the patient and his family.

The vectorcardiogram is also more sensitive than the ECG in diagnosing thickening of heart muscle (hypertrophy). Patients with mitral stenosis may show hypertrophy of some heart chambers. Often we can detect this earlier on the VCG than with the ECG. Bill S.'s VCG showed findings compatible with mild mitral stenosis, and the echocardiogram confirmed it.

The echocardiogram

It is another new non-invasive technique.

Its principle is the same as sonar. The position of objects with different densities can be accurately determined by analysis of the echo—that is, the sound waves bounced off of them.

The echocardiogram is small and portable, again about the size of a small television set, with an oscilloscope.

A small cylinder is pressed against the chest over the heart. It is completely painless. When the cylinder is energized it sends sound waves which then bounce back from the heart. These are detected by the same cylinder and fed into the oscilloscope. Patterns from inside the heart can be identified and recorded.

The signals from inside the heart will inform the doctor about the heart valves, the chambers, the heart muscle, and the *pericardium* (the covering of the heart). If there happens to be fluid in the pericardial sac, it will be apparent. The lungs also send their echo.

Jake K., a 45-year-old auto mechanic was admitted to the hospital with a very rapid heart rate. It was very difficult to control. Multiple medications were tried and finally electric shock plus intravenous medicine stabilized it. His heart was very enlarged. He was limited in his activity: see New York Heart Association Class IV, Appendix A.

Could Jake have a "silent" valve problem? His heart was so enlarged the murmur might not be audible. If so, an operation, though dangerous, would be his only chance. But he was literally too sick and couldn't tolerate a catheterization.

An echocardiogram demonstrated normal movement of his valves. It showed that his heart was enlarged and the heart muscle was very weakened. Unfortunately we couldn't pull him through. After his death an autopsy confirmed the findings of the echocardiogram. No valve problems. Disease of the heart muscle—cardiomyopathy (see chapter 9).

With newer recording techniques, echocardiography is rapidly emerging as one of the most valuable tests of the future. With it we can actually "look" into the heart of a patient painlessly and accurately. In years to come we predict it will be an essential tool in the evaluation of a cardiac patient.

Dr. Tai's report on Bill S.

It was the echocardiogram that confirmed the degree of Bill's mitral stenosis. We put him on a regime to cut down his weight, antibiotics as needed to keep him free of infection that might injure his valve more. Presently, he is doing well. Eventually, he may need valve surgery, but the prognosis is good.

The phonocardiogram

Heart sounds, within and beyond the range of the human ear, are picked up in all their distinctive variations, normal and abnormal, and then amplified and recorded.

The phonocardiogram is about the size of a console television set. A stethoscope with microphone is placed on the patient's chest. It is connected to an oscilloscope, on which the sound signals are displayed. The physician gets a permanent recording on paper. It can be saved and compared to subsequent phonocardiograms, thereby objectively evaluating any change in heart sounds with time.

The combination of the contracting heart muscle and closing of the mitral and tricuspid valves produces what we call the *first* heart sound, the "lub."

The closure of the aortic and pulmonic valves creates the *second* heart sound, the "dup."

All normal hearts produce these two sounds—lub-dup.

Certain valve or circulatory abnormalities may cause additional heart sounds.

If a ventricle is weak or overloaded, it cannot normally dilate to accommodate the inflow of blood. This causes a *third* heart tone, which follows the second one. A third heart sound may be heard in normal young people, but in a person past the age of 40 it is abnormal.

A *fourth* heart sound is also normal in young people, but usually abnormal past middle age.

The third and fourth heart sounds are often referred to as "gallops" because their syncopation mimics the sound of hoof beats from a galloping horse. The third heart tone is called the "ventricular gallop" because it is usually due to a ventricular weakness. The fourth heart tone is called the "atrial gallop" because it occurs in association with atrial contraction.

We use mnemonics to help us remember these extra

heart tones and to help detect them as we are listening to the heart. A combination of the first three heart sounds is called the "Kentucky" gallop because their rhythm corresponds to the timing of the syllables: the first sound corresponds to "Ken-", the second to "-tuck-" and the third to the "-y" syllables.

The "Tennessee" gallop represents the fourth heart sound. "Ten-" corresponds to the fourth heart sound, "-nes-" to the first heart sound, and "-see" to the second heart sound.

When both the third and fourth heart sounds are present in the same patient, we could call them the "Tennetucky" gallop.

• *Murmurs:* When the valves are elastic and pliable with a normal opening, the blood will flow smoothly and the sounds will be normal. If valves are narrowed or close improperly, turbulent blood flow results, causing noises which are called heart "murmurs."

Murmurs, extra heart and valve sounds can usually be heard with the stethoscope. These sounds and murmurs are often distinctive enough to indicate a specific heart condition of one type or another.

With his ear, the physician can detect whether the patient's heart sounds are normal or abnormal, and if they are abnormal to what degree. Then, he can objectively evaluate his findings by this special machine that records sound in graphic form.

On a graph, heart sounds can be precisely plotted. Heart function can be determined with a degree of accuracy that the human ear cannot begin to approach.

• *Pulse tracings:* External pulse tracings are graphic recordings of pulse waves from blood vessels and the heart. They can be obtained via the phonocardiogram by placing transducers against walls of blood vessels or against the chest wall so the heartbeat can be converted into graphic tracings.

Pulse recordings tell something about how the heart pumps blood. This gives the doctor the chance to pick up abnormal changes at an early stage.

In patients with valvular disease, the phonocardiogram is used before catheterization. It is also highly useful in patients with artificial heart valves to discover whether they are working normally or are in trouble. Also, the physician can evaluate changes in heart function over long periods for patients acutely or chronically ill. Bill's phonocardiogram suggested mild to moderate mitral stenosis.

Dynamic electrocardiogram

Occasionally, irregularities of heart rate and rhythm cannot be detected by resting or stress electrocardiograms because they occur at odd times outside the physician's office. This is frustrating to the physician and to the patient. But the answer is simple: a continual recording of the electrical activities of the heart wherever the patient goes.

In the space program, this is done with *telemetry:* the astronauts are monitored from a long distance. We cannot arrange this long-distance monitoring for our patients, but we can approximate it. A miniature monitoring system, with leads taped to the patient's body, records the electrical signals of the heart on a portable tape reel or tape cassette, weighing about three pounds. The patient wears normal dress and can perform normal activities and is monitored while eating, working, or driving, but not swimming. It can be left on the night table when he sleeps or during sexual intercourse.

The instrument records all the changes in the heart rate and rhythm for a specific period of time: usually 24 hours. The patient supplements this record by his own diary, which recounts any dizzy spells, anginal or other pains or complaints.

The tape is scanned in the doctor's office by a machine the size of a portable television. A technician can scan a 24-hour tape in twenty-four minutes, and pick up critical information. He can refer to the patient's diary and the time of day when symptoms occurred, making a note on the strip tracing as it is written out.

If the technician, playing back the tape, sees an irregularity, he then changes the rate of scanning to the normal speed. He transfers the message of the heart from the tape into an electrocardiogram strip tracing. He then refers to the patient's diary, notes the time the irregularity occurred and the complaint. This gives the physician the information he needs to interpret the ECG tracing and the changes in the heartbeat at the moment they occurred.

Bill's dynamic ECG showed only an occasional extra heartbeat corresponding to his symptoms. It was not serious enough to need treatment but we told him to stay away from caffeine and alcohol.

DR. TAI:

"There's nothing wrong with Fredericka," her friends used to say. "She's a neurotic menopausal female."

Freddie K. was in good health and usually in fine spirits. She was a perfect partner for her husband who was in insurance and making an effort to widen his circle of friends. One Saturday night, they were driving into the City with friends, with Freddie at the wheel, because Charles had bursitis. Suddenly Freddie fainted, and the car veered into the guardrail.

The State Trooper thought she was drunk in spite of her protests that she hadn't touched liquor.

"I just fainted," she cried, "can't you understand that?"

On the way home, tearful and exhausted, she admitted to Charles that she had fainted before.

Charles naturally was apprehensive, knowing that Freddie was seeing her gynecologist for menopausal symptoms but he didn't associate fainting spells with change of life. He insisted that she check with their family physician. The doctor found nothing wrong with her but suggested that it would be wise for her not to drive the car until the problem was cleared up. Because Freddie was insistent on tracking down the cause of her fainting, he sent her to a neurologist, who did an encephalogram, which was read as borderline abnormal. She was put on diphenylhydantoin, which is used primarily for epilepsy, and cautioned not to drive again.

The verdict upset Freddie. She was active in the community and her work at the Children's Center involved a good deal of driving. She insisted on seeing another doctor, and her physician referred her to us.

I put her on dynamic electrocardiography. When her tape was played back, it showed clearly that Freddie was having episodes of heart stoppage, but only for a few seconds.

She received a pacemaker (see chapter 17) to regulate her heart's beat, and returned to her civic work with fresh enthusiasm. She now drives again, goes about her routine, entertains and accompanies her husband everywhere.

Dynamic electrocardiography is used:

1. For patients with abnormal heart rhythm, palpitations, skipped beats, irregular rhythms, or fluttering which are missed by the routine ECG in the doctor's office because they occur intermittently.

2. For the patient who is getting treatment for arrhythmia. It is used to test the effectiveness of medical or surgical treatment.

3. To test pacemaker malfunction.

4. To check on patients who complain of being dizzy without explanation of cause. The chance of such dizzy spells being related to the heart can be clarified.

5. For patients with angina or chest pains, who have normal ECGs during a visit to the doctor's office. They experience their chest pains, under stress, in traffic, in rushing for a train, but not at rest.

6. In patients who have myocardial infarctions and who have abnormal heart rhythms. For these people, the incidence of sudden death is higher than in those with normal rhythms. Their threatening incidents might not be detected instantaneously on the intermediate or general nursing floors of a hospital or in the physician's office. At the end of hospitalization, the patient can be monitored at home or even in returning to work.

7. To monitor the heart rate and rhythm while exercising, on a bicycle or tennis court. The tape recorder for exercise monitoring is smaller and can be strapped to the back during a game of tennis.

DR. KRAUTHAMER:

Blood tests for the damaged heart

At times, the physician feels like a crime detective, particularly when he is trying to determine how much damage a heart has suffered. Certain blood tests are vital in his search.

The heart muscle cell contains sodium and potassium, as well as enzyme systems. The enzymes work as catalysts. They initiate, activate, accelerate and maintain a cycle of energy. Oxygen is used to convert food (proteins, carbohydrates, metabolites) into energy that the heart cell can use.

The heart muscle can be injured either by lack of oxygen supply due to narrowing of the blood vessels (heart attack) or any kind of trauma, such as auto accident or knifing. The injured cell leaks enzymes into the blood stream where they can be measured with such sensitive and sophisticated techniques that even a minimal change can be detected.

Normal blood enzyme values are known. If the patient suffers damage to the heart muscle cell, the level of these enzymes rises above normal. Even with a normal ECG, a rise in enzymes tips off the physician to possible trouble.

In the laboratory, the blood sample of the patient is spun in a centrifuge, the red blood cells are separated, and the plasma retained to measure all these enzymes.

It takes 24 hours to get the results.

Creatinine phospho-kinase (CPK) is the most sensitive enzyme. It leaks if there is injury to any muscle, including the heart. Its peak blood level is reached within six to eight hours after the initial insult to the heart. Then the mechanisms of the body bring the level back to normal —unless there is continuing damage to the heart.

The only problem is time. If the patient doesn't come to the hospital until 24 hours after the attack, the CPK level may return to normal by that time. So the physician turns to the next enzyme.

Serum glutamic oxalo-transaminase (SGOT) starts to elevate within 18 to 24 hours, reaches its peak in 48 hours and begins its decline to normal in 72 to 96 hours. If the patient reaches a physician 24 to 48 hours after a heart attack, the physician can still determine the degree of injury to the heart by the SGOT estimation.

Even a week later, another enzyme can carry the news. It is lactic dehydrogenase (LDH), which starts to rise a few days after a heart attack and continues to rise, taking a much longer time to return to normal, sometimes up to two or three weeks.

The physician has different kinds of enzyme tests available to him in his search for damage to the heart. The tests are sensitive, well standardized, and can be done in any general hospital laboratory.

If a heart attack is older than three weeks, it is difficult to judge the damage from the enzymes. The physician's clinical judgment and the ECG are helpful. If the ECG is normal, stress testing is a sensitive indicator of coronary heart disease.

Thermography

The skin emits infrared energy. Mapping of this energy is called thermography. It is safe and non-invasive. It can be repeated as often as necessary. The emission of radiant energy is dependent on various factors—the most important is blood supply. Thermography can tell the difference between cooler areas (with fewer blood vessels) and warmer areas (more vessels). It has been helpful in evaluation of peripheral vascular disorders such as thrombophlebitis and poor arterial flow to the legs or arms. Thermography has also been useful in evaluating cancer of the breast and certain cardiac diseases.

We have described the most frequently used non-invasive tests you may encounter as a patient today. From them we get more information than was possible ten years ago, but less than we will get ten years from now.

Chapter 15

The heart in motion photography: catheterization and angiography

1. Arteriography is the general term for outlining arteries on X-ray film, after dye has been injected into them.

2. Venography is the same but applied to the veins only.

3. Angiography is the same but applied to any blood vessel in the body—artery, vein or lymphatic vessel.

4. Coronary arteriography is a specific term referring to X-rays of the coronary arteries.

5. Cardiac catheterization is the process of passing a catheter, a narrow flexible tube, through blood vessels into the heart. Often it is combined with angiography.

DR. FRANKLIN:
We are in the Special Procedures Room in the hospital. I am about to pass a catheter into this man's heart. When I inject dye, I can see just where his coronary arteries are blocked. What I see here by means of the fluoroscope and camera will give us a roadmap to his future. It will help determine medication or surgery and the patient's future activitics.

Mario G.

Mario is 48 years old, a heavy-set muscular man with thick gray-streaked hair, dark eyes; he is a good husband, a wise father, a man of honor and dignity. He is a landscape gardener with acres of valuable seedlings and fine greenhouses. And he has had two heart attacks.

Yesterday, he checked into the hospital at the suggestion of the cardiologists to whom his family doctor had sent him after the chest pains started again.

Before he was taken to his room, a nurse's aide wheeled him to X-ray for pictures of his chest, then to the laboratory, where they drew blood for tests. Then he was put to bed, and after a while Dr. Franklin came in, sat down beside his bed, and told him what to expect in the test. It didn't sound too bad. This morning, when a nurse's aide took him to the Special Procedures Room, he was nervous but not scared. The nurse had given him a tranquilizer to take the edge off.

There was a good deal of strange equipment in the room. In the center was a table, about the length of a good-sized man. Resting on the table was a contraption that the technicians referred to as a "cradle" and which looked like one.

A nurse wheeled Mario to the table, asked him to step on a small footstool and lean back against the table. The long curved cradle pressed against the small of his back. The nurse touched a button and Mario heard a motor start. The cradle was rotating slightly away from him.

"Now lift yourself up," the nurse said. The motor began again, the cradle moved toward him, and he felt himself supported by the cradle itself as he was eased into a horizontal position in its close fitting framework. He felt them strap him into the cradle.

Someone joined the nurse, and they were speaking to each other. He was the resident who would assist in the test. They attached cardiogram leads to his arms and legs. Mario was an old hand at electrocardiograms; he had had a hundred, it seemed, by now.

The resident placed Mario's right arm on the board which was attached at a right angle to the cradle. It had to be in a rigid position so the cardiologist could work on it. The nurse now shaved a small area on the front of his elbow. Last night, Dr. Franklin explained that his test would be done through the arm, but other times, it may be done through a blood vessel in the groin.

Five minutes later, Dr. Franklin appeared wearing his baggy hospital whites. He pinned on a small badge with his name on it. Mario found out later that it was an X-ray badge that registered the amount of radiation the doctor was exposed to, since he did this test on patients nearly every day. The nurse and technicians also wore them.

The doctor scrubbed his hands and arms and then put on a pair of snug rubber gloves. He approached the small table near Mario, where a number of instruments were laid out. Mario murmured a small prayer.

DR. FRANKLIN:

"Mario, you will be feeling something wet on your arm now. It's an antiseptic solution. It may burn a little, but that's all.

"I will be putting some towels over your arm and on your chest. You can use your left hand, if you need to rub your eyes or scratch your nose. But try to keep your hand away from the area where I'm working.

"You'll feel a needle prick, Mario and then you'll feel a little burning sensation as I put in the anesthetic. For maybe two or three minutes."

It is our practice to tell our patients what they can expect during a cardiac catheterization. We explain the major features of the examination, so they will not be frightened by an unusual sensation they experience during the procedure. We feel this is very important. A frightened patient is nervous and tense, puts out excess adrenalin, which can increase the possibility of problems such as blood vessel spasm, or arrhythmia during the procedure.

We do not use general anesthesia for several reasons. The patient is asked to take a deep breath before each injection of dye. This is to help position the catheter and to lower the diaphragm to allow us to get a photograph of the heart without an overlap of the diaphragm and liver. Then he is asked to cough, which accelerates his heartbeat. We would refuse to do this procedure on an unconscious adult because of the increased risk and difficulty involved. The cardiologist must feel confident, and his confidence will communicate itself to the patient.

"Mario, you may feel an electric shock down your arm in the next few minutes. It's almost like the way you feel when you hit your funny bone on a door. There's a nerve that runs near the blood vessel we're using. If I should happen to touch the nerve while I'm separating it from other vessels, it may cause a shock."

Five minutes later, I said, "Well we have the blood vessel ready for the catheter now and it should be a lot more comfortable for you."

The nurse wiped Mario's face with a damp towel and he smiled his gratitude.

"Now, you may feel a tiny bump in your shoulder or neck as the catheter passes around on its way into your chest. It shouldn't be uncomfortable. If anything bothers you, please tell me."

"Okay, doctor."

"Take a deep breath, Mario. Hold it!" I repeated, and then, "Cough, Mario—a deep cough."

He obeyed. Now I told him the table was going to turn. "It will seem like you are going to fall, but the straps will hold you in place. We need to put you in different positions, so we can take pictures of the heart at different angles."

A moment later, Mario was asked to take a deep breath and hold it. The camera made a whirring sound and again he was asked to cough. This was repeated several times. Then I asked the lights to be turned on.

"Please bring the injector, nurse," I said. And to my patient, "Mario, I've been injecting dye by hand to look at the blood vessels. Now, I'm going to inject it with a special machine to outline the main pumping chamber of your heart. When it's injected, you'll feel a pounding sensation in your chest, palpitations, and then a real warm flash through your whole body. Sort of like 'instant Scotch.' It won't hurt. But if I didn't warn you, it might upset you because it happens so fast."

I gave instructions to the nurse about attaching the machine to the catheter now passing through Mario's heart. Then the lights were dimmed once again.

"Once more, Mario. Take a deep breath. Hold it!"

I turned to the nurse.

"Fire!" I commanded.

When I am doing a catheterization, I feel like a man wearing many hats. I am a juggler, for as I stand at Mario's side, I am manipulating an injection system plus a set of foot pedals. I am a photographer, since I must be aware of the fluoroscope, the camera and the television set, which are helping me diagnose what is wrong with Mario's heart.

I use the individual foot pedals while I scan the television set. One pedal runs the fluoroscope which enables me to watch the dye pass through the vessels. The other triggers the camera when I want a permanent picture of the heart and blood vessels. These pictures will be used later in diagnosis and in surgery, if it is required. I cannot explain the sense of coordination, except to suggest that it comes with experience. You must have a good rapport with your patient, be skilled in catheter manipulation, and be a knowledgeable photographer.

Other equipment in the catheterization laboratory includes a bio-medical monitor with an oscilloscope and nearly as many dials and knobs as a jet plane.

Once we start the procedure, the bio-medical monitor will continuously display the electrocardiogram, and the blood pressure within the circulation, from the tip of the catheter placed in the heart or blood vessels. This is more accurate than any blood pressure reading taken by the customary blood pressure cuff.

At one side of the room is the defibrillator, that emergency restorer of the heart's beat.

If by some remote chance, a catastrophe should occur during a catheterization, the patient is in the most favorable spot for instant treatment. All vital equipment for cardiovascular problems is available here for his care.

Most cardiac arrhythmias can be converted back to a normal state in less than 30 seconds. This is due to the coordination of the staff which has worked for several years as a team.

The technique of cardiac catheterization

Some cardiologists set up the catheterization laboratory as an operating room, with full sterile techniques. Our group is less formal. We use antiseptic wash and gloves and leaded apron, but no cap, gown or mask. We substitute speed of performance, combined with sterile technique, for the prolonged procedure in a complete operating room atmosphere.

The syringe that we use for injection is a 10 cc. syringe. It holds about 2½ teaspoons of the dye to be sent to the heart.

The syringe is placed in a special barrel holder with rings

for the cardiologist's index and middle fingers. There is a third ring for the thumb. It is in turn attached to three stopcocks in a row. These are attached to the pressure transducer (see below) and the solution used in the procedure.

Before we inject any dye the catheter is placed in the heart to record the pressure there.

Pressure is a physical phenomenon and travels like sound waves in water. If you put your head under water

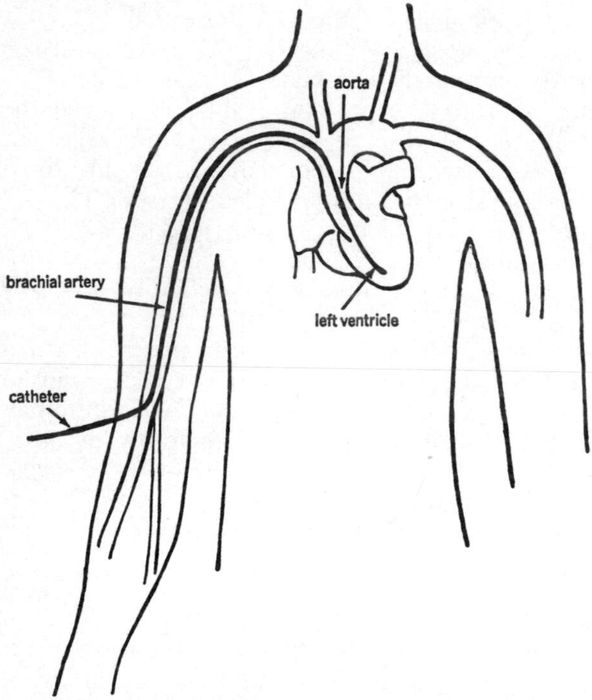

Cardiac catheter

The catheter, inserted into the brachial artery through an incision made in the crook of the elbow, is passed through the aorta into the left ventricle. A fluoroscope allows the cardiologist to see the catheter as he manipulates it. Dye is injected so the heart and its blood vessels can be photographed. The right side of the heart can similarly be studied by passing a catheter through a vein rather than an artery.

and knock two rocks together, you'll hear the resulting click a long way off. The sound passes through the water as a wave phenomenon. So the pressure in Mario's heart is passing through the fluid in the catheter as a wave phenomenon. The wave is sensed by a special measuring device, called a transducer, and is then transmitted to the oscilloscope screen of the bio-medical monitor. It can be recorded on photographic paper merely by the push of a button by the nurse.

Working with the catheter, I frequently inject small amounts of dye as an aid to position the catheter in various places. I keep asking Mario to hold his breath so that as I record film, his diaphragm will stay clear of his heart. If the patient doesn't breathe properly you may get photographs of the diaphragm and liver superimposed on the heart. It's like trying to see in a fog.

After the catheter is positioned where I want it in the heart, I insert the dye by squeezing the syringe. The dye is thick, so it is important to squeeze the syringe hard as the fluid is being injected. The dye is a special organic iodine solution. Iodine blocks the passage of X-rays and therefore outlines any structure into which it is injected.

We also use a dextrose and water solution for flushing out the catheter system and keeping it clean.

During the catheterization, we alert the patient to the fact that he will feel a warm sensation as a small amount of dye is injected.

With a larger injection, a true hot flash may be sensed. The sensation usually doesn't last more than 30 to 60 seconds. Sometimes a patient may have a headache or feel nauseated, but this is rare.

What happens is this: As the dye is injected, it has a tendency to open the blood vessels in the skin. Warmer blood from inner parts of the body rise to the surface so the patient feels the heat. The blood vessels shortly attain their normal pattern again and the heat fades. The patient is really experiencing his own "inner warmth." This is actually the same reason for a "glow" after a nip of brandy.

When the test is underway, a cylinder suspended from the ceiling is positioned over the patient's chest. It is the modern fluoroscope, with a TV camera attached to it. The image of the heart is brightened, and projected on a TV screen through a closed circuit, so that the cardiologist can watch what his catheter and dye are doing in the heart. By using television tape, information can be reviewed by "instant replay."

Patients fear death or serious complications from coronary arteriography. For every thousand cases, we have had less than one death, and less than three serious complications.

A patient with arteriosclerosis sometimes worries that a bit of plaque on the wall of the blood vessel might break off and lodge in his system as the catheter passes through. This is a possibility but it rarely occurs. We usually use arteries that are open. We can tell the artery's condition by the pulse in the neck and wrist and by listening with the stethoscope. Coronary arteries can be blocked. But we don't need the catheter to define the blockage. We need the dye. The catheter takes the dye to the precise spot that we need to photograph.

We ask the patient to cough because that helps restore circulation after the dye has passed through the heart. Sometimes the heart rate does slow down during a dye injection and then a cough will speed it up effectively.

The dye in the body often leads to an urgent need to urinate. We prime our patients to expect it. The table is so set up and protected that if he has to let go, he should, and without any sense of embarrassment.

The procedure on Mario is completed. We have taken enough pictures and measurements. After I slide out the catheter, I sew a small thread around the opening in the blood vessel and pull it tight like a purse string. This keeps the artery from bleeding. Then the skin incision is closed.

"How are you feeling, Mario?" I ask.

"I've had it worse at the dentist's," he says.

A simple catheterization usually doesn't take more than an hour, sometimes less, but a more complicated procedure may take from one to four hours. Often it depends on how easy we find it to advance the catheter tip into those parts of the heart that are being examined.

A nurse helps Mario out of the cradle. He walks back and forth to restore his balance.

"In about 30 minutes, start exercising your arm," I tell him. We have found exercise extremely helpful in mobilizing the arm and decreasing discomfort.

Most patients feel some discomfort at the incision for twelve to twenty-four hours. They may have painkillers if they want them. In the next week, the arm may become a bit stiff after a period of inactivity but a few quick pumps at the elbow will bring it back to normal.

Occasionaly a small non-tender lump may appear under the incision. This is due to some drops of blood trapped in the incision site. In a week or so the blood cells break down into small particles and the lump gets larger. Later, it slowly disappears.

I stitch up the blood vessel used for catheterization in an attempt to maintain a smooth flow. Sometimes the vessel will block up, but this is unusual. If the blood vessel happens to be a vein, and is lost, it has no effect on the circulation or the heart.

If it is an artery, there may be a temporary decrease in blood flow to the arm and hand. But there are plenty of collateral vessels to make up the difference. We need only to allow time for these collaterals to enlarge and accommodate the flow. How long will this take? Anywhere from a few minutes to two years. The takeover by the collaterals can be helped by physical exercise under the doctor's instructions. Cigarette smoking seems to delay this type of collateral formation.

I promised Mario that within twenty-four hours after the catheterization I would see him and call his physician with a report of the findings, and an explanation of what this will mean to his future.

Dr. Franklin's report

One of Mario's three coronary arteries is completely blocked (occluded). The portion of heart muscle that is fed by the occluded artery is severely damaged—the result of his heart attacks.

The remaining two coronary arteries are severely narrowed. But Mario cannot afford to lose the heart muscle that depends on those two remaining arteries.

Each coronary artery feeds a specific part of the heart. The right coronary artery supplies the back wall. The left coronary artery starts out as one vessel—the main trunk—but then it branches into two: the left anterior descending which supplies blood to the front of the heart, and the circumflex, which supplies the side.

It is Mario's right coronary artery that is completely closed.

Mario is getting next to no flow through the circumflex branch of the left coronary artery. The left anterior descending is only slightly better. He is in danger of losing more heart muscle and he cannot afford it. Additional heart damage could lead to further weakening of the heart, heart failure, invalidism, and death.

If the blood flow to the remaining normally contracting heart muscle can be restored, Mario's symptoms can be relieved and he will be able to return with safety to a more normal life.

His former heart attacks make him a slightly higher risk for heart surgery than a man who has had no heart attack. However, the overall function of the heart muscle is still reasonably well preserved, and we feel that he has a 90 to 95 percent chance of surviving the operation, plus an 80 to 90 percent chance of benefitting from an operation. Therefore, we would place his overall "surgical risk" at 70 to 80 percent for success—surviving surgery and obtaining the desired results.

This compares quite favorably with our estimated poor outlook for him if one of his two remaining coronary arteries blocks and causes more heart damage. We feel his risk of not surviving a third heart attack is in the vicinity of 30 to 50 percent, and even with survival, Mario would remain uncomfortable and significantly incapacitated.

In our judgment, more favorable results could be expected from surgical rather than medical treatment. Obviously we felt Mario should have heart surgery performed to improve the blood flow to his heart muscle.

We spoke with Mario and his family doctor and they agreed he would go for surgery. Meanwhile, we were trying to get him on an operating schedule at a good hospital. We felt it should be done quickly and without undue delay. We could not predict that he would drop dead working in his greenhouse the following week, but there was a chance that it could happen. If the remaining blood vessels closed, Mario would not survive.

Our recommendation was that he have two saphenous bypasses. The right coronary was irrigating total scar tissue and there was no reason to bypass it. We hoped to see an anterior descending and a circumflex bypass, saphenous veins connecting both branches of the left coronary artery to the aorta (see chapter 18, "Surgery").

We were in luck. A good surgeon at a nearby university hospital made an opening for Mario. We got word that he came through the operation successfully.

After his discharge from the hospital, we will be following him in our office during his convalescence and will set up a repeat catheterization and angiogram one year after surgery to check the results of his operation.

We combine cardiac catheterization and cardioangiography (the process of filming the heart structure by X-rays) to get precise information about the anatomy and function of the heart. When the diagnosis and treatment of a predictable heart condition can be determined as accurately without it, cardiac catheterization and angiography should not be used. Many valvular and congenital heart disorders are quite predictable and cardiac catheterization and angiography may not be needed at all. Or they may be reserved for critical decisions, such as in helping to decide whether or when heart surgery is needed.

But the illness that is called coronary heart disease seems unpredictable. One patient with severe angina may live for many years while another patient with minimal or no symptoms may have a heart attack or die suddenly, almost without warning.

We feel coronary arteriography makes coronary heart disease much more predictable. We believe that classifying a patient according to what blood vessels are narrowed, how much good heart muscle is left, plus mapping the collaterals, allows us to recognize future risks. It puts us in a better position to prescribe for him, even if he doesn't need a heart operation. It helps us find the patient who is in danger of severe heart damage *before* it happens, and hopefully protect him. *We recommend coronary arteriography for all our patients with angina or heart attack, un-*

less there is a good reason not to. Some life threatening or incapacitating condition other than the heart, or a patient who has had too much heart damage for us to help him.

There are doctors who don't feel coronary arteriography is as helpful or as safe as we do. But we are convinced this approach has been a great help in the care of patients referred to us. We cannot speak for anyone but ourselves and recommend each patient consult a cardiologist of his choice concerning these procedures.

DR. FRANKLIN:
This case might be called "Don't upset poor Laura."

In 1964, I was called into consultation with a family physician for a patient, Laura S., who was then about 63 years old. Laura had a chronic stomach ailment for which surgery was being considered. However, she had been diagnosed as having a severe heart condition, so the surgeon requested a complete cardiologic evaluation before he operated.

Laura had first been admitted to a major university center in the 1940s for chest pains. A diagnosis of coronary insufficiency was made then. Over the next twenty years, she was hospitalized several times annually for recurrence of "angina." A number of consultants in the Northeast had confirmed her indisposition as severe heart disease.

I had just left Cleveland Clinic after training with Dr. Mason Sones in coronary angiography. I was still young and wet behind the ears as far as the local physicians were concerned. And true to character, I questioned the diagnosis in Laura's case.

Laura had been hospitalized many times at a fantastic expense. She had no sex for the last fifteen years of her husband's life. After his death she had often called her physician frantically at night for help. At times the ambulance corps helped by the police would have to break down her door to get to her and carry her to the hospital. She usually had a three-week convalescence. Yet she never had the classic electrocardiographic changes of an infarction. Nor did her blood tests ever confirm a myocardial infarction. Furthermore, her heart was normal in size. A patient with severe coronary heart disease doesn't go on for twenty years without having a heart attack.

It was quite a bizarre case and I began to wonder if Laura wasn't the family cardiac black sheep. Everyone was taking such good care of her that her secondary gains were superb.

I was discreet about suggesting she didn't have coronary heart disease at all. I kept quiet for fear I'd get tossed out of the window from her fifth floor room.

Fortunately, the surgeon wanted angiograms to make certain she could tolerate surgery. I did the studies on her. Laura's coronary arteries were perfectly clean. No coronary disease. No ventricular disease. No heart disease.

But now the trouble started. Laura *knew* she had heart disease. In spite of the fact that the tests proved otherwise. I urged her other doctors to be honest with her, presenting a solid front and telling her that she had never had heart disease.

One doctor insisted she be told that at some previous time she'd had a heart condition but it had cleared up.

"He couldn't fool me," Laura said triumphantly. "I've read enough heart books to know that it doesn't go away."

Laura closed her ears to the good news. A sick heart was her crutch for living and nobody was going to deprive her of it.

Even today, years later, her family doctor is awakened in the middle of the night by Laura, having another "attack." But no ambulance corps arrives. No police break down the door. She hasn't been sent to the hospital since her evaluation.

"Take two aspirin and call me in the morning," her doctor says patiently.

She was irate at the change in her lifestyle. No more coddling, pampering, indulging her. No more "Don't upset Laura. Remember her heart."

Her previous doctors made their conclusions on what was firm clinical ground at that time. A consultant is apt to fall into a trap when several doctors before him diagnose the patient as having coronary heart disease. It's easy to slide right along and agree. But when you have an angiogram, it protects the patient from misdiagnosis.

Laura is an extreme example of a very interesting medical fact. Nearly 30 percent of patients diagnosed as having coronary heart disease in a clinical evaluation do not have it when examined by coronary arteriography. Indeed, most of these patients, like Laura, have no heart disease at all.

Some years ago, when we sent out questionnaires for patient follow-up, Laura's came back with an irate note. She wrote that she had never been so miserable as she was since that damned test. Dr. Franklin had ruined her existence.

I guess I destroyed her secondary gain—her use of illness to gain attention—but at least her family physician is getting more rest now. And so are her family, the police department, and the ambulance corps.

Chapter 16

The delicate balance of medications

DR. TAI:
In the private school where she taught French for 20 years, she was known as Madame LaFarge. Her pupils didn't exactly march to the guillotine while she knitted, but those who took her class directly after lunch complained of a "French stomach." She was a perfectionist with an explosive Gallic temper.

I saw her for the first time when she came to our office with complaints that suggested the classic angina syndrome. She had never had a heart attack. We watched her for the next two years. Then it became obvious to us and to her that her physical strength was deteriorating because of her anginal pains. Because of her age (she was 77) and her generally poor physical condition, we agreed no coronary arteriography should be attempted. It would have been of academic interest only, since there was no problem making a clinical diagnosis.

The ECG was abnormal, suggesting coronary insufficiency. She had no murmurs or other disease to cause angina or a lack of blood supply or a lack of oxygen to the heart. She was not a candidate for heart surgery.

The treatment for Madame was a program of medication to dilate her coronary blood vessels plus control of a mild degree of high blood pressure with an anti-hypertensive drug, and a weak diuretic pill to prevent mild accumulation of fluid (edema).

The results were gratifying. Madame had retired from school and her life was now completely her own. She could walk at a slow pace and without much difficulty to the nearby shopping center and the library. She took great pride in polishing the small fine pieces of furniture in her apartment.

We all got great satisfaction out of treating Madame; she was so utterly different than most of our elderly women patients. About six months ago, I admitted her to the local hospital for a short period. She had suffered a small myocardial infarction from which she recovered quite well. Because of her increasing incapacity, we administered propranolol, which helped her heart tolerate the decreased blood flow through her narrowed coronary arteries. The side effect, however, was a slowing down of the heartbeat.

When her heart slowed to 50 beats per minute, she was free of angina. But she complained of being a bit lightheaded if she overdid.

"Doctor, I am about to surrender my driver's license," she confessed. "I fear that I might faint at the wheel of my car and perhaps inflict damage on another."

She has not deteriorated. She is, according to the New York Heart Association Classification, in Functional Class III (see Appendix A). She gets angina with less than ordinary activity but not with minimal activity or rest. Two months ago, she developed a condition that required minor surgery. We consulted with her gynecologist and with the anesthesiologist. The operation proceeded without complications. She checked out of the hospital two days later and has done well since.

She has been able to take both her practical common sense and her intellectual capabilities and fuse them into a form of life which she can enjoy. She reads, she does needlework, she is well aware of world events and discusses them with the slightest encouragement. Her reputation still lingers at the school.

"My pupils, they truly learned my language," she often says.

On her last visit to us, she told us proudly, "One of my old pupils—she is now a married lady with children of her own—she telephoned me and she asked would I tutor her in French. This *jeune fille* had always complained I gave her a French stomach. Now she comes to me again. Before she takes a trip to Paris."

A patient may have several conditions, as in the case of Madame. She could not have tolerated heart surgery but managed adequately on a combination of medications.

After a patient is thoroughly tested, we are able to evaluate what can be done in his individual case. Each person is different—in age, strength, and stage of disease and each requires a different course of treatment with medication, exercise (see chapter 20), and diet (see chapter 21) devised for him.

The scope of drugs to correct faulty conditions is wide and constantly increasing. Vasodilators, preparations which dilate the constricted coronary arteries, are of major importance in providing blood to the damaged heart. Often we must eliminate excess fluid (edema). We can do this with the help of diuretics. Then there are new drugs to suppress arrhythmias. To help the pumping action of the heart, there is digitalis. We have drugs to reduce the blood pressure, to slow the heart beat, to help the heart tolerate a decreased blood flow.

Choosing the correct medications requires an understanding of a patient's condition, and recognition that patients react differently to the same drug, and to different dosages. It would be impossible to write down all the factors that go into prescribing the individual program for each heart patient. We can, however, explain how some of the more widely used drugs help specific conditions (see Appendix I for generic and trade names).

Nitroglycerine and the nitrates

If there isn't enough oxygen-rich blood to fuel the heart muscle, the heart begins to ache. The patient's chest hurts. Angina. When the supply of blood is increased, the pain eases.

Nitroglycerine is the doctor's first line of defense in the battle against angina. Nitroglycerine and its companion drugs, the nitrates, are a group of related medications that work in two ways. First, they cause the coronary arteries to widen (dilate). A wider blood vessel can transport more blood to the heart muscle. A healthy artery expands and contracts easily, but after a coronary artery has narrowed with arteriosclerosis, it loses some of its ability to dilate. When the body calls for more blood, under pressure of exertion, the narrowed artery cannot deliver. It needs the added help of the nitroglycerine.

Even then, the diseased vessel may not be able to respond fully. If collateral arteries are present, nitrates can be a powerful stimulus to increase blood flow through them. Medication can thus help supply oxygen to the endangered area of heart muscle, even when a severe inelastic narrowing is blocking a coronary artery.

The second effect of the nitrates may be even more important. Nitroglycerine and all other nitrates, in varying degree, lower the blood pressure a small amount and decrease the heart's work load. This effect lasts only for a few minutes. But this is enough. Even a small drop in blood pressure means the sick heart doesn't have to pump as hard.

If a patient is having an argument with his boss, his wife, the kids or an obnoxious neighbor, his chest gets tight and begins to ache He puts a nitroglycerine tablet under his tongue. Thirty seconds later it has melted. Within two or three minutes the tightness in the chest vanishes, his moist brow dries. His blood pressure has lowered a little. His coronary arteries have widened. More blood reaches the heart muscle. Pain disappears.

"It's like a truck going up hill," one patient said. "A truck with a partly blocked gas line. It can just make it on level ground. Well, that nitroglycerine smooths out the hill (decreases the work load), opens the blocked gas line (widens the coronary arteries) and the patient reaches the crest."

Too bad that nitroglycerine works only for a short spell. Patients would find it annoving to be obliged to take a pill under the tongue every half hour. Other nitrate preparations have a longer lasting effect. Some are taken under the tongue, like nitroglycerine. Others are swallowed like any other pill. The doctor decides which medication, and how it is to be taken. Though these drugs may not prevent anginal attacks completely, they often decrease the daily number of such attacks, and increase the amount of physical activity the patient can tolerate.

There is no magical curc. But this therapy does help the

patient to live at what we doctors call "an improved functional level."

Even though a patient is taking a longer acting nitrate, nitroglycerine tablets may be needed for occasional anginal attacks. A sudden scare as a car cuts in front of you on the Thruway, an unexpected drop in temperature toward evening as you climb the small hill on the way to your house —a nitroglycerine tablet will help.

We feel strongly that people liable to angina should carry nitroglycerine tablets at all times. They should have spare bottles around. In their shirt pockets or purses. In the desk drawer. In the bathroom. On the night table. By the TV set. The tablets must always be within reach. If an anginal attack is shortened or aborted, it means the labored heart spends fewer precious minutes without an adequate oxygen supply. The earlier the tablet is taken, the quicker the relief.

Nitroglycerine can grow stale. It can lose its potency. It should be kept in a small, dark glass bottle with a screw cap. Nitroglycerine evaporates. It is absorbed by plastic, cotton and paper. We can't tell you how many patients we have seen with nitroglycerine stored in plastic, snap-top containers filled with cotton and with the paper label inside. After a week or two they might just as well chew the cotton as take the nitroglycerine. Even if properly stored, it should be replaced every three months. Ineffective medication is probably worse than no medication at all. Loss of the burning taste means loss of potency.

And it isn't enough to have a supply of nitroglycerine tablets. They must be used whenever symptoms flare up. It is often difficult to convince a patient of this. The ostrich approach again. "If I don't take a pill, it won't really be an anginal attack."

The doctor is sometimes an unwitting ally to this kind of denial. He may ask at the regular visit, "Well, John, how many nitros did you need this week?"

If the patient reports he is using less medication, it may indicate he is getting better. But we have learned to follow up with another question, "Okay, John, how many anginal attacks did you have that you did not take anything for?"

Nitroglycerine can be used to *prevent* anginal episodes. If the patient remembers to take a pill before an activity that may turn into a stress situation, he may sail through without any discomfort. But not if he is really exceeding his tolerance limits. Then it can be risky.

"What do you mean by the 'rule of five'?" a patient asks.

"Each finger of one hand represents a nitroglycerine tablet," we tell him. "The space between each finger represents a three-minute period.

"When the angina pain starts, you should look at your watch and notice the time. Then you should pop a tablet under your tongue. And wait three minutes. If the pain hasn't eased or is getting worse, you should take a second tablet. Then you wait another three minutes. And ask yourself, 'Is the discomfort easier? Has it gone away?'

"If so, you don't need any more tablets.

"However, if there's no letup in pain or you feel it is getting more painful by the time you take the fifth pill, call your doctor immediately. You may not need a visit. But you do need advice.

"Twenty minutes of continual anginal pain can lead to permanent heart damage."

Propranolol

A new medication has been used now for several years along with the nitrates. It is called propranolol. The combination of the two makes an effective medical program for many heart patients. Propranolol works by slowing the pulse rate and allowing the heart to beat more gently. If the heart beats more slowly and less vigorously, it needs less oxygen. The heart can now function better with the oxygen it is receiving.

Propranolol does this in a special way. Adrenalin is a strong heart stimulant that doctors use only in emergencies. The body always has a small amount of adrenalin and other similar chemicals in the blood stream. Just enough to keep things running smoothly but not enough to set up any problems. Propranolol makes the heart less responsive to adrenalin and its cousins. The pulse slows down. The work load decreases. The pump gets the blood around the body but uses less oxygen to do it.

The doctor must slowly build up the proper dosage of propranolol, watching his patient carefully.

While medication does help a majority of paticnts, it may not help everyone. Unfortunately, the coronary narrowing remains and may worsen. By-pass surgery may be required.

The angina sufferer may encounter other medical difficulties. These supplemental situations may not be dangerous, but they may exacerbate a heart condition, and must also be treated.

For example, a patient who is not responding well to a medical program of nitrates and propranolol might be anemic. Oxygen in the blood is carried by the chemical hemoglobin. If the patient has low hemoglobin and anemia is severe, not enough oxygen gets to the heart muscle.

DR. KRAUTHAMER:
Hal is a bookkeeper, a little overweight, physically inactive and always harried over deadlines. Tax time is always an ordeal for him. On April 13th, he was working over books that didn't balance when he experienced some chest pains.

He forgot about them. The next morning, he found a snowfall had blotted out his lawn and driveway. He had a nine o'clock appointment with his boss, so he set about clearing a path for his car. The ache returned.

Hal was apt to get anxious, so he saw his family doctor the next day, and the doctor wisely sent him to the hospital for an evaluation. His resting ECG was normal. Other tests showed no abnormality. By the time he was discharged from the hospital, April 15th had come and gone, and Hal returned to the office in a much calmer frame of mind.

When audit time came, Hal was stuck in the middle again. He awakened from a deep sleep with a feeling that death was sitting on his chest. He was sweating, faint and short of breath. This time, an ambulancc brought him to the hospital with red lights flashing and siren sounding. His family physician met him in the emergency room, where narcotics and other medications were administered. His ECG showed mild heart damage over the next few days—a subendocardial infarction (see chapter 6, "Angina"). I was called in to see him.

Three days later, he developed a fresh episode of severe chest pains. The ECG showed more damage, which this time showed up in blood tests as well.

"There was a large elephant on my chest, but now she's stepped away, leaving her offspring," he told us. It's strange how many heart patients have a similar feeling. Evidently, they cannot visualize anything more massive than a pachyderm.

"I know I'm going to die," he repeated. "I know I'm going to die."

In reviewing his case, I felt that although he wasn't on the verge of death, it certainly looked like he was heading for a massive heart attack.

"Just *do* something," he said.

We scheduled him the next morning for catheterization and soon saw on the screen of the fluoroscope the dye outlining his coronary arteries. Hal had an extreme narrowing near the origin of his left anterior descending. Certainly a Widow Maker if ever there was one.

But Hal had something else. He had a definite set of collaterals. They weren't big, but they were definitely there. We felt they would grow larger. The left ventricle showed only mild damage, and we felt these collaterals would improve with time and give Hal the protection he needed. We asked him to wait before deciding on heart surgery, to see how he would respond.

We placed him on a treatment program of nitrates and propranolol. That would slow down his pulse and lessen the oxygen demand of his heart. Nitrates would help lessen the angina.

Within five days, he was out of his hospital bed and walking the corridors with only mild symptoms of angina. Ten days later, he went home. He was still scared, but he admitted freely that the pain was lessening week by week.

Back at work, he took his medicines faithfully and was able to accept the stressful aspects of his job without precipating serious symptoms. He embarked on an exercise program. A mile to two miles walking when the weather was good and his exercise bike when the weather was inclement (see chapter 20, "Exercise and the Return to Action").

In six months, there was a remarkable change in Hal. He was working full time. He was exercising as well. We lessened his dosage of nitrates and propranolol. When the next audit came around, he was able to fight back when the boss turned the pressure on.

"I even told the boss he was wrong," Hal said, and you could sense the new pride in his voice. There was a little tiger in him now, the result of his cardiac experience. If he could lick that, he could tackle other problems with success.

A year later, I repeated his coronary arteriograms. The left anterior descending, the Widow Maker, was now totally occluded, but the area was entirely served by many new collaterals arising from his other coronary arteries, neither of which was blocked. The left ventricle had returned to normal.

During the time between the two catheterizations, Hal had had a total coronary occlusion *without* a heart attack. This had happened while his symptoms were decreasing and his exercise tolerance improving. It was possible because his collaterals were more than keeping pace with the coronary artery blockage. So when his occlusion happened, the collateral flow was so good that he didn't even burp.

Hal, with unjeopardized collaterals, avoided surgery.

Cautiously, we continued a low level of medications.

DR. FRANKLIN:

Digitalis

Digitalis is one of the oldest medications in the cardiologist's black bag. It was first described by Dr. William Withering in 1785 as an extract from the foxglove plant. A woman in Shropshire had a secret recipe, that included twenty herbs, for the treatment of "dropsy." An expert botanist, Dr. Withering quickly spotted the foxglove as the active ingredient. Of course the preparations today are purified, and dosages are more exact than they could be in the eighteenth century.

Digitalis' most important action is to improve the pumping ability of the heart. It does this by strengthening each heart muscle cell so that it contracts more vigorously. The strengthened heart can then better handle the work load of an abnormal valve or a congenital cardiac problem. When the heart's wall is damaged by a heart attack, digitalis can assist the remaining muscle to compensate for the scarred area.

A person without heart damage or an extra work load on his heart may still have a digitalis preparation prescribed by his doctor. It has a second action that Withering just barely suspected. It can help stabilize the heart's electrical system and is important in the treatment of some irregular heart rhythms, especially atrial fibrillation.

Digitalis must be given carefully. If a patient gets too much, the side effects, including changes in the heart's rhythm, can be harmful, even catastrophic. Digitalis overdose often results in an upset stomach. The first symptom may be loss of appetite or nausea. If it is ignored and the drug is continued, irregularities of the heartbeat may set in, and the patient may require immediate attention. To be in exact dosage, blood level tests can be done. But this is not necessary in the majority of patients.

DR. TAI:

Anti-arrhythmic drugs

All medicines used in treating arrhythmias (irregular heartbeats) affect the electrical activity of the heart, either directly or indirectly.

There are three general types of arrhythmias: 1) Tachycardia, the heart beats too fast; 2) Bradycardia, the heart beats too slow; 3) Irregular heartbeat.

• *Quinidine and procaine amide:* Used to correct irregular heartbeat. Quinidine may cause a bleeding disorder. Procaine amide may cause an arthritic condition. Most common toxic effects are uncomfortable but not serious. Stopping the drug corrects the toxic effect.

• *Lidocaine:* This is effective in certain conditions of tachycardia and irregular heartbeats. Must be given by injection and therefore, primarily used in the hospital, especially in CCU. Toxic effects occur only with very large doses.

• *Epinephrine (adrenalin) and isoproterenol:* Stimulates the heart to beat faster and improves conduction through heart's fleshy wires. Helps heart muscle beat more forcefully. Must be given by injection and requires careful supervision by trained personnel. These drugs are also important in the treatment of cardiac arrest.

Graham P. was sent to us by his family doctor, and was on one tablet of digitalis a day to help his weakened heart muscle. He was concerned that it was not enough. He also took water pills.

"It is sufficient," I told him. "When digitalis is taken by

mouth or injection, a large part of it is stored in the heart muscle and improves its functions. However, if a patient has a kidney problem or is elderly, we prescribe smaller doses of the drug."

"Is there anything I should watch for?" Graham asked apprehensively.

"If you also take water pills (diuretics), you should know that they not only remove excess fluid from the body, but unfortunately also remove vital chemicals, especially potassium. It is important for you to maintain a normal level of potassium to help avoid the toxic effects of digitalis. If potassium is removed, it should be supplemented in your diet or by medication. Spironolactone and triamterene are weak diuretics which do not remove potassium, and they are often teamed with stronger diuretics. In that case, no extra potassium is needed."

"Well, what is the reason for my taking quinidine too?"

"Graham, your heart has shown a tendency to beat irregularly (see chapter 8, "Short Circuit"). When the upper chambers become rapidly irregular, we call it atrial fibrillation. Instead of beating 72 to 80 times per minute, the upper chambers may suddenly send impulses at 300 or more per minute. Most of these extra impulses are stopped at the A-V node and the ventricular chambers receive only some of them. But the ventricles may still beat irregularly at 100 to 120 times per minute. Digitalis will slow the heart by increasing the block at the A-V node. But it can't make your upper chambers beat in proper sequence. Quinidine helps that. You should continue on this drug—it will keep your heart beating regularly."

"Is it like the quinine used in the army for malaria?"

"It's similar to quinine, but with some chemical or structural difference."

DR. FRANKLIN:

Medication for high blood pressure

Medication for high blood pressure depends on the level of the pressure, and its stage of severity, starting with mild drugs, and going on to stronger ones. High blood pressure is not a dramatic catastrophe like a heart attack, but can be just as serious in its future implications. Treatment can be difficult, frustrating and prolonged, and may be needed for years. The rewards are often not apparent, since the aim is to prevent damage to the heart and blood vessels, rather than to treat something already there which can be felt by the patient. He needs constant encouragement to continue on his medical program so that his blood pressure can be maintained as close as possible to normal limits.

When to treat high blood pressure?

Life expectancy decreases with any rise of blood pressure, especially if above normal levels. Lowering normal blood pressure has not been proven to lengthen the life span. Lowering high blood pressure to normal does seem to improve life span.

The most severe form—untreated accelerated high blood pressure (see chapter 10)—causes death in 90 percent of its victims within one year, and 99 percent within three years. But if the patient is treated for accelerated hypertension before the onset of severe kidney damage, the death rate is reduced to 30 percent in one year, and 60 percent in three years.

It is important to start therapy before damage to other organs has occurred.

• *Diuretics:* We start with diuretics. They remove sodium (salt) which retains fluid, from the body. One of the benefits is that sodium and fluid may be removed from the blood vessel walls, thus increasing their size and lowering blood pressure. Even more important, diuretics help other anti-hypertensive drugs lower blood pressure. If diuretics aren't doing the job alone, we go on to stronger drugs. One of these is *reserpine*, an extract of the roots *Rauwolfia Serpentina*, a plant known as "Snake Root." It works through the central nervous system.

Psychic depression is a common side effect in patients taking high doses. Suicides have occurred. So we watch their moods carefully. Side effects include lethargy, weight gain, increased gastric acidity. We are especially cautious with a patient who has a peptic ulcer or ulcerative colitis.

• *Methyldopa and hydralazine:* These are other "second stage" drugs to be used in combination with diuretics for patients with more elevated blood pressure. Methyldopa works indirectly and hydralazine directly on the blood vessel wall. Hydralazine can cause tachycardia, but used with propranolol it is very effective.

• *Guanethedine:* Reserved for severe high blood pressure,

it is very potent. Patients who use it may feel weak and faint when they rise from a lying down position. Their blood pressure falls after exercising. Some male patients become impotent, but not all of them. This drug may decrease blood flow to the kidney and allows waste products (urea) to build up in the blood. In our opinion, it should be used in combination with a diuretic and a stage two drug which doesn't have similar effects.

• *Diazoxide:* A new and potent drug, given intravenously that requires close observation by doctor, nurse, or paramedic. Used only for extreme cases of high blood pressure for emergency control.

• *Paragyline:* As potent as guanethedine, this drug acts in a different way to block the reactions of the sympathetic nervous system. It is dangerous because it leaves the body supersensitive to the effects of adrenalin-like substances. These substances are found in some cheese and alcoholic beverages, which can then cause severe high blood pressure. Also, cross reactions occur with other drugs such as antihistamines and barbiturates. Certain pain products also cause problems. Because of these idiosyncracies, many doctors prefer not to prescribe the drug, despite its excellent effect.

Certain tranquilizing drugs interfere with the actions of some high blood pressure drugs. It's wise for the patient to tell his physician if he is taking tranquilizers.

DR. KRAUTHAMER:

When I saw Frank E. for the first time in the Emergency Room, he looked to be in cardiovascular shock—cold and sweating, little output from his kidneys. But instead of low blood pressure, his was 160/110. He complained of an excruciating, tearing pain in the chest and back. There was a family history of high blood pressure. His family physician told me that he'd given Frank a prescription for his blood pressure, but Frank didn't follow directions because he hadn't felt sick until this attack.

"He's too busy having a swinging life to take care of himself," the physician said.

His chest X-ray showed a bulge in his aorta. The findings suggested a dissecting aneurysm. A tear of the inner lining of the aorta had allowed blood to get between the layers of this large vessel. The force of the heart's pulse pushed blood further into the tear creating a "pocket" in the wall of the aorta. I promptly admitted Frank into the Intensive Care Unit, started an intravenous, injected powerful drugs (in this case nitroprusside and propranolol) to bring down his blood pressure and decrease the force of his heartbeat. Once his blood pressure came down to 100/80 he was more comfortable. But his kidneys were not working properly. He was not producing any urine.

An angiogram revealed that the dissection had extended into Frank's abdomen. The renal arteries, leading to the kidneys, were blocked. Waste products were present and increasing in his system. Surgery would be necessary to re-establish the blood flow to his kidneys. We arranged for his transfer to a larger university hospital as our own wasn't equipped to handle this kind of emergency.

As sick as he was, Frank made sure that the nurses would forward his mail (get-well cards in feminine handwriting) and telephone calls (all social) to the new hospital. He was a tall, attractive man, with dark hair, a heavy mustache, and a winning way with women. Even the nurses responded to his deliberate and calculated charm.

I rode the ambulance with Frank, regulating his medication. He was feeling better now that the pain was gone.

"I don't want any operation," he informed the surgeon. We tried to explain the dangers of his condition. When told about the lack of urine and what it might do to him, he retorted, "Just as long as the other part works."

"Frank, you've got to have this operation or you'll never be able to have sex again."

Sex played a major part in his life. His family doctor had told me confidentially that Frank was married to an older woman who tolerated his infidelities as long as they didn't cause her embarrassment. He had a pad in midtown, and his girls were frequent visitors. He had boasted to his doctor about his sexual vigor and if his reports had any basis in truth, he was remarkable for a man approaching fifty. Life without women would be a true catastrophe for him.

So he finally agreed to the operation. The surgeon entered the abdomen and focused on the aorta. He created a "double barreled" aorta allowing blood to flow through the true aorta and the false "bulge" channel as well.

The kidneys now could receive blood again. But they had gone without adequate blood flow for such a long period that they had shut down temporarily. He required treatment with the artificial kidney until urine production returned.

Frank was obliged to stay in the hospital for two months before he returned home again. Now he had to take care of himself. Potent drugs controlled his high blood pressure —so potent that his sexual abilities were just about gone.

"I wouldn't have had the operation if I knew this would happen," Frank complained. "That damned surgeon promised me I could have sex again if I had the operation."

"He was right," I told Frank. "But you'll have to stop taking the medicine. And if you stop taking the medicine, you'll run the risk of having the same thing happen to you all over again. In the near future, we might have a medication to control high blood pressure without that side effect."

"Side effect. I call it the main effect," he commented bitterly.

Frank suddenly realized for the first time he had to choose: sex or life. "I'll think about it."

We've been seeing Frank for two years now. He's still thinking about it—and taking his medication.

DR. TAI:

Anti-coagulants

These are important drugs in heart disease. Normally, blood clots when you have a cut. While the blood is circulating in your body, it doesn't clot. But if there is stagnation of the blood or even damage to a blood vessel, it will clot.

There is danger that a clot will detach itself and prove dangerous, even lethal, depending on where in the body it lodges.

Anti-coagulants are drugs that forestall clotting.

• *Heparin:* Given only by injection, preferably intravenously. In its usual dose, it is effective against clotting for four to eight hours. Injected intramuscularly, it can act from twelve to twenty-four hours. Unfortunately, it can cause large bruises at the site of the injection. Since heparin must be given frequently, injections can be inconvenient.

For recurrent blood clots entering the blood stream because of mitral stenosis or phlebitis, oral medication is a better choice.

• *Warfarin derivatives:* These and similar drugs affect clotting factors produced by the liver. Doses must be regulated by special blood tests. Even after the dosage is stabilized, it may be necessary to repeat blood tests every few weeks.

Other drugs taken simultaneously can increase or reduce the effect of these anti-coagulants. Aspirin can induce major bleeding. Some tranquilizers and sleeping pills can modify the effect of the anti-coagulant dose.

Since the purpose of these drugs is to keep the circulation free of blood clots, it can cause bleeding if taken in excessive amounts, bleeding in the stomach, rectum, kidneys, nose, or even in the brain.

The patient should carry a card with him always, stating he is on an anti-coagulant. In case of accident, the anti-coagulant effect is counteracted by giving Vitamin K or whole blood. For surgery, anti-coagulants must be discontinued for twenty-four to forty-eight hours before an operation.

• *Aspirin, clofibrate, and dipyridamole:* These decrease the stickiness of blood platelets, the forerunners of clots in the arteries. At present, their use as anticoagulants is experimental (see below for more on clofibrate).

Drugs that lower cholesterol and triglyceride levels

Most patients can reduce their cholesterol and triglyceride levels by proper diet (see chapter 21). If this fails to bring satisfactory results, various drugs are available. Many others are still being researched.

• *Cholestyramine and cholestipol* bind cholesterol in the intestine and excrete it in the feces. They are very effective for Type II cholesterol patients (see Appendix D).

• *Nicotinic acid:* A derivative of Vitamin B-2 is effective in lowering both cholesterol and triglyceride levels and can be used in Types II, III, IV, and V. It has to be given in large doses, and has shown some serious effect on the liver in rare cases. Side effects include a flushing sensation.

• *Clofibrate:* Extensively used, although its effect on cholesterol is not as profound as on the triglycerides. Has some anti-coagulant effect but other side effects are minimal, mainly stomach upsets.

Chapter 17

Pacemakers: temporary or permanent

DR. KRAUTHAMER:
We allow our patients to cheat on their diets once a month (see chapter 21) and we allow ourselves the same privilege. Which means lunch at an Italian restaurant near our office. We seldom see Mama Carlucci, because she is in the kitchen with the pots of spaghetti, savory meat sauces and her marvelous lasagna. However, one day she was brought to the hospital with edema (swelling) of the legs and extreme shortness of breath.

Her family physician had given her medications, including digitalis and diuretics without effect. Since her pulse was slow, digitalis was discontinued. But this slow heart rate persisted even after the drug was stopped. There was retention of fluid both in the lungs and legs (edema), and X-rays showed enlargement of the heart. After a complete evaluation, an artificial pacemaker was recommended and inserted. The heart returned to normal size in a period of weeks. With its rate maintained at 70 beats per minute, the edema cleared. Her breathing was normal. Mama Carlucci was back in her restaurant, preparing her pastas for the neighborhood.

An artificial pacemaker is a small device that sends electrical impulses to the heart muscle, causing it to beat regularly. The instrument is fueled by batteries, and emits a spark which reaches the heart through a connecting wire.

Pacemakers are a recent innovation in medical science.

Yet the knowledge that electrical energy could cause a muscle to move goes back to the 18th century, when Volta and Galvinius found that frog muscles would contract when stimulated by an electrical impulse.

Dr. Paul Zoll was among the first to employ an *external* pacemaker system in the late 1950s. He connected wires to needles or tiny plates and pasted them on the patient's chest, and then hooked up the patient to a machine that was plugged into the wall. Electricity, modified by the machine, was thus passed through the patient and caused the heart to beat. It was a painful process. Dr. Zoll was forced to give his patients medication to ease the pain of the muscle contractions of the chest wall.

How is the pacemaker inserted today?

Over the years, the process of inserting an artificial pacemaker has been refined. One technique is a chest operation in which wires are actually sewn into the surface of the heart, then guided out through the ribs and into a pocket created under the skin for a battery pack, which is, incidentally, about the size of a hockey puck.

In the other method, a wire is inserted in a vein and then is passed into the heart chamber, reaching the right ventricle. This technique was pioneered by Dr. Seymour Furman of the Montefiore Hospital and Medical Center in New York. The cephalic vein is usually used. It is a small vein that runs between the muscles of the chest wall and the shoulder. If you run your right finger from the top of your left shoulder down for two or three inches until you reach the chest wall, you will feel a small depression. The vein is in this area. An incision, usually four to six inches long, is made *below* the collarbone but *above* the breast region.

Once the vein is isolated, the wire is passed through it, and the cardiologist positions it in the heart with the help of a fluoroscope.

Placing it in the proper location is essential to the pacemaker's success.

When the position is right, the wire is tied into place by several small stitches. The pacemaker itself, with the batteries and electronic components, is attached to the wire and slipped into the same incision. It is buried beneath the skin and lies on top of the pectoral or chest muscles. The entire operation is usually done through the one incision. If the vein is too small to allow passage of the wire, another vein in the neck can be used. But another small incision of one to two inches will then be necessary.

We usually use heavy sedation plus local anesthesia in our elderly patients who need pacemakers. This avoids the risks, however small, of general anesthesia. The entire operation consists only of an incision in the skin. No entry is made directly into the chest cavity. Post-operative care is simplified and risks reduced.

Initially, there was considerable competition between the two techniques. The simplest one was adopted. Now the majority of pacing is done with the wire sent through the blood vessel.

Still, in certain rare cases, the open chest operation is needed. In this procedure, an incision between the ribs exposes the heart. The wires are sewn directly to the exterior of the heart (rather than slipped inside it). They are then led out between the ribs. The attachment to the pacemaker and insertion under the skin are the same as described previously. But the risks are somewhat higher and the convalescence is longer.

The pacemaker can do only *one* job. That is to guarantee an electrical impulse to stimulate the heart muscle. People have a wrong idea about its purpose. They tend to believe it will strengthen the heart. This is not true. *The artificial pacemaker only guarantees a certain heart rate.*

The number of beats per minute it will send out is decided by the patient and doctor. It can be built to send out 40 to 140 beats per minute. Usually an artificial pacemaker is set at a rate of about 70 beats per minute. The pacemaker is the answer for certain electrical problems of the heart. But it is not the answer for the problems of the heart muscle, valves or coronary arteries.

The pacemaker's most frequent use is in patients who have deterioration of the heart's conduction system, as in Stokes-Adams attacks, usually a result of aging. Often the rest of the heart shows no malfunction. Pathological studies have made it clear that this need for a permanent pacemaker is usually *not* due to arteriosclerotic coronary artery disease.

Yet at times it will be used for patients with coronary

disease. For a patient whose heart attack has damaged the heart muscle in which the conduction system lies. Sometimes, in the first few days after a heart attack, temporary damage to the conduction system may cause the heart to beat slower.

If medication doesn't help, a temporary pacemaker may be needed. A vein is punctured with a needle and a wire is passed through it. It is guided to the heart (right ventricle) usually with the help of a fluoroscope or an ECG. The outside end is attached to a battery pack strapped as a temporary unit to the patient's chest.

Pacemaker therapy is also an aid in controlling certain irregular heart rhythms. As in Stokes-Adams attacks, there is usually no significant problem with the other parts of the heart. But in this case, the *natural* pacemaker is at fault. At times it beats very quickly or very slowly. A combination of potent medications is needed to prevent the episodes of rapid beating (tachycardia). The medication will make the slow part of the cyclic pattern even slower. So a pacemaker will be put in to help the heart return to normal, while the medication is used to control the tachycardia. The end result for the patient can be the ability to work again. And not be at the mercy of the caprices of his "temperamental" sino-atrial node.

Not all patients react as well and as quickly to the artificial pacemaker as Mama Carlucci did.

Some do not consider the insertion of an artificial pacemaker as minor surgery. The fact that a mechanical device helps to keep the heart running troubles them, almost as though they feel their heart is no longer entirely their own. Even though the cardiologist prepares the patient and his family for the adjustments of living with a foreign instrument in his body, it takes many patients considerable time to be able to accept it.

The patient often goes through various stages until he is reconciled to the hardware in his chest. After the operation, he may feel isolated from other people, like some mechanical toy wound up in order to perform its duties. He may be overly afraid that if the battery wears down, his life will go down with it. In this stress situation, he may be beset by emotional upheavals. He suffers from inertia.

"I have to whip myself to get going," a patient reported. "I could just drift into nothingness."

Then gradually there is a change. The feeling of helplessness disappears, and he is ready to rejoin the mainstream of life. His attitude is helped immeasurably by the greater feeling of well-being the pacemaker frequently provides. The physical lift helps him handle the emotional problems. He finally accepts realistically the fact that he is dependent on the artificial pacemaker. He loses his anger and suspicion about this strange mechanism tucked under his skin. His moodiness lessens as his confidence returns. His self-image improves. He has traveled the cycle from the helpless infant to the adult ready to face the world again.

DR. KRAUTHAMER:
Two basic types of pacemakers are in use today. For the patient with a constant unchanging heart block—fixed pulse at about 40—there is the *fixed-rate* pacemaker. It is pre-set to work at a certain rate and has nothing to do with the heart's natural rhythm. It cannot detect the heart's own beat, should the conduction system recover and compete with it. Therefore, it is used only in patients who are known to be in complete heart block.

The second type is a *demand* pacemaker. It is equipped with a circuit that can sense a spontaneous heartbeat. When the natural beat occurs, the pacemaker does not fire. But if a spontaneous beat is absent, the demand pacemaker will fill in for it. It steps in whenever the patient needs help. But is shut off every time *the patient has a heartbeat of his own*. It is used when the block in the conduction system is intermittent. Most importantly, it is used for those patients who need control of irregular heart rhythms.

The artificial pacemaker is a sturdy object.

Once implanted in the patient's chest by a skilled team, it will create no problems in over 90 percent of the cases, until its battery begins to fail.

"What happens when my pacemaker batteries weaken?" the patient asks.

"When will the batteries fail?"

This is now the major concern of both physician and

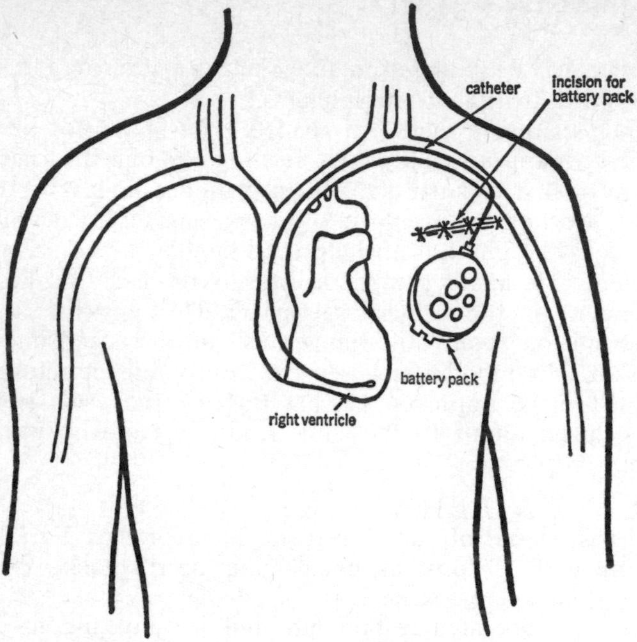

Permanent transvenous pacemaker

An incision is made in the chest. The cephalic vein is exposed and the electrode catheter is passed to the right ventricle. The cardiologist observes the catheter on a fluoroscope screen as he guides it.

The catheter electrode is then tied in place, and the "battery pack" is buried in the incision, the skin is sewn and heals.

patient. *When* should the unit be replaced? Do it early and lose some battery life? Or wait and take the chance of a Stokes-Adams fainting spell if the batteries should fail completely before the replacement?

Replacement involves another operation, shorter this time. The older batteries and the electronic components (all are actually sealed together in the one unit called the battery pack) must be removed. The incision must be reopened, the new unit attached to the old wire (which is usually not changed), and then nature's healing process again closes the incision.

Each time this is repeated, the doctor is operating on scar tissue. Healing the second or third time may be slightly slower. There may be a greater chance of infection. The long-range goal is to replace the battery as infrequently as possible, getting as much out of each unit as possible without endangering the patient.

Batteries weaken slowly over a gradual period of time. Only toward the very end of their life span is there an acceleration in their downhill course.

To help solve this problem, new pacemakers have a built-in special circuit. As the battery strength decreases, the rate of the pacemaker also decreases ever so slightly—say from 70 beats to 69.5 beats per minute. Then to 69.4 and so on. Now we have a way to tell when to replace the unit. A decrease in pacemaker rate, greater than the normal variation, that persists for a few days, means battery replacement is due.

How do we detect this change in the pacemaker rate?

"Count your pulse each day and report any changes to us," we tell all our pacemaker patients.

But the pulse test is not sensitive enough. It can tell gross problems, but not gradual battery failure. The next step is monitoring the patient with electrocardiograms. The cardiogram records the pacemaker impulse as well as the heart's beat. Again not quite accurately enough in a number of cases, although it can measure as small a change as 40 milliseconds (40/thousandths of a second). We would like to be able to detect changes in the pacemaker rate as small as 1 to 5 milliseconds. To do this an electronic gadget called an "interval counter" is needed. With the necessary technical equipment, the cost of an interval counter ranges between $600 and $1,000. Plus a technician's salary to operate the machine. The average physician doesn't have enough of a pacemaker caseload to warrant such an expense. So pacemaker clinics have become routine in hospital centers.

Next, how often should the pacemaker be checked? Right after it's been put in, several visits to the doctor are necessary to establish the particular unit's "basic rate." Thereafter, checkups can be less frequent until the anticipated time of battery failure approaches. Then checkups must be more frequent, perhaps weekly.

For the elderly person, infirm with arthritis, possibly without transportation, weekly visits to the doctor become a difficult problem.

Science has come to the rescue once again. A device is now available that can detect the pacemaker impulse when the patient holds two pieces of metal (electrodes) in his hands, or attaches them to his wrists with elastic bands. Just like an electrocardiogram, these detect the electrical impulse of the pacemaker. Instead of producing a strip with squiggles, they convert the impulses to sounds, which can be sent over a regular telephone to a center that has an interval counter. An immediate analysis is available to the doctor, and the patient is never further from a pacer check-up than he is from his own telephone.

It is easy to check the fixed-rate pacemaker because it is always working. The demand pacemaker occasionally may be shut off by the patient's own heartbeat. Its battery may also fail. But it can be converted briefly to a fixed rate system by holding a magnet over it, directly against the skin. In this way, its signals can be counted and its battery life evaluated. This too may be done by a telephone monitoring system. The patient is simply given instructions when to place a special magnet over the pacemaker and another telephone transmission is recorded. Once the magnet is removed, the unit goes right back to being a demand pacemaker.

DR. KRAUTHAMER:

"What about exercise?" our patients with pacemakers often ask us.

"You can swim, play golf, walk. You can even drive a car. And of course, you can have your shower or bath as soon as the incision heals."

We remind our patients to avoid body contact sports. No football, for instance. No hunting either, since the rifle stock is held against the shoulder and the kick of the recoil might throw the pacemaker off. If the patient is right-handed, we try to place the pacemaker on the left side, and vice versa. It then may be less of an encumbrance (and he can still go skeet shooting).

We remind our patients always to wear a medallion and to carry a card which identifies them as users of a pacemaker. These ID cards are issued by the manufacturers of the instrument. The patient's family should also know the make, the model number and the rate of the unit.

"Doctor, I'm taking a world cruise in January," a woman

patient told us recently. "What about the battery in my pacemaker?"

"If you won't be home by the time you may be due for a replacement, we suggest that you have a replacement *before* leaving on the trip."

Earlier pacemakers were subject to outside electrical interference. There are actual records of a pacemaker shutting off momentarily under such circumstances. The new units are protected by shielding but we still suggest the patient avoid close exposure to microwave ovens, Ferrari spark plug coils, direct radar beams.

The fixed-rate pacemaker is much less sensitive to electrical fields than the demand unit, with its sensing or input circuit. To protect against this danger, it has a fail-safe system that is activated when the sensing circuit is swamped by a burst of electrical energy, from a close-by radio station for example. It converts the demand pacemaker to a form of fixed rate pacing at 80 to 120 beats per minute. The pacemaker now ignores all other signals and goes merrily on working until the interference stops. Patients do not have to worry about accelerated or stopped pacemakers because of manmade electrical storms.

Women who have pacemaker implants usually placed just at the upper margin of the breast find that with time and gravity, the pacemaker will sink a bit, so they may be more comfortable with a firm-fitting bra.

The cost of a pacemaker system is about $800 to $1,000. This does not include hospital and physician charges. When replaced, an identical unit is usually used.

The high cost is part of the reason for active research to extend battery life span. New developments in circuit design now allow us to use what we call "low output" pacemakers in certain cases. The batteries are the same, but the electrical impulse is shorter and not as strong. It still does the job, but the battery lasts longer. Some of these units have been operating for as long as thirty-six to forty months. Hopefully, further steps in this direction will be possible in the future.

The artificial pacemaker has radically changed the outlook for the patient with heart block. Heart block without the help of a pacemaker means a 50 percent mortality within one year. Today, the mortality of the patient who has been paced and is properly watched approaches the actuarial statistics of other people in his age bracket, with the difference of only a few percentage points at most.

Many people are inclined to think of the artificial pacemaker as a crutch for the older heart. But it is also used frequently in children with congenital heart block.

Insertion of an artificial pacemaker in a child is a bit different than in an adult. The size of the pacemaker is smaller. As with an adult, the battery pack must be changed almost every two years. This means that the young person can anticipate thirty to forty battery changes in his lifetime.

Two years. Seventy beats a minute. Four thousand two hundred beats an hour. Thirty-six million, seven hundred and ninety-two thousand, two hundred beats a year. Replace it in eighteen to twenty-four months. Two years. New battery. Hospital visit. Incision. Replacement. Stitches. Healing. Is it worth it?

Ask any person who's been restored to life.

On April 27, 1970, in France, a 58-year-old woman received the first atomic-powered pacemaker. How long it will last is beyond our ability to estimate. Five years, ten, maybe even fifteen. Power source is estimated at twenty years. But it is likely the electronic components won't make it for that span of time.

The atomic power supply for the nuclear pacemaker is an isotope—radioactive plutonium 238. It is "hot" both in the sense of heat and radioactivity. A thermo-electric unit converts its heat to electricity. This is then fed to a regular pacemaker circuit and wire system. One fuel cell is manufactured by the *Société Alcatel* of France in conjunction with France's Atomic Energy Agency. Another by an American company which makes the pacemaker portion as well.

In the United States, the first nuclear-powered pacemakers were implanted by physicians at the Veterans Administration Hospital in Buffalo, New York, in July 1972. By the time this is published, there will surely be others.

The question asked most frequently about the atomic pacemaker concerns its safety. Is it radioactive? How well has it been tested?

Both the U.S. and the French Atomic Energy commissions insisted on extensive qualification testing. Simulated auto, airplane and train impact situations were used. The unit was evaluated under temperatures as high as 2,400 degrees Fahrenheit, and crush loads up to 40,000 pounds. Rifle shots were fired without shattering the unit. Under all of these circumstances, it performed creditably. At the surface of the pacemaker, under the patient's skin, the radiation emitted is about that of a wristwatch with a luminous dial. Over a year, the exposure is equivalent to the amount a person absorbs by having a routine chest X-ray. There is no danger of significant radiation for anyone in proximity to the patient.

The atomic pacemaker is costly. The unit comes to between four and five thousand dollars. But at its estimated life span of ten years, it will cut down the cost of pacemaker therapy by 50 percent. At the present time, because of this high cost, they are being used predominantly on the younger patients.

Meanwhile additional research continues in attempts to prolong battery life in the less costly mercury cell units currently in use. Newer and longer lasting non-nuclear batteries are inevitable. One using lithium is currently being tried. It may be able to supply power for as long as six to eight years.

Considerable strides were made in the early 1960s, shortly after pacemakers were first introduced. Then, a plateau in pacemaker technology was reached in the late 1960s. Now it may be time for another jump forward. The atomic-powered unit, and the lithium battery may be the first offspring in the second generation of pacemakers.

Chapter 18

Surgery

BEN W.:

I was a logical candidate for a heart attack. I was addicted to cigarettes. I'm a compulsive worker. I'm forty-two, and my father died suddenly at the same age of a heart attack.

My work as a medical photographer brings me in daily contact with physicians, surgeons, and psychiatrists. Like many others who do not separate work from leisure, I am intensely interested in my profession. My photographs, both color and black and white, appear in the general magazines as well as medical journals. I also teach medical photography at a nearby college. Drug companies use my photographs as guidelines for their artists, and a recent book on the heart, whose artistic illustrations will become classic, is based on my work. I know a great deal about the heart. I ask innumerable questions. Doctors are intrigued by my total absorption in my work. They don't know about my background.

We're more conscious of the influence of genetics these days, and the awareness of my father's death at an early age is always with me, a kind of presentiment.

Janet and I have been married fifteen years, and our daughters, Lee and Julie, are fourteen and thirteen years old. We live in the Lower East Side of New York City, in a converted loft on Houston Street that has space and light. I have my studio and Janet has room for her loom and her sewing machine. She teaches in a school for retarded children, and has had extraordinary results, in terms of their response to color and pattern.

Fatigue has been a part of me since I went through college on part-time jobs and a meager scholarship. Since I've started teaching, it is often midnight before I climb the five flights to our loft. Janet always has a hot meal for me, something nourishing and not too heavy. Since she is employed full time herself, she has the grace to let me rest before we catch up on each other's day.

When symptoms began to show, I ignored them. From my work, I should have known better. I had a sense of fatalism about my father's death. I dreaded the approach of my forty-second birthday, though I knew what could be done medically for those who inherit a tendency to arteriosclerosis.

Denial is not only a part of our inner defense, it is the rope we clutch in order to hold on to life. I learned as much from Dr. Daniel R., a psychiatrist who is my consultant in all my medical work. He has become a friend and is helping me understand myself. Say it isn't so and it won't be. My father died within a half hour after he was stricken. *It won't happen to me,* I kept repeating to myself, but the echo in my mind said *It will happen to you.*

One Saturday night, late in January, Janet and I drove out to North Stamford to visit a friend of ours, a nurse. Over tender roast beef and Yorkshire pudding, we were discussing the wretched conditions of many emergency rooms. I was talking, Janet remembers, with considerable emphasis and animation.

It started as a burning sensation—hot, intense, pressing. A few seconds later, it was clawing down my arm. As it radiated, I knew I was having a heart attack. It was the quality of the pain, the shooting of the pain, the sweating. None of these symptoms had ever been present before.

Janet said I turned white.

She drove me to the hospital. The Emergency Room physician cared for me and telephoned Dr. Samuels, our family doctor in New York, who said, "Have Ben stay there." I was taken up to the hospital's Coronary Care Unit. By that time our doctor contacted Dr. Tai for a consultation.

Denial is persuasive, I admit it. Dr. Daniel R. had taught me that, and it was reinforced by my reading.

"Denial is one of our most primitive defenses," Daniel

told me again when he came to visit me in the hospital, this time as a patient. "As we grow, we learn to defend ourselves against painful stimuli in complicated physical and psychological ways. The most primitive defense which the infant uses is the prototype of denial. He does it first physically. He actually turns his head away. As he develops, he does it psychologically. He refuses to recognize it. This is different from repression, when something is blocked out of the conscious mind and remains blocked."

Confronted with a life-threatening situation, I found myself denying. The ECG and the enzymes in my blood showed something. When Dr. Samuels drove up from New York to visit me at the hospital, he made a casual offhand mention of the possibility of heart surgery. But I passed it over without recognizing it. My ears heard but didn't hear. Denial.

In the Coronary Care Unit, I was hooked up to a monitor. I knew, of course, what this equipment was, and realized that some patients felt the monitor exerted some magical influence on the heart. It wasn't merely recording the heartbeat, it was the causal agent keeping me alive.

"During periods of regression," Daniel said on one of his visits, "the monitor is experienced as an extension of the body. You regard it with the same respect that the child feels for the omnipotent mother, because the mother is the life-saving force."

My attack happened on January 30th. I spent ten days in the hospital and during my stay, Dr. Tai did a cardiac catheterization.

DR. TAI:

The catheterization and X-rays showed a hazardous heart condition requiring a saphenous vein by-pass. Recommended treatment: heart surgery. He was an excellent candidate in every way.

It never gets any easier to sit across the desk from a patient and tell him he needs heart surgery. Just as no operation is without risk, no surgery is 100 percent successful. The success for by-pass surgery ranges from 80 to 95 percent. When there is failure, it is because blood clots close the by-pass. The reasons are still poorly understood.

If the patient is properly selected, like Ben—and the procedure is properly done, most of these operations are successful. This means a dramatic decrease in symptoms and, we feel, protection from future heart attack.

THE SURGEON:

When a coronary artery in the heart is blocked, the blood cannot course along briskly. It slows down at the narrowing, much like traffic slowing down at a toll booth. The coronary artery may be clean, except for the short segment where it is narrow because of fatty deposits. But the narrowing makes him vulnerable to a fatal heart attack.

So surgeons devised an operation which eliminates the danger of the narrowing. It may even close off entirely and yet the patient can be saved. It is called a saphenous vein by-pass.

The saphenous vein by-pass is one of the most dramatic aids in the history of heart disease. The surgeon cuts a vein from the patient's leg or arm, sutures one section of this healthy vein to the coronary artery beyond its point of obstruction. He carefully sutures the other end to the aorta. The displaced vein is now part of the artery and passes around the obstruction. If there are more narrowings, the surgeon may by-pass them with two or more saphenous veins.

It's not like replacing a section of rusty pipe with a clean piece. Rather, it's like putting a new piece of pipe beside the rusted part until you get past the rust. Then you hook the new piece to the old pipe by-passing the rusted segment.

The saphenous vein by-pass operation is about seven years old. It was devised by Dr. Rene Favalaro at Cleveland Clinic. It has provided a kind of rebirth to many patients who suffered from angina or coronary heart disease and were unable to lead normal lives. We have seen hundreds of patients in our practice who we feel have benefited greatly from this type of operation.

The success of these operations has been made possible partly by the development of the heart-lung machine.

If the heart must be opened or stopped for an operation, circulation to the rest of the body, especially the brain must be maintained. This is accomplished by by-passing the heart and lungs with a special apparatus—heart-lung machine or "pump." Attended by specialists called perfusionists or the "pump team," it works like this:

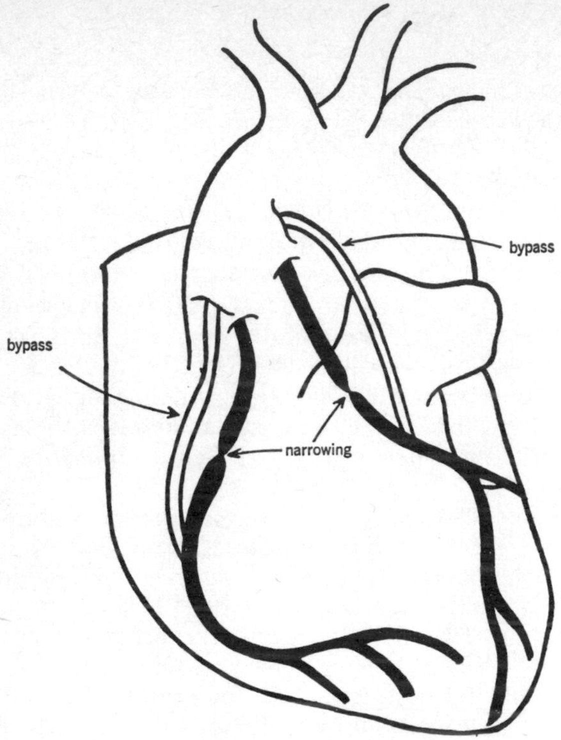

Coronary by-pass surgery

The left and right coronary arteries have severe narrowings. Segments of vein, removed from the patient's leg, have been sewn into the aorta and then connected with the coronary vessels beyond the narrowings. The blockage has been by-passed.

The heart surgeon puts large tubes into the two large veins (vena cavae) that bring blood back to the heart. All this blood is diverted into the pump. It is carried through a chamber where carbon dioxide is exchanged for oxygen, just as in the lungs. The oxygenated blood is then gently pumped back to the body through a tube which the surgeon places in one of the large arterics. In summary, blood is *taken* from the veins, diverted to the pump where it is oxygenated, and *returned* to the arteries. This supplies oxygen to the brain and other vital organs while the surgeon operates on the heart. When surgery is completed and the heart is pumping again, the tubes are removed and the normal circulation restored.

Nowadays most heart-lung machines are made in two parts. A mechanical, reusable pump and a plastic exchange chamber (the "lung") which is totally disposable.

Most patients having open heart surgery need blood transfusions. The patient's blood is typed and crossmatched to prime the heart-lung machine, and to replace blood loss if needed. With improved techniques less transfusion is needed and in some cases can bc done with no blood transfusion.

For anesthesia a tube is inserted through the mouth into the windpipe. The endotracheal tube. During surgery, while the patient is on the heart-lung machine the anesthesiologist pumps air in and out of the endotracheal tube to keep the lungs pliable. When the patient is relying on his own lungs again, the breathing can be controlled more easily with the tubc in place. Brain function is monitored by electrodes on the scalp. Of course the cardiogram is monitored as well.

Operations are performed on many patients not to save their lives, but to make them more comfortable, since they find it impossible to function with the discomfort and pain they experience.

To prepare a patient for cardiac surgery, we spell out the purpose of the operation: Heart surgery usually does not cure. It compensates. So the patient who goes into the operating room convinced that he will come out of the surgical procedure fully cured may sometimes have an unhappy awakening. He may discover during his convalescence that there is no miraculous cure. This disillusion can lead not only to depression, but to anxiety, anger and distrust of the physicians who are caring for him.

Therefore, number one on the list of priorities is to give the patient some insight into his heart condition and the way in which the surgical procedure will alter it.

He must understand that one risk is being played against another: the basic risk of having his heart condition treated with medications versus the risk associated with surgery.

The patient must be informed and understand that he has to give his consent before he puts himself on the operating table. The patient is the boss. The body is his. He must know whatever risks there are, and make the decision.

The physician is the servant, the professional who does the job. It is his obligation to inform the patient what procedures are available to him and which he recommends. This is how we handle our practice.

Ben was a good pre-operative patient and followed advice faithfully.

"Cut out smoking," we warned him again. Cigars used to be his weakness. Good lung function and adequate oxygenation are so important to a swift recovery from surgery that giving up smoking beforehand is absolutely essential. Smoking adversely affects the bronchial tree. It may delay recuperation. It can even cause pulmonary complications, such as an excess of secretions piling up in the bronchial tree, blockage of the bronchi, infections.

Reducing is also important for the overweight patient. Surgery at the ideal weight will greatly help post-operative care and recovery.

Liquor is on the taboo list for several weeks to a month before surgery. If a patient has been drinking over the years, his liver may be affected. It requires adequate liver function to detoxify the anesthesia. If there is alcoholic cirrhosis present, the body's ability to heal will be altered and recuperation delayed.

The psychological effects before and after vary from person to person. Arthur Godfrey had a lung removed and came through superbly. Yet another person has hemorrhoids removed and is convinced that his world is coming to an end.

The frightened patient always needs much reassurance, particularly if he's scheduled for heart surgery. A tranquilizer is almost routine therapy for heart patients coming into any hospital.

But one must understand that no matter how much the physicians try to ameliorate post-operative reactions, it's still going to hurt.

BEN W.:
The films of my heart showed a narrowing in the left anterior descending and an almost complete blockage in the right, which made it a critical situation. But beyond the narrowings, the arteries looked good.

Because of my medical background, Dr. Tai allowed me

to see the films; I marveled at them. I had worked on coronary arteries in my photographs, but never thought of questioning the state of my own arteries. He offered to show me films of successful results. His enthusiasm, his obvious knowledge and his optimistic references to ". . . and after surgery" kept Janet and me in a state of confidence.

Looking back, I begin to appreciate how tactful yet honest the doctors were during the entire experience, taking us slowly from one step to the next, with a very measured sense of urgency. Their timing was wonderful.

Even before they knew of the extent of the disease, Dr. Samuels had mentioned saphenous vein by-pass surgery in an offhand way. Then the cardiologists spoke of it, but always kept open the possibility that an exercise program or medication might be the answer.

It wasn't.

We had decided on a particular heart surgeon, Dr. Martin F. Dr. Tai was enthusiastic about this surgeon and showed me catheterization films taken after he had operated.

During the waiting, there were the times I had recurrent angina and with each pain we had the suspense of wondering whether it would last and become a full-blown coronary.

The surgeon was a gentle man, and spoke to us about the work he had done, the risks, the followups, how many people he had operated on. He was extremely calm and matter of fact, which Janet and I found most reassuring.

"Doctor, if you were in my situation, what would you do?" I asked.

"I'd have surgery," he said quietly.

Then we knew. There was no equivocation. The decision to go ahead came as a relief and a very positive solution.

But after it was decided, there was a long wait. There are long waiting lists at the various cardiac centers around the country. Janet says now that she was astonished at my patience.

I had the benefit of talking to my consulting psychiatrist, Dr. Daniel R., and that helped. Control and humor were the saving qualities, and fortunately Janet shared them with me. My great curiosity helped too. It seems to me I began to master trauma through learning. It was congruent also with my work. Janet, though somewhat less sophisticated about medicine, read with me, and researched articles. And just the fact of her knowing made me more comfortable.

Dr. Tai put me on an exercise program that made the waiting manageable. Work, activity, structured exercise. I would soon be inactive for a relatively long time, so he wanted me to build up as much cardio-vascular reserve as possible. I walked and used the exercise bicycle, working up to a good level. No doctor gave me this advice, but I put myself on a special vitamin regimen with massive doses of B-complex, C and E. I was already on a low cholesterol diet, and taking clofibrate and aspirin which help reduce the danger of clotting.

"The procedure doesn't scare me," I told Dr. Tai, "but what does is the heart-lung machine."

I knew that transient anoxia (lack of oxygen) can lead to psychosis or possible brain damage. I had read about some people who are completely disoriented, even psychotic. And I told Dr. Tai so.

"It's a perfectly natural fear," Dr. Tai agreed, "but heart-lung psychosis with residual brain damage is rare." The surgeon agreed that the dangers were very minimal, though I couldn't entirely shake off the sense of dread.

Our first impression of the exterior of one of Manhattan's great hospitals was depressing. It looked austere. We paused a moment at the entrance.

"Let's go," I said to Janet.

The staff was warm and competent. They moved a cot into my room for Janet and she stayed there the night before I went to surgery.

I slept during the night. That Janet was nearby was comforting but in an abstract way.

I had a pre-op shot of a sedative. Part of me is the fatalist. I knew that very few patients die during this operation. I was furious at my doubts that I would not make it, even though death in itself didn't scare me. It was night-time jitters.

JANET W.:

We made very intriguing plans for communicating after the operation—a detailed list of questions and answers that we'd use while Ben was in the Intensive Care Recovery Room. Since he would be on the respirator and wouldn't be able to talk, we had arranged signals, eye blinks, the raising of eyebrows and so on.

Waiting is the usual course of events in a hospital, of course. In the waiting room at off-visitor hours, you see the people who are on an emotional precipice for the long, tedious unrelieved vigil. Friends came to sit with me. I talked to them and tried to comfort them (so they said), and don't remember a word of what I said. What sticks in my mind is the big ashtray at my elbow, gradually filling with stubs, and a woman friend bringing coffee in a soggy container, and the clock that held my attention.

It was noon, and he had been in surgery for five hours. Another hour dragged by. Six hours. Suddenly I saw the surgeon, and in spite of my determined control, I felt such a great relief, that it showed.

"All went well," the surgeon said as he approached. "We had a little trouble with the left anterior descending coronary artery because it was buried under muscle."

My friends brought me more coffee and we waited for Ben to be wheeled into the Intensive Care Recovery Room.

The doctors had explained about the operation. Yet nothing quite prepared me for the sight of Ben on the rolling stretcher, bottles suspended above him. Nor for the way the respirator looked. This was the most terrifying sight, because of the endotracheal tube connected to his mouth. Ben's face was puffy. His eyes were half-closed and swollen. His body twitched from the respirator. None of the attending nurses was concerned about it, and Ben told me later that he was conscious and it wasn't uncomfortable, even though it evidently looked gruesome.

BEN W.:

The suction from the drainage apparatus.

The respirator.

The vaporized oxygen steaming into the oxygen delivery system.

Tubes from my body lead to bottles in the air and on the floor. I am still hazy from anesthesia. I look at this room, which is like something out of science fiction. I feel kind of detached, in a fog tent, unable to move or to ring for a nurse. People wander in and out, less interested in me than in the tubes and equipment.

Sometime during the drifting, I hear a voice, "You are in the Intensive Care Recovery Room. I am your doctor, and as you know, these instruments are to help you breathe . . ."

Janet is holding my hand.

"A truck ran over me, backed up and is sitting on my chest," I tell her hoarsely. They smile. Janet, the house physician, the nurse.

Every patient is extremely uncomfortable for a couple of days after the operation. But don't listen to me or anyone who has gone through heart surgery. We tell you the *wildest* tales.

DR. MARTIN F., the surgeon:
Ben knows the importance of following instructions. In the Intensive Care Recovery Room, they watch his blood pressure and oxygen carefully. Sometimes complications occur in the lungs if the patient will not or cannot breathe deeply. One post-operative complication (atelectasis) is due to an accumulation of mucus put out by the bronchial tree. The patient is apt to get into real trouble. He may experience tachycardia, either high or low blood pressure; and he may suffer a heart attack as well.

It's also important to get the patient on his feet early. If we don't, blood clots from leg veins can be a killer.

Many patients cannot track down memories of the initial period after cardiac surgery. To block out memories is perhaps the best defense against the trauma. The patient may speak to the nurses, the doctors, his family, and yet later, not recall a word of it.

The recovery room staff was pleased at Ben's quick recovery from anesthesia and the shock of surgery.

Within two weeks he was convalescing at home.

The scar on the chest after heart surgery is usually about twelve inches long with multiple stitches. A patient with a midline incision in the front of the chest will have in addition, a cut separating the breastbone (sternum). This is held together by wires which are not removed. When, during recuperation, the skin stitches are removed, the patient may feel some of these wires in his chest, but there is no reason for concern. The wires are sterile and will not harm him. If they do cause definite irritation, they can be removed. However, this is rarely required.

BEN W.:

I've always been athletic. Played basketball. Worked on the exercise bicycle. Maybe that's why my convalescence was so rapid.

In the year since my operation, I have seen Dr. Tai for routine followups, not because I've had a return of symptoms or pain. The only pain I had is the result of the opening of the chest wall for surgery. It is bad, especially in damp weather. The fact that the doctors warned us that there would be considerable post-surgery pain was very important. One shouldn't be under the delusion that there is no pain after surgery, and if you do have it, that something is wrong. It is difficult to separate chest pain of the incision from chest pain of angina. They can both be in the same place. But in time, you learn to distinguish between them.

I have no painful memories of the Recovery Room. Having to breathe deeply and to cough was unpleasant but not all that painful. And of course, the IPPB (Intermittent Positive Pressure Breathing) machine was helping to force oxygen into my lungs.

Soon after I came home from the hospital, I started exercising. Very gently at first, perhaps twenty-five revolutions of the wheel on the bicycle. I walked also, gradually building up my strength.

I was operated on early in March and went back to a full working schedule in August. I'm back on my old routine, with five or six hours of sleep a night. But I exercise every day.

I'm careful about food. And I take clofibrate. It may help the body to handle fats better. I'm not smoking.

It requires a severe emotional readjustment to the new life. A fellow patient confided to me that he felt his heart surgery was punishment for old sins. Some surgeons today are asking psychiatrists to counsel their patients before and after surgery.

Yes, I would certainly do it again. A year after open-heart surgery, I know I made the right decision.

Artificial valves

Valve surgery was attempted for the first time about 40 years ago, with poor results. But it was revived 20 years later by a group of courageous surgeons.

Their patient didn't die as had been anticipated. Instead, the patient improved, as did others who underwent the operation. Most of the surgery was confined to mitral stenosis valve opening. Since there was no heart-lung machine, the procedure was done by closed method. The chest was opened, and the surgeon made a tiny opening in the left atrium, inserted his finger and "cracked" the valve. Later it was done with a knife attached to the end of a finger. Today, the valve is still opened simply by cutting the edge which allows the blood to flow more readily.

The operation described above does not cure the basic defect. But it does produce symptomatic improvement in patients with mitral stenosis. Since the opening is greater, the blood flow to the left ventricle is greater. There is less backlogging of blood to the lungs and therefore less congestion.

Mitral valve replacement

When the operation is not successful or the valve thickens again, valve replacement may be considered.

"Are artificial valves safe?" one of our patients asked Dr. Franklin.

A tremendous amount of research has been done on artificial valves. Scientists have tried to imitate normal valve function and achieve one-way flow. At first, they tried to imitate the normal valve cusp. They attempted to duplicate its resiliency as well as its tenacity. But if they used very durable material, it hampered blood flow by its very toughness.

So instead of copying the moving cusp of the normal valve they went to what we refer to as the ball valve. It is a metal ring with two hoops and a ball imprisoned between them. A ball in a cage. As blood is pushed through it from the bottom, the ball lifts and blood flows around the hoops and ball. Then the ball falls back closing the opening and preventing backflow or leakage.

Plastic materials were tried but discarded because of secondary problems. Researchers turned to metals used in the airplane industry. Now the ring, hoops and ball are usually made of titanium.

Since the material is foreign to the human body and mostly of metal there is a chance that blood may clot on its surface. A blood clot would interfere with the movement of the ball. More important, it might detach from

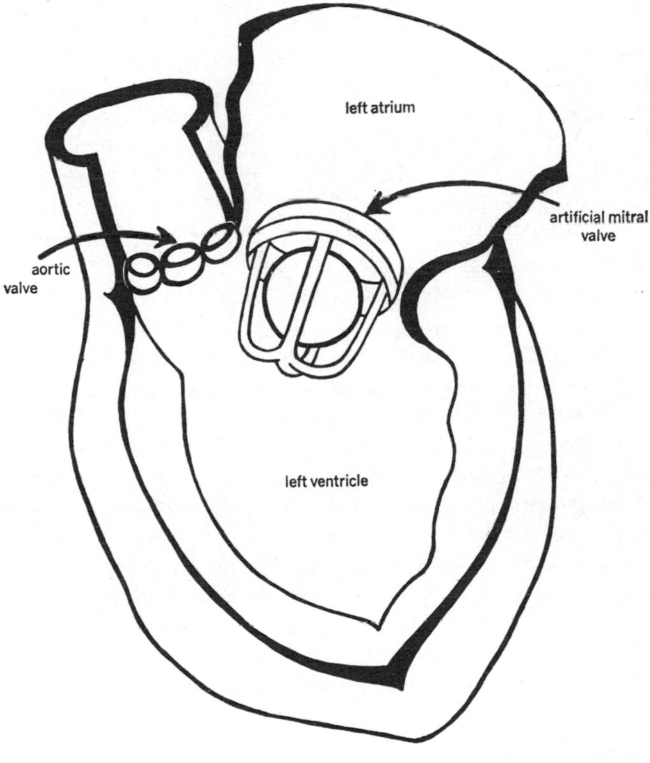

Artificial Valves

An artificial mitral valve of the ball and cage type. The patient's own valve has been replaced. The ball drops down when blood pressure builds in the left atrium, and blood flows easily into the ventricle. When the ventricle contracts, the ball is forced upwards and fits snugly into the cage, preventing backflow.

The aortic valve in the illustration is natural.

The two artificial mitral valves below are a disc valve (top) and a pivot disc valve (bottom).

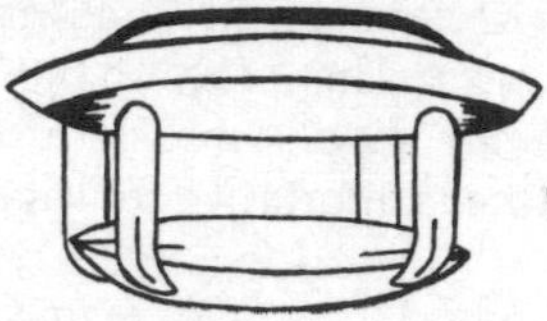

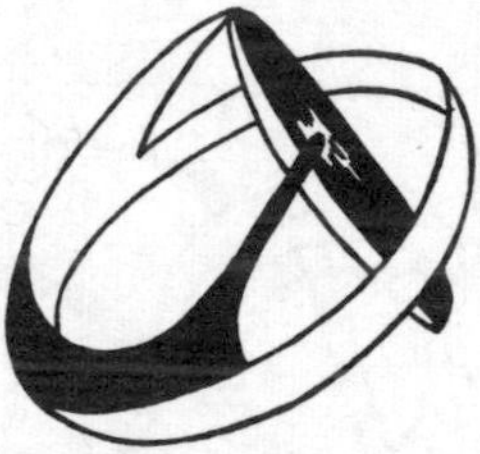

the valve and travel through the circulation. If one were to lodge in a blood vessel it would block it and can cause damage to the organ supplied by that vessel. That would be an embolus. If the organ was the brain or another vital structure it would be serious. Therefore patients with these valves are put on anti-coagulants so their blood is less likely to clot.

The medical profession has made progress in creating different materials which the body will accept. The material also must be able to withstand the wear and tear of almost continuous motion. Your heart beats about 100,000 times each day, and the ball valve must open and close each time against high pressure.

Recent valves have been developed that are much improved. In some, the metal parts have been covered with cloth. This has decreased the clotting problem. New types of metals and plastics are being used as well. Now we don't have to put all patients on anti-coagulants for the rest of their lives.

DR. FRANKLIN:
Reid R. was 51 when he came to us in 1969 for evaluation of a heart murmur. He recalled having "growing pains"

when he was twelve years old, but he had never had any heart symptoms until a few years ago.

Since then he had noticed a slight increase in shortness of breath especially when he lifted heavy weights, and worked long hours in the garden of his farmhouse in up-state Connecticut. In the summer of 1969, while spending a weekend at the farm, he woke up in the middle of the night with increased shortness of breath. He thought it was due to the dampness, and perhaps to fungus and mold. He sat up in bed and the symptoms gradually subsided. He was not unduly disturbed. But the following weekend he had a similar discomfort. At his wife's request, he went to see his physician, who referred him to us.

After taking a careful history, I came to the conclusion that his condition had worsened in the past year. He had a very responsible position, and so he had ignored it, and continued to work as hard. He had taken neither family nor friends into his confidence.

Cardiac catheterization showed aortic valvular disease, and surgery was advised. He thought for a while and said he'd call us the next day. He didn't talk with us directly, but left a message with the secretary that he was not prepared to go for surgery at this time. On a business trip in Ohio six months later, again he had shortness of breath, in spite of his program of medical treatment. He thought it was a result of traveling, and irregularity in food and sleep. However, he did see his own family physician on his return.

A few weeks later he had a respiratory infection. He developed increasing shortness of breath, even at complete rest. His heartbeat became irregular. He was now incapacitated.

Again he came around with medical treatment and even at this stage, he was not prepared for surgery. However, he was very faithful to his program of medication. He was readmitted to the hospital four months later, this time critically ill, severely short of breath, with evidence of failure on the right and left sides of the heart.

We urged him to consider surgery, and told him that without it, his life expectancy would not be more than one to two years. This time he agreed.

Because he was so highly motivated, he was fully active

three weeks after open-heart surgery for a single valve replacement. A year later, we got a card from him from the Bahamas: "Spending second honeymoon with my wife. I do feel younger and wish I had listened to you earlier."

We recently saw Reid in the office for a followup. He can swim approximately a half mile without getting fatigued, enjoys his work, and is no longer apprehensive when traveling. He is not worried about his heart. Because the valve is an artificial one, he has been on "blood thinning" medication (anti-coagulants).

There are three types of valve operations.

1. For the narrowed (stenotic) valve, which is not calcified and which is still freely movable. In this operation, the cusps of the valve, which stick to one another are separated either by cutting or are forced apart by the surgeon's finger, a mechanical dilator, or scalpel. This allows the valves to move more normally without obstructing the blood flow.
2. Valve replacement. When there is no other way to correct the patient's valve, it is cut out of the heart and replaced by a man-made substitute.
3. For the "leaking" valve. In a small number of cases, plastic surgery can be done on the patient's own valve to correct the leakage so that it closes tightly and does not leak.

Coarctation (constriction) of the aorta

To correct this condition, a narrowed segment of the aorta is cut out and the two healthy ends of the aorta are sewn together. If the narrowed segment is too long for the healthy ends to be brought together, a Dacron graft is put in to replace it.

Aortic aneurysm

Here the bulging portion of the aorta is removed surgically and healthy remaining ends are connected by a plastic sleeve, again usually of Dacron. This can be done for aortic aneurysms in the chest and in the abdomen.

The most common type of heart surgery today is the saphenous vein by-pass. Surgery on heart valves is next and congenital heart surgery probably the least frequent. This just happens to be an exact reversal in the way heart surgery began. The first successful heart operations were for congenital heart diseases (see page 302, chapter 23), later valve surgery, and only recently surgery for coronary heart disease.

Post-cardiotomy syndrome

DR. FRANKLIN:
The post-cardiotomy syndrome can appear anywhere from ten days to several months and even a year or two after heart surgery. The patient develops what seems like a viral infection. It is often attended by pleurisy, a sticking pain in the side that hurts when he breathes, and he may have fever.

This condition is thought to be due to a special virus. It happens, fortunately, to very few people. It always requires medical attention for diagnosis and treatment. Cortisone-type drugs are used in treatment. It has a tendency to recur, alternating in intensity, sometimes in a mild form, other times in a more severe form.

Lester Q., one of our patients, had this condition. A severe initial onset was preceded by a very mild premonitory syndrome. He was treated for several months with cortisone-like drugs and the dosage was gradually tapered down and then discontinued. It recurred in a very mild form at which time we put him back on the drugs. But every time we tried to withdraw drugs, he would have a return of symptoms in a mild form. We kept him on a low dosage of these drugs for a couple of years. We finally were able to taper off the dose and stop it completely. He recovered and is in good health.

Chapter 19

The future of cardiology

DRS. FRANKLIN, KRAUTHAMER and TAI:

We hope that a newspaper of the future will carry an article like this in its pages:

Dateline: The Future; Any Town, U.S.A.

John D. escaped a nearly fatal heart attack today. He awakened last night with severe chest pains and was resuscitated within three minutes at his home by a roving paramedical team.

Diagnosis of his heart condition was made by computer analysis while John was in transit to the hospital. Emergency removal of coronary blockage with a cardiac catheter was performed within five minutes of his arrival at the hospital at 4:00 A.M. John returned home at 3:00 this afternoon and expects to go back to work tomorrow.

When we interviewed John D. at his home this evening, he told us, "Everything happened so fast, I hardly had time to think about it. The paramedics told me I nearly died but I feel so good now it's hard to believe."

Review of John D.'s available records show that he saw his paramedic and doctor three days ago for "indigestion." Analysis of his symptoms were inconclusive, so the doctor attached monitoring equipment and a radio transmitter to him. The roving paramedics are automatically informed in such cases.

John D.'s alarm signal went off in the Central Monitoring Station at 3:30 A.M., even before he was awakened by his pain. The roving paramedics record their arrival time at his house at 3:33 A.M. His cardiac arrest occurred at 3:35 A.M. He was promptly defibrillated. Heart-preserving medication was injected at 3:36 A.M.

Hospital arrival is marked at 3:55 A.M. and coronary cleaning performed at 4:00 A.M. The patient, aged 48, is a machine operator. His father died at the age of 45 from a heart attack. John D. remembers his father died at home in his bed at night, after awakening with some chest pain. That was 25 years before the development of the equipment and techniques used today.

We believe these projections of the future will come to pass. But there is one piece of newsprint we would prefer to see:

Dateline: The Future; Any Town, U.S.A.

Hypertension and arteriosclerosis can be prevented.

The 25-year analysis by the Cardiovascular Institute has shown that the vaccine developed and administered by the research group is a success. Of the original 500 test cases, not a single instance of high blood pressure or arteriosclerosis has been reported among those who followed the prescribed program.

The original group consisted of 100 people in each 10-year age group, from 20–29 years through 60–69 years; the oldest patients were a group of 10 patients 69 years of age. Three hundred and eighty of the original group are still alive. Of the 120 who died, not one died of a heart attack, high blood pressure or its complications.

The vaccine was not attended by any complications.

The immediate goals in cardiology—the major areas to be conquered in the future—are these:

Arteriosclerosis

Much research attention is being given to prevention. Some studies have suggested that arteriosclerosis might be reversed with special diet, possibly with new medication.

We must find out a lot more about the importance of cholesterol and triglycerides and their relation to arteriosclerosis. We may pinpoint the precise cause of arteriosclerosis, and learn how to treat it.

The portable hospital

Today, some cities and towns already have mobile coronary care units that bring all of the expertise and vital equipment to the patient in his own home or even on the street. Such mobile cardiac units will become commonplace, and prevent many fatalities in acute heart attacks.

Telemetry

Telemetry in the hospital will help patients be up and around faster, with shorter recovery time. Some of this equipment is now in use. A patient need not stay in bed, fastened by wires to his oscilloscope. With a battery-powered transmitter, he can walk where he wishes while Intermediate Care nurses monitor his electrocardiogram, just as they do when he is in his bed.

The next step is to monitor him after he leaves the hospital. Today, wild animals in Yellowstone National Park have been equipped with radio collars that beam their location and heartbeat via Nimbus satellite for the study of their life habits. A heart patient, carrying a radio unit that monitors his heart, will in the future leave the hospital with a portable battery unit (not in a collar!) which will project the condition of his heart on a screen in the hospital. At an automatic signal, the hospital nurses will be alerted—*before* a heart accident—that the patient is about to suffer a reverse. He will be located wherever he is by a mobile ambulance unit for treatment before the heart attack or heart accident occurs. The heart gives warning. We should heed it.

We believe telemetry will be used on many patients, particularly high-risk individuals, outside the hospital, either before or after heart attacks. These patients will be monitored at home and at work with automatic alarm systems to warn of impending heart accidents. All heart patients will be equipped with portable telemetry units before they return to work. These units will send the patient's electrocardiogram signals from the unit he wears to a hospital receiving station, where they will be monitored by computer. If there are any irregularities of the heart, a warning would sound, alerting medical personnel and the patient. Research on this procedure is now going on and is at present workable. It will not only save lives but restore the heart patient's confidence in going back to work. It should increase dramatically the number of heart patients who will be able to return to their jobs.

"Walkie-talkies" for transmission of the electrocardiogram, blood pressure and other reports of the circulation should permit the patient to be examined by short wave while he is having his symptoms. The heart patient would receive even better care than the hospital bed patient receives today.

Survival kits

Patients with known heart conditions will learn new techniques to administer emergency treatment to themselves. We will have a "do-it-yourself" kit which will help the heart patient until professional help arrives. The United States government has already funded a drug company to make up such a kit, containing two emergency drugs. It will be initially distributed to research centers for testing.

Pacemakers

With time all essential components of a pacemaker may be miniaturized and inserted in a metal capsule small enough to be injected through an intravenous. It will be positioned in the heart with a magnet over the chest. A fluoroscope will be unnecessary and it will be done in the doctor's office. A transmitted telemetry signal will activate barbs within the capsule which will emerge and anchor it to the heart wall. Power beamed from central broadcasting stations will keep it going continuously—battery changes will be a thing of the past.

Cardiac arrhythmias

Most irregularities of the heartbeat can be controlled by medication. Many others require electrical devices called *cardioverters*.

Cardioversion today is used only by trained medical personnel. We believe special cardioverters will be made that patients will be able to use by themselves. The shock-dispensing cardioverter changes dangerous irregular heartbeats into normal and/or safe heartbeats. Scientists are now experimenting with automatic cardioverters triggered to correct cardiac arrythmia as soon as it starts.

Of patients who die from heart attacks almost 50 percent do so before they reach the hospital. This is because of electrical problems within the heart, ventricular fibrillation. An automatic cardioverter-defibrillator implanted in high-risk patients and triggered by the onset of the fibrillation is already under consideration.

Diagnosis of heart conditions

In place of cardiac catheterization, equipment applied outside the body will be developed to record precisely the stage of arteriosclerosis and other heart conditions.

High blood pressure

More curable causes of high blood pressure will be recognized. Medications will be developed that are more effective with less side effects. Early diagnosis and treatment of even mild high blood pressure will become the rule rather than the exception. Primary or "benign essential hypertension" of unknown cause, will be diagnosed and treated more precisely. The patterns that predispose some people to high blood pressure will be recognized and treated, stopping high blood pressure before it even begins.

The cardiologist

Doctor will be talking to computers and computers back to doctors. Diagnosis, care, treatment, medication and special procedures will "print out" as the cardiologist feeds data to the computer. We will be riding the crest of a fantastic information explosion, almost too much for the human mind to absorb. We expect the computer to be a necessity for the practice of high grade cardiology within the next ten years. It will lead to quicker diagnosis and better treatment.

Cardiac evaluations will probably be completed in less than a single day, perhaps within a few hours, without the patient being admitted to the hospital.

With simplified diagnosis, the family doctor will be better able to detect all heart conditions. The cardiologist will help with special procedures. Both will depend more heavily on the paramedics for the treatment. Less time will be spent on diagnosis, and more time explaining each patient's condition to him.

The non-doctor doctor

Paramedical technicians will be trained to handle many cardiac problems, complicated as well as simple. Computers will print out precise information for individual patient care, medication, diet, exercise program, and followup after release from the hospital.

Heart surgery and transplants

With every passing year, heart surgery improves remarkably. Artificial heart valves are becoming less complicated; the by-pass operation of blocked coronary arteries is becoming commonplace. 60,000 have already been performed in the United States. Heart transplants and artificial hearts will become equally successful.

Dr. Christiaan Barnard, as we know, performed the first heart transplant. The ensuing publicity was good for him but bad for medical science. Optimism concerning transplants soured. At present, there are perhaps four or five teams capable of doing a transplant, and caring for the patient afterwards. Problems arise, as physicians have learned from kidney transplant, the pioneer project in this new exciting field.

It is widely known that the problem with a transplant is usually rejection. Not only because blood groups but tissue groups are different. If they are mismatched, the body rejects them. Rejection can produce the same result as an acute heart attack and the patient can die.

To avoid rejection, the patient must take drugs. These drugs work by blocking the defense mechanism of the host. Patients therefore are susceptible not only to ordinary infections but to unusual ones. They must be kept in isolation and fed antibiotics while they are treated with drugs powerful enough to paralyze the immunological system.

The surgeon also cuts all sympathetic and para-sympathetic nerves. This means the recipient can experience no heart pain. As a result, if he gets a heart attack at some time in the future, he will have no warning pain. The best way to evaluate for trouble in a heart transplant is by stress testing. With recent improved methods of treatment, heart transplant patients have begun to survive for longer periods of time. As of this writing, the longest has been five years.

At Stanford University, Dr. Norman Shumway is at present improving the survival rate in his heart transplants. He and his associates are selecting good donors with young hearts, and are now putting their survivors on a low cholesterol diet or giving them a cholesterol-lowering drug.

The heart transplant patients who died previously (in spite of controls and drugs) died of coronary heart disease. In post-mortems, it was discovered that their coronary arteries were loaded with cholesterol.

Followup coronary arteriograms have been done on heart transplant patients who are doing well on cholesterol-lowering drugs and a strict low cholesterol diet. The studies have shown no increase in coronary artery disease. The research group feels that by controlling the cholesterol level, they are prolonging the lives of these patients. For how long, they don't know. But they have eliminated one major factor that was responsible for the death of transplant patients.

Heart transplant is still experimental, but once the rejection reaction is overcome, it may become a standard method of treatment for hearts that have been severely damaged by valve disorders, congenital heart disease, heart muscle disease (cardiomyopathy), and coronary heart disease.

The artificial heart

This is a realistic hope. It may take more than five to ten years to develop, but we will see it eventually. The major problems with present day models are heat, damage to the blood, size and the necessity of a portable power supply. These will have to be overcome before the artificial heart is more than an experiment or a short term helper.

It is anticipated that the nuclear heart will be generally available by 1980. This device simulates the real heart and will function like it. It has four chambers, valves, and is powered by nuclear energy which is stored in the device. The nuclear energy is adequate to allow it to work for a thousand years. We'll have to see what parts wear out first.

Heart surgery

The role of heart surgery in patient care and the way heart surgery is done will change in the future. As better medical treatments are developed, less heart surgery will be needed.

Some heart surgery will be simplified. It is probable that some will be done without opening the chest. At present, one form of heart surgery in newborn infants and children can be performed by a modification of heart catheterization technique. It reduces the risk to the patient dramatically.

Tomorrow's diet

We expect artificial foods to be developed. These will have the good taste of the high cholesterol-high carbohydrate diet while contributing to the health, rather than the downfall of the potential cardiac victim. An artificial egg preparation is already on the market containing only 1 mgm. of cholesterol compared to the more than 200 mgm. in an ordinary egg yolk. There are other such products available, including a cheese, with low fat content.

We do not know what part new foods will play in the diet of the future in terms of prevention and treatment. But if people can be re-educated to use what we already know about diet, exercise and prevention, and if we can lick the inherited gene, there is hope that our children will be free of today's foremost killer. In the following chapters we will talk about what each person can do for himself.

PART V

WHAT THE PATIENT DOES

Chapter 20

Exercise and return to action

DR. TAI:
The dozen men pedaling their bicycles through the park are as unlikely a group as you'll ever see together outside of a far-out movie. The broad-beamed white-haired fellow in sweat shirt and shorts may look like the warden of Sing Sing, but he is actually the general manager of a six-billion-dollar mutual fund. The dark-haired man with handsome features and the shadow of a retreating beer belly is a local plumber. The others range from section manager at a local department store to a podiatrist who is also an authority on geriatrics. A wide range of men who pedal with expressions that vary from smiles to stoic determination. And in their faces, sunburned and ruddy, you catch the look of men who have glimpsed the other shore.

They are victims of serious coronary heart disease.

They are dedicated members of a cardiac exercise group which is part of a program for prevention, post-care and rehabilitation.

We hear so much about the negative aspects of heart disease that we fail to appreciate the positive side. Patients —and their families—are usually surprised to learn that they can restore themselves to a state of reasonable health, well-being and dignity. If anyone robs a man of these reachable goals, he robs him of his reason for living.

Work is included, along with diet and exercise, in any overall restoration program. We have found an almost euphoric, and certainly a therapeutic, value in having our patients go back to work.

Let us tell you about Sal D. Through hard work and a reputation for integrity in dealing with his clients, he had built his plumbing business from a one-man operation to a big organization that installs plumbing equipment in large office buildings and housing complexes.

Sal never allowed business to swallow him completely. As a hobby, he did ballroom dancing, an art in which he and his wife are nearly professional.

One Saturday afternoon, he went to visit his aging mother in a nursing home. As he sat in the waiting room, he became aware of an acute chest pain and broke into a sweat. A nurse saw his discomfort, called the physician, and he was taken to a nearby hospital. His own general practitioner took care of him and finally told him, "Sal, you have a severe heart condition. You must not go back to business. If you want to live, you've got to retire. You may need a heart operation."

Sal agreed, submitting to his doctor's decree and the emotional pressures of his family. But he was dejected. This man who had always had a lusty appetite for living was suddenly condemned to a form of life that to him was no better than death.

He was referred to us. I did the evaluation. The coronary arteriograms showed that one of his three coronary arteries was completely blocked, but the other two were wide open. He should have had a large heart attack, but fortunately, he had collaterals coming from the two open vessels, feeding the blocked one. He had had chest pains but not a heart attack. Instead of heart surgery, we recommended a program of cardiac rehabilitation and then return to his work full time.

Before setting up his exercise program, a treadmill stress test was done. He tolerated 2½ minutes of mild exercise before he complained of chest pains and the ECG showed changes. An exercise program was prescribed for him. Initially, long slow walks, the pace gradually to be increased, as well as a stationary bicycle regimen.

After three months he could walk at a rapid pace on the treadmill for 12 minutes without chest pain or change in his ECG. I was able to calculate his energy expenditure and determine when he would be ready to return to office work. I felt he could start dancing again.

The news delighted Sal, and he continued to carry out our rehabilitation suggestions with enthusiasm. And most important for his sense of well-being, he was able to take his wife dancing again. He learned how to protect himself. If he begins to suffer chest pain while he and his wife are on the dance floor, he leans against her, maintains the rhythm and slips a nitroglycerine tablet under his tongue. When the pain subsides, he begins moving again. And he always rests between dances. He has improved so remarkably that now he can put in a day's work in his office and go dancing from eight to midnight.

When Sal felt normal again, this discipline began to lapse. He began to find excuses for skipping his exercise. "I haven't got all that time for walking—there's an early morning appointment at the office," he'd say to his wife. Or, "I'm taking a few days rest from that damn bike."

He can get away with it for a while. But then the chest pains recur more easily because of his reduced exercise tolerance. Once he goes back on the program, his activity level is restored. I have been seeing him now for three years and his condition remains stable.

The more you exercise to reasonable capacity, the better your heart will function.

Then there's Charles S., tall and lean, who is careful about his diet, exercises conscientiously, but is cardiac prone. He is in a high-pressure job and woke one morning with severe chest pains—acute myocardial infarction. His recovery afterwards was uneventful, but neither his friends nor other physicians helped his state of mind by telling him to retire.

"What is your advice?" he asked us.

We believe that the purpose of rehabilitation is to return the man to his functional capacity.

His cardiac catheterization showed one vessel was blocked, the other two clean.

"You can return to full-time work. We will set up a program for you."

He embarked on an exercise program and became able to do a mile in fourteen minutes. He now can run from three to five miles every day and at 49 years of age, has normal exercise tolerance. He should continue this for the rest of his life.

As long as he continues the exercise program and his arteriosclerosis does not progress, he can continue working.

DR. FRANKLIN:

I recently checked a man who came in and insisted he was in the best of health, though his doctor was concerned about a recent collapse. At 55, Eric R. looked ten years older. He was thirty pounds overweight. After doing his physical and taking his history, I spent an hour with him discussing his condition. But we were not communicating.

"'I'm in great shape," Eric said bluntly. "And I'll tell you something. I'm not gonna cut out the booze, and the steaks and the broads. This is the way I want to live. And if I die a little sooner, what the hell. You come through this way only once. You might as well enjoy it."

It was impossible to get him to take further tests or to change his mind. Of course, he was going on the assumption that he could live as he chose. He wasn't interested in finding out whether a heart attack might jeopardize his life. He would not listen. We have talked to such men before who have had a first attack and a second, all the while chipping away at the heart muscle, damaging it more and more with additional smaller or larger attacks, some symptomatic, some non-symptomatic, until their lives become extremely limited—cardiac cripples. That kind of life would be torment for Eric R. The end result is not always sudden death, but may be a gradual and progressive disability that leads to a very uncomfortable end.

Eric was a difficult man to treat. He secretly believed himself invulnerable. Yet he was typically coronary prone, and would do nothing to help himself.

Physically fit people are less subject to heart attack than those in poor physical condition. Many patients who have recovered from heart attacks embark on an exercise program, under a physician's care, that will strikingly improve their health.

Regular and increasing levels of exercise also give the

patient a renewed sense of pride and strength and a sense of well-being, which in turn helps him to maintain control over his weight.

Old habits are discarded, new habits taken on, and after a while the new habits became ingrained.

"I used to growl about walking," a patient told us. "I'd take a car down to the corner newsstand for a pack of cigarettes and a paper. But after walking became a habit, I've gotten to like it. Even on the golf course, I don't use a cart."

We tell our patients: Any activity that involves pleasurable exertion is good, just as long as it doesn't prove severely tiring. Walking is great. The more, the better. A healthy person should easily walk at the rate of three miles an hour. Even in our cardiac patients, we strive for the twenty-minute mile and go on from there. It's very good exercise.

In physical conditioning, we are trying to interest parents in teaching their kids to be physically active every day.

Every kid gets ample exercise, playing with his friends. But if you can get him interested in a regular daily exercise program, either aerobic calisthenics, jogging, running, riding a bike, you are helping to insure his coronary vessels and future health. Once an exercise schedule becomes part of his daily life, much as washing and brushing his teeth, it is apt to carry over into his adult years.

It will help him to better tolerate a heart attack should it ever strike him. And the onset of coronary heart disease symptoms are delayed in a physically active person.

People who were active children, particularly in sports such as long distance running, seem to have larger coronary arteries than their peers who were more sedentary. The *New England Journal of Medicine* ran an interesting autopsy report of a man who died in his 90s. He had participated in the annual Boston Marathon for nearly all of his adult life. He was reported to have had absolutely huge coronary arteries. They were so large that it would have taken a great amount of arteriosclerotic material to block them off. The highly active youngster, therefore, may be insuring himself of a healthy maturity by exercise that enlarges the coronary arteries.

However, an adult over 40 years of age and perhaps

thirty pounds overweight, should not go into a reconditioning program before he has a medical examination. We feel this must include a resting and exercise electrocardiogram, so that a man with a potentially hazardous condition is not thrown into a rigorous exercise program.

If both his exercise cardiogram and physical checkup are normal, he can then go into a graduated exercise program. Minor activities at first, building up to the more stressful ones. This program should be initiated on a daily basis, or at least five days a week. After he becomes physically conditioned, which means that *his pulse does not rise excessively when he exerts himself and comes back to resting level three minutes after he stops his exercise,* he can go on a three-day-per-week exercise program, and he will remain physically fit.

Exercise that uses the legs is better than that using the arms.

Swimming? An excellent sport that involves use of both arms and legs.

Weight lifting is fine for the "healthy" person, not good for the cardiac patient.

"Skip isometrics," we tell our cardiac patients. "That is tension against tension without producing motion." Think of it as a compression kind of exercise, with one side pushing against the other side, and the heart is stuck in the middle. This kind of exercise has a great tendency to raise the blood pressure. Elevated blood pressure places an excess workload on the heart which isn't good. We recommend aerobics. This form of exercise produces motion with less tension through the use of large muscle groups.

Carpentry is a good hobby. You are using gross movements. You are moving around, lifting things—a feeling of creativity is an added bonus.

Gardening is great. You stoop, you bend, you dig. There is tension and motion as a result of tension—this again is aerobics.

DR. TAI:

Six of our male patients were sitting in the doctors' conference room, discussing the cardiac exercise program.

"Doctor, just what do you mean by *cardiac* rehabilitation?" Ken F. asked. "How can you rehabilitate a scarred piece of your heart?" Ken was convalescing after a mild coronary and expected to be discharged from the hospital by the end of the week.

I chuckled, "You're right Ken. We don't rehabilitate a piece of scarred muscle. By cardiac rehabilitation we mean a program that rehabilitates the cardiac patient. An exercise schedule tailored to your physical capacity and structured within the limits of your cardiac status. Exercise to improve that status. Education in proper eating habits, emotional support, and answers for the many questions you have as you return to your roles as wage earners, fathers and husbands."

"Who are candidates for this?" Monte L. asked.

"All of you," I said. "Patients with angina. Those who've had a myocardial infarction, and sometimes those with other forms of heart disease. Especially patients who are suspected of having coronary artery disease, even though we don't have definite documentation, or are incapacitated for psychological reasons."

"Doctor," Ken asked, "how can we join this program?"

"The patient's doctor is the ideal person to screen him and recommend the program."

"But almost everybody who's had a heart attack or is suffering from coronary artery disease could benefit from such a program," Carroll B., an older, white-haired man, said. His mottled skin suggested that he had been incapacitated for some time, but his eyes had a glint of stubbornness.

"Yes. It is also a general physical fitness program. The normal adult population can take advantage of this regimen. Your wife and children, for instance."

I stood up and went over to one of the charts that was on an easel.

"Let's see how we measure the ability of the heart to work and its reserve capacity. The body uses foodstuffs, especially carbohydrates, to produce energy and keep things going. To convert the carbohydrates into energy we need oxygen as well. By measuring how much oxygen is used by the body we can accurately determine how much energy the body needs. This energy is measured in terms of heat production by the body—calories are really units of heat.

When resting, the body normally needs 250 cubic centimeters (about one cup) of oxygen each minute. This in turn produces 1.3 calories of heat. So the resting person needs one cup of oxygen to make 1.3 calories each minute.

"Physiologists, to make all these numbers easier to work with, have developed the Metabolic Equivalent Unit—the MET. One MET is equal to 1.3 calories in one minute. Or putting it another way, at rest the body uses one MET per minute.

"During exercise we use energy and need more oxygen. If oxygen consumption doubles (2 cups of oxygen per minute) the energy cost of that exercise is 2 METs per minute. Now we have a system we can use in relating different physical activities to one another and their energy cost to the body.

I explained how exercise testing on the treadmill or bicycle ergometer makes it possible to measure a person's exercise capacity. The energy cost (MET) of nearly all common activities—leisure, sport, work—is available and can then be correlated with an individual's tolerance as found by the testing (see Appendix B).

"Hasn't this principle something to do with aerobics?" Ken asked. He had been doing aerobic exercise before his heart attack.

"It has. In aerobic exercise there is a balance of oxygen supply and the demand of the body. It has been demonstrated in physical fitness programs that a trained athlete has a capacity of 20 METs per minute, while a healthy, but untrained young man can only generate 12 METs per minute in aerobic exercise."

"How does this fit in with the New York Heart Association classifications?" Monte wanted to know. He knew that he was in Class II (see Appendix A), and he was already busy with plans for his rehabilitation.

"If you're in New York Heart Association Class I, your capacity is in the range of 6 to 9 METs per minute. That means you can undertake all physical activities except participation in competition.

"For Class II, the maximum expenditure is 4.5 METs, as long as it doesn't produce distress.

"For Class III, it is 3 METs.

"For Class IV, it ranges from 1.0 to 1.5 METs maximum."

I explained exercise testing on the treadmill or bicycle ergometer makes it possible to measure the aerobic capacity. That is, the ability of energy expenditure can be shown and a specific exercise program can be prescribed.

When patients are confined to bed, their physical fitness deteriorates, even though they were fit prior to their enforced bedrest. The myocardial insult can make the situation even worse. So in our patients with heart attacks, the rehabilitation program, if properly instituted, improves the performance of the heart and builds up reserve strength for more normal living.

"Just how does exercise help?" Ken asked. He had always been a great walker, which kept him thin, but like many midwesterners, he was partial to ham and eggs and marbleized beef, which had contributed to his dangerously high cholesterol level.

"Strangely enough, if you exercise on a regular schedule and have a regular program, your heart rate *becomes slower* and your blood pressure *lower*. Because this happens, the oxygen need of the heart is reduced. The heart is able to function more effectively with less oxygen supply."

The half dozen men, ranging in age from forty to seventy, listened intently, knowing that their future might depend on what we were discussing. Even Monte, who had been depressed by finding himself back in the hospital for his second heart attack, looked less glum and nodded whenever we stressed a point which seemed pertinent to his case.

"This is our plan, gentlemen," I said. "We feel that this program should be started in each case shortly after the patient's admission to the Coronary Care Unit for treatment of a heart attack. Once he is stable, we begin with passive movement of his limbs. Several days later, some walking at a predetermined pace. This could be started on patients outside the hospital who have angina and who have not had a myocardial infarction. In patients who have recovered from heart attacks and are convalescing, the exercise capacity should be measured sometime before they leave the hospital.

"This exercise evaluation must be done by a physician knowledgeable in cardiology.

"After hospitalization, a meeting place is chosen for your exercise group. It's the same idea as Weight Watchers and

Alcoholics Anonymous. In an open session the patients are able to direct their questions to the physicians who explain the program's goals. Each group is limited to about twenty people. The physicians are part of the team which participates in the exercise program. They teach patients how to condition themselves and work better with the least oxygen available."

"How soon after a heart attack can you join such a program?" The young man who asked was in the hospital with anginal symptoms. He was already on a 1,000-calorie diet program that had in ten days subtracted eight pounds from his ample body.

"About three months after an episode of a transmural myocardial infarction. Earlier in a subendocardial (non-transmural) infarction. And even earlier for you, Paul, once you lose more weight."

I explained that the program was effective for patients with stable angina and then listed the types of patients who would be advised not to join the program.

Among them: patients with severe rheumatic heart disease or certain congenital heart problems. Patients with unstable angina or uncontrollable hypertension. Patients with recent transmural myocardial infarctions. Or pre-infarction angina. Patients on a drug program with electrolyte imbalance. Patients with congestive heart failure and ventricular aneurysm. Patients with known arrhythmia problems. A patient with premature heart beats at rest should not embark on an exercise program unless he is completely checked out by his own physician. If during this exercise program, extra heartbeats are noted and they become more frequent or in multiples, he should drop out of the program. And it doesn't matter whether these beats are picked up when the person is taking his pulse or whether he senses the palpitations and confirms it by the pulse.

"Exercise should be undertaken five times a week. A short period of exercise followed by rest in repeated cycles of three minutes each, to tolerance, for a period of 15 to 30 minutes. With time and proven tolerance, continuous exercise periods of 15 to 30 minutes may be followed only three times a week.

"The patient should be tested for improvement or

deterioration in his function by stress testing on a treadmill or bicycle approximately three to six months after the beginning of his program.

"We start the exercise program according to the patient's condition. We exercise-test all patients before prescribing for them, but this isn't always possible. Therefore, we divide our cases in two groups, those who have not been exercise-tested, and those who have been exercise-tested.

"The key to our rehabilitation program is the pulse rate. Each of you will be taught to take your own pulse. As your rehabilitation program goes along, you will be informed of certain 'target rates' that are specific for your condition.

"The target rate will change as you go along. We calculate the target rate for you either from the results of your exercise test or from a table of values appropriate to your condition if you haven't been tested.

"There is a table called 'Maximal Predicted Heart Rate for Age' (MPRA). The values on this table are adjusted for age and note the fastest rate a normal heart can safely tolerate.

"In youngsters—teenagers and younger—this rate is about 220 beats per minute. Once you pass the age of twenty, this rate decreases.

"You can count the beats by feeling your carotid, which is a blood vessel in the neck. Calculate your own maximal predicted rate simply by subtracting your age—in years—from 220. But none of you in this room has a normal heart. Therefore, we must talk about allowable percentages of the MPRA for each of you. To be on the safe side, we readjust the MPRA using 200 rather than 220 minus the age.

"For those we cannot exercise-test, we allow 60 percent of the adjusted MPRA during the first six weeks of reconditioning."

I picked up the chart of one of the patients.

"Jack, you are fifty years old. Let's calculate your target rate. Two hundred minus 50 equals 150. Sixty percent of 150 is 90. Therefore, during the first six weeks of convalescence, you shouldn't do anything that makes your pulse go faster than 90 beats per minute. After that, if your condition allows, you may go to a pulse rate equal to 70 percent of your adjusted Maximal Predicted Heart Rate for Age (MPRA)."

"About 105 beats per minute," Jack calculated.

"Exactly," I said. "For those of you who can be exercise-tested, we don't use the charts except to know what your MPRA should be. We don't like to let any heart patient push his pulse rate beyond 90 percent of that. For those of you who can be tested, we talk about a 'Critical Heart Rate.' This is the pulse rate at which you develop angina symptoms or certain ECG signs of your heart condition.

"We then allow you to exert yourself to 70 to 75 percent of the Critical Heart Rate and feel safe in that range. Furthermore, by exercise testing, we can tell you how many METs you can safely tolerate.

"We have a chart (see Appendix B) that you can refer to which tells you what household, recreational and vocational activities correspond to your METs rating. You can then go directly to doing these things and simply double check your pulse to make sure you're not over-extending yourself.

"Each exercise program is preceded by a warmup period of calisthenics, followed by your individual program."

Isometrics are bad for the heart patient. Aerobics are good for him. Isometrics set the force of one muscle against another, for weight lifting, pushups or pullups. Isometrics have a greater tendency to increase blood pressure and the need for oxygen.

Aerobics involve motion without tension. Exertion comes from movement, rather than fighting resistance. Consequently, there is less rise in blood pressure.

Exercises that produce the least amount of tension are the best for a continuing program. Slow walking, slow bicycling (particularly on an exercise bike with low tension), arm exercises. As the exertional program progresses, the walking pace can be increased, the bike rate can be increased with a change of tension. The patient can progress to jogging or to fast pedaling on the bike, within the limitations of his tolerance.

Exercises which extend or bend the arm several times per minute produce mild degrees of exertion. They can be done standing, sitting or lying down. If leg exercises are done lying down, they produce slightly more exertion than that required for arm exertion, as long as the person doesn't get into the inverted bicycling position, which puts too much of a strain on the heart.

The next series of exertional activities involve truncal movements: rotating the hips, or bending at the waist to touch the toes. Then leg exercises, standing up, or seated, or propped up by one's arms and swinging the legs back and forth. And finally, deep knee bends, and the like.

After a patient reaches a good level of physical condition, he can determine his progress by any changes in his exercise tolerance. If there is a significant decrease, it is a signal for him to see his doctor.

The patient who knows the background of his heart condition, its characteristics, dangers and complications is in a better position to engineer his future without creating any new problems.

The charts for diet, exercise and work tolerance should be obtained from the physician who is caring for him.

Do's and don'ts for travel and vacation

DR. KRAUTHAMER:
Why is it that so many of our heart patients long to climb the Swiss Alps or ski in Aspen? Why can't they choose tranquil sea level spots like Southern Pines or Sea Island for their travel and vacations?

Ortego J., a patient of ours, who has at 77 lived through two heart attacks, telephoned us one day with the casual announcement that he was off to mountainous Chile, to look after his mining interests.

"Hold it," we said, describing exertion in high altitudes, but he took off anyway. He suffered a third myocardial infarction in Santiago, but bounced back, lively and chipper. When we chided him, he responded briskly that he'd rather wear out than rust out and the life of "sittin', starin' and rockin' " was definitely not for him. Ortego has a talent for not hearing what doesn't appeal to him. He is too busy trying to outsmart the Chilean government on tin mines, and he might make it through another attack, but he probably won't. A vacation should be a restful change, not an endurance contest.

Tom D. suffered his first heart attack at 46. He was a big fellow from Montana, who spent most of his life supervising the construction of a network of Federal highways. A heart attack put an end to his outdoor work. He had saved enough money so that it wasn't necessary for him to find a job right away. Throughout their married life, his wife, a totally feminine woman, had dreamed of the time that she and Tom would travel together around the world. Now was the time.

They pored over travel folders intrigued with the photographs of gay, fun-loving young and handsome couples. The fantasy world.

The fantasy world of new places and new people can be the heart patient's if he follows his own tolerance schedule. Tom and his wife Elise signed up for one airline's fabulous Group Tours.

"The only trouble is that it may be too much for Tom," Elise said to us. "He goes overboard once he's interested. How can we moderate the trip so that he gets only the good and not the fatigue?"

During a consultation, we worked out a schedule.

"You'll be going by plane," we said. "You should tolerate air travel quite well. You can arrange for extra oxygen on board by checking with the airline medical director or the airline itself.

"During a flight, every passenger has some anxiety. The airline stewardesses pacify the anxiety by feeding you. If you go first class, you'll have a problem. You can eat and drink yourself into a coma."

We warned him that in spite of new places, new experiences, new foods, he was to follow the rules for his post-heart-attack life.

We could not help being apprehensive while they were gone. A series of postcards with mountains, valleys and Greek ruins marked their itinerary. Since none came from a hospital, we were assured that all was going well.

On their return, Tom came in for his checkup, deeply tanned, less five pounds and with a jaunty manner.

"He followed all your directions," Elise reported with pride, "juice when drinks were served and at dinner, he skipped rolls, butter and dessert. Instead of jamming into the group bus, when he was tired, we splurged on taxis to and from our hotel. Instead of going out, sometimes we called Room Service. Tom always took naps while I unpacked. We decided that the trip to Versailles by bus was worth taking, but that afternoon we stayed at a little inn after lunch and they let Tom lie down in a small sitting room. We saw nearly as much as most of our companions on the tour, but we paced ourselves." In four weeks, they had visited Paris, London, Rome, and the Greek Islands.

"Paris is for walkers and that's how Tom got all his exercise. If he grew tired, we stopped at an outdoor cafe. You know, it was really easier for him to follow his new way of living on the trip than at home."

Not all patients are able to control themselves as well as this couple.

The recent travel trend is to herd forty to fifty people on a chartered bus, and feed them rich lunches and dinners at first-class hotels. The goal of the guide, following instructions from the tour office, is to give his charges what they have been promised: six countries in two weeks and as many miles and sights as their endurance will allow. It's rush, eat, pack, unpack, pack.

About half of our patients are able to travel without problems. Nevertheless, for the patient who has had a heart condition, a few reminders are essential:

1. Know how much you can do without symptoms appearing and don't exceed it. Have full knowledge of your condition, so you can discuss it with a strange doctor, in case you run into problems.

2. Carry a summary of your condition with you. It will be a great help if you need medical attention. If your electrocardiogram is abnormal, carry a copy with you. Some patients wear an identification bracelet or dogtag on a chain around their necks, with the red caduceus, and on the reverse side, their illness or condition engraved.

3. If taken sick, contact the American Embassy or Consulate. The International Association for Medical Assistance to Travelers has a directory of English-speaking physicians around the world.

4. Carry a small medical kit with all your medications,

as well as routine travel pills for headache, upset stomach, etc. Take enough for the whole trip, plus a little more in case an emergency detains you.

5. Know your diet. When you are hungry, eat small portions, just enough to tide you over. Don't indulge in a heavy meal while sightseeing. Instead, skip food and have a small meal on your return to your lodgings.

6. During sightseeing tours, particularly on buses, don't force yourself to join the crowd. If tired, let the crowd trot off without you. Remain seated in the empty, air-conditioned bus. Rest. If determined to see a particular site, go back later in a taxi. It's cheaper than getting sick. Even healthy people become ill on tours, and must sacrifice some good times occasionally.

On a formal tour, stick to your own schedule, based on your own sense of well-being. If the morning is tiring, forego the afternoon's sightseeing. Travel agencies are elastic in their arrangements. As a cardiac patient you need only to explain your problem, and they will accommodate you.

7. Commercial airliners are pressurized to an equivalent of at least 7,500 feet. People with heart conditions can tolerate this altitude at rest, as long as they aren't overly anxious or upset. But get some activity on the airliner. Get up every hour or two, to keep the blood from stagnating, particularly in your legs. Wiggling your toes is no help, since their muscles are predominantly located below ankle. Flap the whole foot back and forth at ankle level, exercising the large muscles in the leg. This simulates walking; leg muscles work on the veins and act as a peripheral pump, squeezing the blood out of the veins so it can be recirculated.

If during an air flight, you experience chest pains or other indication of heart trouble, take care of yourself as you would at home. Some airliners will have oxygen for you if you need it. Never be afraid or ashamed of asking. Ring for the stewardess for help.

8. Stop frequently when traveling by automobile. Long stretches of driving on thruways can result in an ailment called "turnpike phlebitis." Commercial truck drivers, who drive anywhere from twelve to fourteen hours without a break, are particularly sensitive to this

affliction. Driving in one position for many hours can lead to blood clots and phlebitis, particularly the veins of the legs.

9. Cruises are ideal for the heart patient, no flights to catch, no buses to fret about, no missed connections to raise your blood pressure. Stewards are usually helpful. Prior to the trip, write to the catering department of the cruise line and explain your diet requirements so that they can be sure to put aboard any special foods you may need. Once aboard the ship, arrange with the chief steward for your special diet. On a cruise, there can be many temptations for the cardiac patient; sightseeing on shore, over-eating, pre-dinner cocktail parties, rich food, a busy social atmosphere and late nights. As a cardiac patient, you can't let your guard down.

10. Vacationing in high altitude places such as Denver, Mexico City, the Swiss or Italian Alps, can have complications. The patient's exercise tolerance is decreased because there is less oxygen in the air.

A person who already has some inadequacy of blood supply to the heart muscle may suffer from the decreased concentration of oxygen in the blood (hypoxemia) that develops in high altitudes.

It makes a lot more sense for the cardiac patient to choose a vacation spot close to sea level.

11. Hot and cold climates: If traveling in an extremely warm climate, remember that the hours between 11 A.M. and 3 P.M. are the hottest and can cause physiologic stress. Tour either in the early morning or late afternoon. Follow the pattern of the natives who appreciate the hazards of their climate.

It's just the opposite on a jaunt to the Land of the Midnight Sun and fjords. In Norway, Sweden and Denmark, the warmest part of the day is between 11 and 3, and that's when you should be sightseeing. Stay inside during the cold mornings and evenings.

12. Taking children along is a dubious idea. Anxiety adds a burden to your heart, whether you are on vacation or at home. Disputes over where to go, what to see, when, often arise. An explosive scene is enough to send the cardiac patient back to CCU, if he gets there at all. We see it happen all the time.

13. If walking a good deal, go where the footing is firm and easy. Avoid long walks in soft sand, deep snow, mud, or water above your ankles.

DR. KRAUTHAMER:
One of the most encouraging factors today is that when a man suffers a heart attack and is rehabilitated, there may be state agencies that can give him concrete plans for a new kind of work.

Peter G., a man of 39, was employed at one of our local factories, which has a reputation for excellent employee relations. He smoked a pack and a half of cigarettes a day; he was a heavy beer drinker; he was overweight; he had a family history of heart disease. In 1969, he came to our office, complaining of chest pains. His family doctor had notified his employer that Peter now was totally disabled because of a heart attack. He was shattered, for he had a family of nine, and pride would not allow him to go on welfare.

After I did a complete cardiac evaluation, we were convinced Peter was perfectly capable of returning to work, but his old company wouldn't hire him, nor would any other firm.

We put him on an exercise treadmill. At the end of five minutes, he complained of chest pains. But he went into the exercise program and worked at it. Now he does thirty minutes of exercise without any chest pains and he runs five miles in an hour.

We wrote the State Rehabilitation Department about his unfair plight, and he was evaluated by them. He was given a financial grant and after a period of study, he became a dental assistant, and he is now completely self supporting.

Peter had been terrified because he had had a heart attack; it took time on our part to build up his self-confidence so he could begin a new kind of work and remain the head of his large family.

DR. FRANKLIN:
There is a difference between clinical medicine and insurance medicine.

In clinical medicine, a doctor sees the patient and makes a judgment from his physical presence.

In insurance medicine, judgment is made from reports sent to the insurance company and insurance is either given or denied on the statistical analysis of that information.

The life insurance company has built up a wealth of statistics based on how long the average normal person should live. They know, for instance, how long a normal 5-year-old should live beyond his fifth birthday. They know how long a 30-year-old should live beyond his thirtieth birthday.

Individuals who have had heart disease may be faced with an increased risk of death at their age level. The insurance company has been able to compute how much greater than normal is the risk of death in various diseases. They express their findings in terms of percentages. The risk of death in a certain illness may be 150 percent of normal, or even 200 percent of normal, or 300 percent or even 500 percent. In this way, they can pro-rate the cost of insurance to an individual based on his own risk compared to the normal expected rate of 100 percent.

If he is 100 percent, he receives an insurance rate normal for his age. If his risk is 200 percent, his insurance premium is greater. Beyond a certain percentage, he is uninsurable. The company won't give him a policy at any price.

It isn't surprising therefore, that the cardiac patient will be offered a different insurance cost than his healthy neighbor.

Certain illnesses are totally curable. Patients with a congenital illness, such as inter-atrial septal defect, that has been corrected, will be insurable without increased risk or premium. But if they have developed enlargement of the heart, abnormal ECGs, abnormal blood pressure, or permanent heart damage, they may remain at a higher premium rate despite the fact that they had a total surgical correction of their illness.

Patients with valvular heart disease aren't so fortunate. Even after surgery, they are not in the normal insurance risk level, no matter how successful the surgery may be.

People with coronary heart disease are also rated in keeping with the size of the heart, the ECG changes, clinical symptoms and the presence of myocardial infarction. The longer a patient with coronary heart disease carries on, following a heart attack, without symptoms and without additional ECG or X-ray changes, the less costly his insurance premium will be.

If he is alive and well fifteen years after a myocardial infarction, some insurance companies may accept him at no increased risk.

There is no standard approach to these illnesses by the insurance companies. But insurance companies have evaluated various features related to the heart: blood pressure, ECG changes, heart size, irregularity of the heart beat, heart murmur, etc. Each factor contains a "risk" associated with it based on statistics that have been carefully drawn. If you happen to have one of these findings, it does not necessarily mean you have a severe or critical heart condition. However, it does mean that you fall into a category of an increased insurance risk for which the insurance company feels it must charge you extra.

The insurance company is not your doctor and does not handle you in a manner similar to the way a physician would. The insurance company is an insurer and must place a risk on certain patterns of information it receives. It is these patterns that determine your insurance rate.

Chapter 21

Diets for survival

DR. TAI:
"We're meeting here today to talk about getting rid of calories you'll never miss. But most important, we will talk to you about what you should eat so you won't damage your heart further."

The six women patients meeting with me in the doctors' library of the hospital all had heart disease and all were about to be discharged. Before they departed for home, I wanted to discuss food with them. Not diet as diet, but how they could create new eating habits which would mean literally a new life style as well as the loss of extra pounds.

On the end of the sofa sat Edwina L., who was 59 years old and twenty pounds overweight. She had diabetes and recently had developed chest pains which, we had discovered, indicated the onset of angina. Her resting ECG was normal, she had intermittent high blood pressure. Her treadmill test was abnormal. She was catheterized and found to have a severe narrowing in one coronary artery and moderate narrowing in the remaining two. She was lucky to have good collateral vessels, so we could treat her with a medical program, which includes medication, exercise, and diet, rather than surgery. But she would have to follow the rules to improve her chances.

Sitting beside her were two young women, both tense and nervous, both suffering from valve disease but not yet needing valve surgery. The other three women, seated around a small table, were post-menopausal. The drop in estrogen hormones, combined with high blood pressure, made them vulnerable to heart attacks. Avery R., wife of a local judge, was fiercely fighting weight. Beulah F. was principal of a private business school, a victim of angina and stress. Maisie, a Texas woman whose husband was on the board of directors of half a dozen corporations, had blood pressure up in the danger range, even after an hour's rest.

All were diet-conscious. Most of them had tried out the "miracle diets," and two had had sensational weight losses, but found themselves fat-bound again in six months.

My object was to explain the mechanics of body chemistry not always included in diet books. Although my partners and I had discussed with them their individual cholesterol or triglyceride levels, I felt it important to go over this again.

"Living with your diet won't be so difficult," I said, "if you learn the danger of too much cholesterol or triglycerides in your blood. We all have a normal amount but four of you make more cholesterol or triglycerides than is good for you. We don't know the reason—it may be genetic. Studies suggest that both cholesterol and triglycerides contribute to a buildup of plaque which can block coronary arteries. People with high cholesterol levels are likely to get coronary artery disease at an earlier age and in a greater percentage than those with low levels."

"But one of my husband's legal friends just had a coronary artery attack and his cholesterol was absolutely normal," said Avery.

"That's possible. Normal cholesterol doesn't guarantee immunity from a heart attack. But the incidence is higher in people with high cholesterol."

I pointed out that a low cholesterol diet should include 70 to 80 grams of protein each day, and that protein should come, preferably, from fish that have fins and swim, chicken, and turkey. The breast is best, with all the skin removed. Between the flesh and skin of poultry, there is a fine penetrating layer of animal fat, which is poison for people with high cholesterol. Non-creamed cottage cheese, farmer cheese and non-fat yogurt are good, too.

"Why protein from fish and chicken only?" Marie, one of the young women, asked.

"Because they are low in cholesterol and saturated fat," I said. "Two-thirds of the fat you serve should be polyunsaturated."

"You mean the vegetable oils," Edwina said. She read a good many health books, so she was knowledgeable if not a practicing health addict.

"Not all. Coconut oil is a saturated fat and should be avoided. Peanut and olive oil neither raise nor lower the cholesterol level. All animal fats are saturated. This includes not only meat and chicken fat but butter. Most vegetable fats are polyunsaturated. They don't raise the cholesterol level and better still, they may lower it by causing it to be excreted. Of the vegtable oils, we find corn oil and safflower oil the best."

"What about margarine?" Lola asked. "I've been using it because it's so much cheaper."

"Many solid margarines and shortenings are similar to butter," I said. "The best kind to use is made from corn oil. But if the oil has been hardened by hydrogenation, it becomes a saturated fat. Margarine made from liquid polyunsaturated oil is better."

"What about diet margarine?" asked Marie. She was partial to pasta and a rigorous change of eating was a drastic step for her.

"Diet margarine contains less fat than you find in regular margarine—it can be used as a spread. If you use it for cooking, don't be concerned if the margarine separates."

"We're great milk drinkers in our family." Lola said. "Can I continue to have milk?"

"You'd be wise to serve yourself and your family skim milk—"

"The kids wouldn't touch it."

"Keep after them, they'll get used to it. Especially if you tell them that it will help their bodies to grow strong. Are they athletic? We've found with kids that you can't say 'No, don't have French fries and thick chocolate malteds.' We tell them about foods that will improve their athletic ability. They listen. Skim milk and buttermilk are 99% fat free. Cream, of course, is out for the heart patient."

"Cheese?" Avery said, looking plaintive. "My husband is a connoisseur of cheese."

"Since most cheeses are made from butter fat, they have

a high percentage of saturated fat. Some cheeses like cheddar, Swiss and cream cheese are much higher in saturated fat and cholesterol. Uncreamed cottage cheese is low in saturated fat and so is mozzarella. Synthetic cheese is available now. It's made with corn oil instead of butter fat and is very palatable."

The talk turned to eggs. It seemed that nearly all of them had at some time dieted on hardboiled eggs for lunch.

"I hate to be a spoil-sport," I said, "You're allowed 300 milligrams of cholesterol a day. One egg yolk has between 250 and 275 milligrams. You may have the equivalent of two eggs per week, and it's usually in bakery items. But you may use plenty of egg whites, if you like. The white is free of cholesterol and high in protein."

"You're not leaving us much," Avery said, "I suppose steak is out, too."

"Not entirely. You may have beef or lamb three times a week, a medium portion. A sirloin or round steak is best, if the fat is trimmed away. Round is preferable. Pork is entirely out. The other nights you may have fish, poultry or veal for dinner. Fish that is white is low in cholesterol. Fresh salmon and fresh tuna are higher in cholesterol than other fish. But canned tuna has the fat processed out of it. Shellfish, lobster and shrimp are definitely limited. They contain too much cholesterol.

"You may serve any bread, as long as it doesn't contain egg yolk, solid shortening, dried eggs, lard or cream."

By this time, the women looked glum. And now I was coming to desserts, which meant even more deprivation. Fresh fruits, sherbets or ice milk, gelatin, angel food cake are allowed, I told them. Even mince pie, if it is made with egg whites and liquid shortening. As for other desserts, you must forget them. The choice is *not* whether or not to have a piece of chocolate cream pie. The choice is between sickness and health.

"Cocoa has a lower fat content and is preferable to chocolate. Whenever a recipe calls for chocolate, you can substitute 3 tablespoons of cocoa plus one tablespoon of polyunsaturated margarine in the place of every ounce of chocolate."

We talked about mayonnaise which is so essential to

perk up a summer salad. For each egg yolk, there is usually a cup of corn oil, sometimes more. But if you serve one teaspoon of mayonnaise you aren't getting too much cholesterol. And diet mayonnaise is available.

"Try mixing your own salad dressing, using polyunsaturated oil and vinegar, with spices. You'll get used to it and I'm told it brings out the salad flavors better than the heavier salad dressing."

"That might be all right for me, but not for my husband." Avery said.

"Perhaps he will get used to it if you try." I said. "When it comes to soups, we recommend clear soup or broth rather than cream soups." I went on. "Vegetable, chicken soup and chowders, if not creamed rather than meat soup. If you do make a meat stock soup, let it stand overnight in the refrigerator and skim off the solid fat the next day.

"We ask our cholesterol-prone patients to abstain from spareribs, gravy, hamburgers, hot dogs, fish roe, caviar, duck, goose and sausages. However, you may substitute one egg yolk for two ounces of shellfish or two ounces of organ meat or two ounces of cheddar cheese."

"But what can you eat in a restaurant?" Beulah asked. Many of her meetings were business lunches.

Beulah's hands were distorted with knobs of cholesterol deposit; they looked like an arthritic's.

"I know that avocado and sweet potatoes are higher in cholesterol than other vegetables and should be avoided," she said. She had already learned a great deal about her problem in her short stay in the hospital.

"I still don't understand about triglycerides," said Maisie, whose devotion to Bloody Marys interfered with her blood chemistry.

"We should be as knowledgeable about triglycerides as we are about cholesterol. Triglycerides are probably just as dangerous as cholesterol, and just as much to be avoided in our diet and drinking. A percentage of carbohydrates—sugars, alcohol, breads—is converted into triglycerides and deposited as fat.

"But what has weight got to do with it?" Maisie asked.

"People who are overweight have a much higher level of cholesterol or triglycerides. By diet and weight loss, they can decrease the levels. For heart patients, the loss of weight is essential, even when they do not have high cholesterol or triglyceride levels. It's important to eat only the foods that are listed in the diets we are giving you. And eat just enough to maintain your proper weight."

I continued to talk about triglycerides, because all of them seemed largely unaware of the dangers here. The basic principle in triglyceride dieting is to avoid starches. Refined sugar is very easily converted into triglycerides and partly stored as fat. If you've eaten food high in starch or sugar, your triglyceride level goes up, so it is wise to skip starches and sweets. All cereals are high in starch.

"All grains and potatoes are starch," I said. "Eat too many slices of bread and you add weight."

"I suppose," said Maisie, coming back to her particular problem, "that alcoholic beverages are out since I know they raise the triglycerides."

"Yes," I said. "Any person with high levels of triglycerides or a Type IV hyperlipoproteinemia should never have more than one cocktail a day. One ounce of rum, brandy or hard liquor is equal to 1½ ounces of sweet wine, or 2½ of dry wine or 5 ounces of beer. Large amounts of alcohol raise triglycerides, supply 'empty calories,' and cause other problems.

"Patients with high triglyceride levels should also avoid muffins, pancakes, pastas, and breads. These add weight as well as raise triglyceride levels. And they also may raise cholesterol levels, especially if made with eggs."

I knew about Maisie's love of sweets, as well as drinking. Her triglyceride level had been extremely high, before she entered the hospital suffering from chest pain. She looked distressed.

"No cocktails before dinner, no ice cream and cake. I know."

"Ice cream is forbidden," I said, "but you can have a little sherbet and ice milk. Most non-dairy creams contain coconut oil, unless it is otherwise specified. This is true also in frozen puddings and non-dairy whipped dessert toppings. They are not good.

"You can have melon or fresh fruit cup (not canned which has sugar added) or fruit juices, consomme, a salad with a simple oil and vinegar dressing, non-shell fish or chicken or lean meat that isn't fried, gelatin, angel food cake or sherbet. Just stay away from chocolate."

"We should talk about salt, in these few sessions we will meet together," I said. "The normal person usually takes in about ten grams of salt per day. (Salt is a combination in equal amounts of sodium and chloride.) Sodium is retained in the body, holding onto water and this expands the blood volume. It puts an extra load on the heart and is responsible for swelling of the legs.

"When a patient has congestive heart failure, sodium must be rigidly restricted in his diet. (He should get drugs to expel the sodium as well.) His sodium intake should if possible be held down to 1 gram per day.

"You'll see on the diet list we give you the foods high in sodium which you must avoid: Any vegetable, fresh or frozen, processed with salt. Artichokes, sauerkraut, spinach are relatively high in sodium. Most other vegetables, especially if fresh, are very low in sodium. So are all fresh fruits. Many instant cereals, salted popcorn, potato chips, snack chips, waffles, pretzels are high in sodium. There is an artificial egg substitute. It is high in sodium. Organ meats, ham, canned meats, koshered meat, luncheon meats or smoked fish, shell fish—all are high in both sodium and cholesterol."

"Don't you think, Dr. Tai," said Lola, the young lady who had valve trouble and had to watch high blood pressure, "that it will be almost impossible to remember all this while we're cooking?"

I knew the question would come up and I met it in the only way I could. "Not at all," I said. "If it's important to you, you absorb the information, just as you learn anything else." I turned back to the charts.

"You have your diet lists. Now there's only a little more on sodium—salt and all the salty snacks. Bacon, olives, commercial salad dressing, salted margarine, salted nuts are high in sodium. (Cashews and macadamia nuts are also high in cholesterol.) And beware of boullion cubes, garlic salt, meat extracts, tenderizers, pickles, relishes, Worcestershire sauce. But even sweetened puddings and gelatin desserts have sodium. You should always read labels."

I lifted a cup of orange juice. "Now we come to potassium and foods that contain it."

Potassium is an essential part of the heart's muscle cell. The loss of potassium can disturb the cell's function. Drugs used for heart conditions, including diuretics, also have a tendency to deplete the heart cell of potassium. This means the patient is more prone to arrhythmias or electrical irregularity of the heart. So it is vitally important for this patient to replace the lost potassium.

Fruits, especially bananas, cantaloupes and apricots are high in potassium. Fruit juices, especially orange and grapefruit and prune, and vegetables like sweet potato, squash and lentils have a good amount of potassium. (Sweet potatoes are not for patients with high cholesterol.)

"A glass of orange juice, a medium-sized banana, a half dozen apricots, figs, dates or prunes, half a cantaloupe, two tangerines, one-third cup of lentils and a potato, white or sweet, each would provide some potassium to replace that which is lost by taking water pills. If you are taking large doses of medications, your doctor may prescribe potassium in a liquid form. Potassium chloride is better than other forms."

Our discussion had lasted an hour. I wanted to sum up, but we would have several more sessions before they were discharged from the hospital and I knew there would be more questions.

"You are about to embark on a new way with food," I added, "If you feel deprived, if you brood about it, sticking to certain foods and avoiding the harmful ones will be more difficult. But if you can accept the fact that you are making a choice—choosing to get back your health and well-being, you will in time accept the change with resignation. It won't be easy at first, but if you stick with it, you'll soon see the good results."

And then I added what we allow all of our patients—a little leeway. "If you stick to your diet, you may cheat, twice a month." (For diets, see appendices.)

Changing his food pattern is a trial to a patient who has just been discharged from the hospital after a heart attack. He needs to regain his strength, but his nourishment should help his body, not harm it. During his hospital stay, he has learned to eat either the low fat, the low sugar, or low salt foods his doctor has ordered and the dietician has arranged in the most palatable combinations. But everything still tastes different from what he is accustomed to. "It tastes like nothing," he says of a serving of breast of chicken, skin removed, and lightly seasoned with herbs. He tries a light sprinkling of salt substitute. It helps a little.

His complaint requires a re-education of his taste buds. If he can discipline himself enough to eat prescribed foods for a week, not only his taste buds but his mind will be prepared for the change to safer dishes. Some of our patients have found various ways to deal with this.

"I found that just talking to myself wasn't enough," Tess R. told us, when we suggested that a change in diet would lower the level of her triglycerides. "I'm a compulsive sweets eater. While my friends are enjoying martinis, I'm busy with a hot fudge sundae. I talk to myself the last thing at night. As a matter of fact, I incorporate it in my prayers. I say, Please God, help me to get through tomorrow without sugar. I know it sounds silly, but it helps me. And if I slip, I don't get too disheartened and go on a sweet binge. I just start over again the next day. You know, your group talks are like Alcoholics Anonymous."

She is right. It is easier to fight against temptation in the company of other people who have the same problems.

Another patient, Vivian M., who is overweight and should lower her cholesterol level confessed, "My mother died of a stroke. I never gave it much thought in relation to my own problems. But now, when I am tempted by a cup of coffee and a piece of cake at bedtime, I close my eyes and visualize my mother, in the hospital bed, her left side paralyzed by a stroke. I say to myself, 'Do you want to be like that?' I push away the cake and pour the coffee down the drain—sometimes. But the sometimes is getting more often now, which gives me the strength to say no, even more."

We play tricks with our minds and appetites in order to get started, although sometimes a doctor's warning is frightening enough to shake off the old damaging habits. Often the time of crisis for a patient comes when he has lost some weight, his blood pressure, cholesterol or triglyceride level is lower, and he is feeling good. Then he takes a drink or pie a la mode, and says to himself, Why not, I feel good.

But he hasn't licked his problem, and as he reverts to old patterns, his former symptoms may return.

Food is usually arranged more easily by the woman patient or wife of a patient. The kitchen is her habitat. She can create new eating plans for herself or her husband, while still feeding her other members of the family in the old familiar pattern. It is simple enough for her to take a portion of vegetables out of the pot before she butters them. Or use very lean chopped meat for her own hamburger while she prepares a complicated form of meat loaf for them. As a matter of fact, her family would do better to eat as she does in order to save themselves from future hazards, but this isn't always easy and must be done with tact and skill.

It is more difficult for the man who is recovering from a heart attack to eat his plainer fare, while the family is enjoying their typically rich American dinner. To him, there is something unmasculine about this fuss and he resents it as much as taking pills. Paul B. was forty-five when he became our patient.

In his youth, Paul was a big fellow, a former All-American from Michigan, who weighed about two hundred and ten, and had the frame to carry it. But after marriage, and a career as public relations chief of a clock company, he began to accumulate pounds. The memory of his training days didn't help. Steak and eggs and whole milk for breakfast may be fodder for tackling the West Point backfield, but superfluous and even dangerous when you are attending a Rotary Club luncheon to bring fresh industry to your hometown.

Paul had recently become a full-fledged gourmet, an expert on fine wines. When he and his wife Mimi moved to a new home on Long Island Sound, he supervised the remodeling of the kitchen according to his interests, not Mimi's. He and three other men had formed a small eating club, meeting every fortnight at one of their homes, where the host prepared an extraordinary gourmet dinner. Wives were not allowed in the kitchen until after the brandy and cigarettes.

This was real fun. Paul and his pals were written up in the food pages of local papers. By now, Paul had added thirty pounds to his frame, there was too much ruddy color in his cheeks with their dewlaps and his mouth had a juicy look.

He went to his physician at the first sign of severe chest

pains and was referred to us. "I'll do whatever you say, doctor," he said to me. "I want to live."

That day, before we could get him into the hospital, he suffered a severe coronary artery attack. He had known subconsciously how near to catastrophe he was. He came through well, considering his weight and blood pressure. On his return home, after we had given him his new regime, he said to Mimi, "I'm building a new kitchen."

"What? What for? she exclaimed, "All this food nearly killed you."

"That's just it. I'm on a diet and I intend to stick to it. The only way to be sure is to do the cooking myself."

There are no signs of butter, cream, heavy cheeses in Paul's Spartan laboratory, but he has collected all the scientific booklets available and has experimented to get a maximum of taste while using a minimum of what is poisonous for him.

"I wish I could persuade my friends to try it," he said recently. "I had them over for a low sodium, low fat, low sugar meal, but they weren't buying it. I suppose they'll have to wait until they reach the hospital like I did."

We all know that sometimes wisdom comes late.

Chapter 22

The sexual comeback

DR. KRAUTHAMER:
We, as cardiologists, must often serve as a cold shower.

Sex, yes. It's good for heart partients. But preferably with your spouse. Statistics show the chances of cardiac catastrophe are greater in extra-marital sex.

"It isn't my minister who's kept me faithful," a patient said recently, "it's my cardiologist."

In a study done on people who were having sexual intercourse, each one had telemetry to monitor her/his physical reactions. The general heart rate increased from 82 to 118 beats per minute.

The tests were taken when the patient had sex with his spouse. If he had sex with a lover, the pulse rate and demand for oxygen probably would have been greater and could have resulted in angina.

It's been found that sudden death is more common in extra-marital affairs than with one's legal spouse. Recently a patient of ours, a doctor who had suffered a myocardial infarction, was found dead in a hotel room with his girl friend. He had informed us that he would let nothing interfere with his obsession for sex. And he had told us that she insisted on acrobatics, and that she was something of an Amazon. He wouldn't try to change her. So he brought on his own fatal attack.

Most patients are allowed sex six weeks after a heart attack if they want it and can tolerate it. But no bacchanals. Many wives and husbands are worried that sexual stimulation may trigger another heart attack, but this is less of a risk than they fear. If the man isn't allowed to have intercourse and remains sexually excited, the frustration may have a greater detrimental effect on the heart. During the excitement stage, there is an increased secretion of adrenalin and a greater chance of irregular heart rhythms. And some husbands of female heart patients are so solicitous that they are incapable of intercourse.

Sexual intercourse is like a mild-to-moderate exercise and is good for patients, both male and female.

"Sex is a contact sport, but it can be gentle," we tell our post-heart-attack patients. "If you can climb two flights of stairs, if you can walk three blocks briskly, you can have sex. Non-acrobatic."

The requirement of the heart for oxygen is predicated predominantly on three facts: (1) heart rate; (2) blood pressure; and (3) the vigor of the heart muscle's contraction.

All of these increase during the act of intercourse. The greater the excitement, the greater the response, the greater the need of the heart for oxygen. Therefore, the person with a massive heart attack will need more recuperative time before resuming sex than the one who's had a small uncomplicated heart attack. But the fact that sex two or three times a week is about par for the average couple and that it is such a pleasurable activity makes it a highly recommended exercise.

Most marital sexual incidents usually consume about fifteen minutes, much of which is spent in foreplay. The greatest expenditure of energy, of course, takes place at the orgasm. It is at that moment that irregularities of the heartbeat (cardiac arrhythmias) are most likely to occur.

We have found in our own practice that 80 percent of our post-coronary patients can return to sex. "Just as you go back to work part-time," we tell them, "so you go back to sex the same way."

During convalescence, about 20 percent will develop angina when they first return to intercourse. Eventually, less than 10 percent will experience anginal symptoms while enjoying sex. A nitroglycerine tablet under the tongue may help a patient have sexual intercourse without pain.

During their rehabilitation, we have to reassure our

patients that they can exercise on the treadmill, and later in walking, jogging or other activity up to the very beginning of angina. This should not cause an infarction, and they will gradually build their stamina until they reach normal goals without angina. We're happy to tell them that this is also true when they begin to have sexual intercourse.

DR. FRANKLIN:
Sometimes, nitroglycerine tablets (which dilate or open coronary arteries and have other beneficial effects on the heart) can have an unexpected effect on a couple's restored sex life.

I'm thinking about one particular couple, who had a very happy marriage. Walter was ten years older than his wife, Juliet, but the age difference didn't interfere and they worked at keeping their union happy. Both were health nuts, too. Yet, it wasn't surprising that Walter had his first myocardial infarction at the age of 40. He was definitely a Type A personality (see chapter 12, page 154), a hard-driving man who felt that even one moment spent in contemplation was a waste of time. He often said, "We go through this way only once, and I intend to enjoy every minute of it."

Enjoy it, he did. He was an executive in a company that manufactured detergent and soap products. The competition in the field was cannibalistic, but Walter had an instinct for selling and the naïve belief that his laundry flakes were the best. Whenever he attended sales conferences or conventions, he took Juliet with him. "Why should I pick up a call girl, when I've got a wonderful wife?" he said.

Juliet is the kind of young woman that invites healthy sexual attention. She is thoroughly engaging, with a kind of lusty, uninhibited freedom of motion that had captivated Walter, and everyone else who sees her. They had no children, which didn't seem to disturb Juliet. They were inseparable. Friends couldn't believe they'd been married eight years. They had retained the passion, the dedicated interest in one another that they had had during their courtship.

His heart attack came during the promotion of a new

product. It was also a trauma for Juliet. And she realized that there must be a drastic change in their life style. She sat by his bedside as he improved, or by his chair, or walked with him down the corridor as he tested his strength. But she managed with great discretion to keep his pulse stabilized. "Darling," the nurses heard her say if his hand started roaming, "Take it easy—" The nurses never had to be concerned about Juliet upsetting him.

What she didn't realize was that Walter was frightened about resuming sexual intercourse. In the discussions before leaving the hospital, he confided to me that he didn't anticipate with pleasure joining his wife "in the sack."

"What happens if I get chest pains?" he asked.

"Take nitroglycerine before you sleep with her," I suggested. "If you take it beforehand, it will improve your tolerance."

A month later, Walter reported that the touch of his wife after such a long respite started angina, and he was obliged to stop without completing the act. Juliet was understanding. She did her best to keep him reasonably calm, but her obvious allure was too much for his self-control. And for his chest.

"Are you taking your nitroglycerine right before your sexual activities?" I asked.

"Not exactly."

"Well, look. Take it just before the action begins."

He shook his head. "I don't know if it'll work, Dr. Franklin. I'm afraid I've become a loser."

I became concerned. A few failures were enough to cause Walter anguish and anxiety, which he certainly didn't need. I dismissed the idea of talking to Juliet. She seemed to be handling the situation well.

Several days later, Walter told me what happened after he took my advice. The first night, there was success, so they planned a gala second night. Champagne for Juliet, and even a sip for him. He felt not only urgent sex, but consuming love for her, for her kindness, her loyalty, her femininity. Juliet lay back on the pillow, her extraordinary red hair spread fanlike around her head. The small box of nitroglycerine was sitting on the shelf above the pillows, and as he reached for it in the dark, the box opened and spilled.

Whereupon, there was a mad scramble in the dark for the pills raining down into Juliet's hair. Everytime he thought he had a tablet, her hand would break loose and grab it. And suddenly they realized what was happening and their laughter broke the tension. They never consummated their sex that night, but they ended up hugging and kissing each other and absolutely hysterical at the ridiculous situation. They decided the easiest way to get all the nitroglycerine tablets out of Juliet's hair was to take a shower. Together, naturally. And then they gave each a rubdown in the tub and finally went to sleep, locked in each other's arms, and actually got a fine night's sleep.

It was the kind of fulfillment lovers understand.

The percentage of heart attacks in young people (mostly in young men) is rising. As a result, sex comes up more often than ever, and sometimes less pleasantly.

One of our recent patients was a junior partner in a Wall Street firm specializing in corporate law. Dennis T. had originally planned to join a group of his law school friends who had rejected Wall Street and were practicing storefront law in the ghetto. His marriage to Lois changed that. She wasn't destined to be the wife of a young man who fought for civil rights. As a result, Dennis played golf and tennis with clients, and there wasn't a gala or charity ball in Manhattan that he and Lois turned down.

On his thirty-third birthday, he was stricken with a heart attack. He didn't make an uneventful recovery as we expected, which was puzzling. His wife, Lois, seemed utterly devoted. She was at the hospital every day with books, puzzles, amusing imaginative little gifts for him. After he was transferred from Intermediate Care to the general nursing floor, she was even more attentive. The nurses spoke of her devotion, but with a quizzical air. Then the night nurse related that when she had walked into the room with Dennis' sleeping pill, she found his wife in bed with him.

Their family doctor told us that Lois demanded a hyperactive sexual life, but that she was completely loyal to her husband and never strayed.

"It'll be a problem if he can't satisfy her now," her physician said. "If she turns elsewhere, it'll destroy him."

During Dennis' third week in the hospital, Dr. Krauthamer stopped in to see him. Dennis, in pajamas and robe, was sitting in an armchair. Lois, in a halter top and mini-skirt, was curled up on the bed in a most suggestive pose.

"Doctor," she said, "isn't it about time we talked about our future?"

Dennis was looking away from her, his face strained.

"Look, Dr. Krauthamer," she said directly, "I'm a healthy female and I have certain needs."

"I'm sure Dennis will be able to take care of you adequately in the foreseeable future," Dr. Krauthamer replied.

She hadn't the vaguest notion of what such a remark could do to set back her husband's recuperation and did not have the common sense to discuss her own anxieties in private. As it was, the anxiety created in her husband might be emotionally irreparable even after he recovered from his heart attack.

Such a problem, we know, must be handled with great tact and sensitivity. Most wives do handle it superbly. A husband's brush with death usually brings out the streak of tenderness in his wife, and also a fierce determination not to become a premature widow.

Few of our arteriosclerosis patients are women, unless they are beyond the menopause or have some inherited predisposition. When a woman is the patient, the cardiologist must be particularly sensitive to the sexual problems involved. He suggests to a fearful or reluctant woman patient, who dreads penetration, that many other parts of the body respond to sexual play. If her anxiety is extreme, he may suggest that therapy with a psychiatrist would be beneficial. Two of our patients now in analysis are doing well. What we try to impress on the patient is that her problems are seldom different from that of other women; only the details are different.

We all try to speak of sex with a minimum of embarrassment. Most married people who have a cardiac condition are apt to tense up when the problems are first discussed.

"But then they relax. After a while, the shyness vanishes with relief, and in these sessions, some have worked out their intimate problems," says Dr. Tai. "Many discover for the first time that touching can be enormously gratifying, not only as part of the play before sexual intercourse, but as a source of comfort, a kind of physical renewal, if one of the partners is not yet able to consummate the act. We've only now begun to appreciate the importance of touching, of demonstrative affection for the ill person."

One of our patients, Corinne C. has shown considerable sexual resilience under difficult family circumstances. She was admitted to the hospital complaining of crushing chest pain over the breastbone spreading to the left arm and shoulder. She was sweating heavily. Her blood tests for enzymes were abnormally elevated and her electrocardiogram demonstrated a small heart attack. Her cholesterol was normal.

Corinne was 34, and had two children. Her husband was an incurable alcoholic, whom she would not divorce. Their sex life was very erratic but satisfactory when he was sober.

She felt unable to cope with her children, since he was of no help to her. The older of the two girls was seventeen and the problems of adolescence were compounded by the girl's friends, who were all in rebellion against the middle class way of life.

In spite of her emotional problems, Corinne was an ideal patient. Before she was discharged from the hospital, we did coronary angiograms and found a severe narrowing near the origin of the left anterior descending coronary artery. There were no collaterals for natural protection. Therefore, we felt she was in danger of a large heart attack if this vessel should close and such an infarction very possibly could lead to her death.

We recommended surgery, and it was scheduled in two months' time.

While she was waiting, we began to learn of Corinne's secondary, but perhaps major problems at home. An elderly aunt who raised her was living with the family and there was constant bickering among them. Her aunt was always nagging the girls, complaining about housework, their dates, and even went so far as to suggest that if Corinne died of a heart attack, the girls would be to blame. This aroused hysteria in the girls and after a bitter confrontation the aunt stalked out.

"The girls try hard," Corinne told us, "but they bring

home hamburgers dripping fat and chocolate malts and potato chips. They don't seem to realize I can't touch those foods."

The generation gap extended beyond nutrition. They stayed out late, or overnight with friends, and made no sercet of smoking marijuana. There was no way Corinne could communicate her anxiety, and sleepless nights took their toll.

She had a second small infarction in the same area as the first, and came back in the hospital.

"I'm so alone and so helpless," she said, trying to control her tears. "If my husband would help me—"

She was critically ill now. If her vessel should close off without collaterals, there might be no way to save her. She had to have immediate surgery.

Another good surgeon whose schedule was not full, promptly accepted Corinne. A saphenous vein by-pass was done, she convalesced, and has done well ever since.

On her return home from the hospital, she found that her husband had left home for another woman.

"If I'd had this news before my operation," Corinne said candidly, "I might have dropped dead."

With the help and guidance of her family physician, she managed to come through this family crisis with no further damage to her heart. Corinne found she could take a firmer hand with her daughters and at the same time file for divorce.

Corinne came to our office recently, looking well and happy. No more cardiac symptoms. She has now returned to normal activities. Her emotional reserve is stronger and she can face her circumstances and function.

During her last visit, she confessed that one of her problems was sex. She missed the good sexual relationship with her husband. There was no reason, as far as we were concerned, that her life couldn't be fulfilled in all areas including sex. We told her, as we have told so many patients, that sex would be good for her. The postscript to her story was the announcement of her forthcoming marriage. The odds are with her.

Certain physical factors can inhibit sex in the newly recovered heart patient: angina or dyspnea (shortness of breath) during intercourse, physical fatigue, and sometimes palpitations.

Fear or lack of interest are just as real.

Most physical complaints are based on physiologic or structural abnormalities which can often be treated with medication (see chapter 16, "Medication").

Angina is countered by nitroglycerine and related drugs, and by the drug which renders the heart contractions less vigorous, propranolol. Palpitations are treated by anti-arrhythmic drugs.

Early in a patient's recovery, the major cause of fatigue may be lack of physical conditioning. It will improve with an exercise program. The couple shouldn't be too concerned about the patient's inability to attain sexual fulfillment until he is well into his physical rehabilitation program (see chapter 20, "Exercise and Rehabilitation").

Many of our women patients have responded well after treatment for these problems after their heart attacks. But we have had a few failures.

One of our patients, Maida, was a partner in every area of her husband's life until she developed a "virus" with a cough and shortness of breath that just would not go away. She went to her physician who found a severe mitral valve problem and told her that her shortness of breath and cough were due to congestive heart failure. Her symptoms required digitalis and diuretics. Later, a cardiac catheterization pointed up the need for surgery. She went for surgery and recovered, but it was a long tedious convalescence.

After six months, she detected a change in her husband's attitude toward her. He was more tender, perhaps, but less like a man who had unsatisfied sexual needs. Finally, he couldn't keep his secret any longer. He confessed he'd been having an affair with a girl in his office. He put himself at her mercy saying quietly, "It's up to you, Maida. I still love you, but I can't in all honesty make excuses for my behavior. It's rough for a man like me to be without sex for such a long time."

She forgave him, for she needed to cling to something permanent at that time and marriage was the only thing she had. But the anger remained and festered.

"I can't forget that while I was so sick—practically at death's door—he was in the hay with some babe," she said. "Just thinking about it makes me hurt—" she touched her hand to her breast.

She made a choice finally, and it was divorce. She settled in Palm Springs and made a new life for herself. It took considerable adjustment and help from a counselor, but she is now on the way to a happier and healthier future.

Fear and lack of interest are also major problems for the cardiac patient.

"All of these books on sex have made a great change in the woman's outlook," a family physician told us recently. "Women are demanding better performances from their husbands. I don't know how to handle this. I'm not an expert on sex."

Impotence frequently appears to be emotional, since we seldom find a physical reason. Some patients actually lose interest in sex without becoming impotent. We cannot explain why this happens, at least not on a physical basis.

Impotence and the fear of impotence may stem from a kind of primitive fear. The doctor assures his patient that an erection begins in the brain, but it does not allay his anxiety. He wonders if his damaged heart really can take the strain of making love.

How well he can perform sexually also depends on the emotional effect of his heart attack. And you can't do after a heart attack what you couldn't do before. The patient who has previously enjoyed sex is likely to return to the pleasures.

There can be, of course, certain physical reasons for impotence. A patient with coronary arteriosclerosis can also have arteriosclerosis of the aorta and the blood vessels that supply the legs and pelvic area.

Although such an organic cause of impotence and frigidity is infrequent, the Leriche Syndrome is a definite physical condition. It is characterzied by blockages at a point where the aorta divides into two large blood vessels that go down to the pelvis and legs. The physician can often spot the trouble by an examination of the femoral pulses (the pulse in groin area that goes into the legs). If the pulse is absent, there is a distinct possibility that the Leriche Syndrome is present.

Clinical symptoms of the Leriche Syndrome are intermittent claudication—that is, pain or discomfort in the legs or buttocks, which is precipitated by walking and relieved by rest.

Surgery can often correct this condition by improving the blood flow, but there is no guarantee that sexual function will return.

There are multiple ways in which diabetes mellitus can affect the sex cycle. But most diabetics have had their disease for some time before they become impotent.

Patients with diabetes are predisposed to future coronary arteriosclerosis. They are subject also to peripheral vascular disease with obstructions in the same iliac arteries.

Diabetes mellitus attacks the autonomic nervous system which supplies the nerves that control erection of the penis and ejaculation.

Transient impotency in men and frigidity in women are common even in the absence of organic illness and do not necessarily imply physical or psychological disorders. Nor need they be related to heart disease even in a heart patient. A lessening of sexual need can accompany anxiety, fatigue, depression or other problems associated with living in our tense, hyperactive world.

We advise our patients that the testing period, when the patient is returning to sex, should be as relaxing as the healthy partner can make it.

If sex was good before a heart condition developed in one partner, sexual rehabilitation should become a simple and joyous experience afterward. If the husband is the patient, his wife will, no doubt, exercise tender and considerate concern for him, using her womanly instincts to preserve his masculinity without draining his physical strength. If the patient is the wife, the husband should exercise a kind of tender protectiveness as he may have done on their honeymoon.

The threatened loss of one partner makes the other more acutely sensitive to the finality of death. We have discovered among our patients that many couples find a rededication of love after a cardiac catastrophe. As sexual activity returns, it is accompanied by gratitude, joy, and renewal—making it an experience that is meaningful far beyond sex.

Chapter 23

Pregnancy, the pill and children

DR. KRAUTHAMER:
Pregnancy usually causes a good many changes in the body's functions. These have been translated into various myths that are handed down from mother to daughter. In former times, the prospect of childbearing in a young woman with heart disease was considered hazardous. It was questionable whether she could survive the pregnancy and if she did, whether there was danger of the child inheriting the disease.

It was found in two studies that the coexistence of heart disease in pregnancy ranged from only 1.5 to 2 percent, based on 80,000 pregnant women.

How does pregnancy affect the heart?

Many pregnant women have sudden weight gains. They are troubled by fluid retention, a water and sodium imbalance because of the increased level of certain hormones. The work load of the heart is increased, the heart rate is slightly raised and the output of the heart itself increased.

The enlarged uterus presses on a large vein (the inferior vena cava) returning blood to the heart. This means the return of blood from the legs to the heart is delayed and the veins in the legs become dilated. Varicose veins are not infrequent in pregnant women; sometimes they will have fainting spells.

Emily, a 26-year-old woman, consulted us because of fainting spells in the seventh month of her pregnancy. She had been told she had a heart murmur. Because of her family history of heart disease and these episodes of fainting, her obstetrician had warned her family that she might not be able to carry the baby. Her pulse was irregular at times.

Our examination showed no abnormalities of cardiovascular disease. Her fainting spells always occurred when she stood up suddenly after lying down for a while, clearly due to compression of the inferior vena cava by the enlarged uterus.

"Get up slowly," Dr. Tai suggested, "and when you're in bed, lie on your left side."

Her fainting spells became much less frequent. She carried to full term, had a normal delivery, and no more fainting spells.

Most (95 to 99 percent) cardiac problems in pregnant women are due to rheumatic valvular disease.

If the patient is in Class I or Class II of the New York Heart Association classification (see Appendix A), her pregnancy can usually be continued to full term and the child delivered normally.

If the patient is in Class III, proper medical management, often combined with prolonged bed rest and early hospitalization, will help her to carry to full term and even deliver normally. She may be two to four weeks premature, depending on the size of the fetus. But if the Class III patient develops congestion of the lungs which becomes difficult to treat, she may need valvular surgery—if her pregnancy has gone beyond the first four or five months.

Women with aortic valve disease who are in Class III and IV are usually aborted because it is difficult for them to carry to full term. Even when they are in Class II, these potential mothers require more precautions than those with mitral valve disease.

If a pregnant woman is in Class IV, we advise abortion, which should be performed during the first three months of her pregnancy.

Each case must be judged individually, regardless of classification. For the woman with mild heart trouble and good reserve, pregnancy is usually no problem.

When a woman goes into prolonged labor, there is a greater chance of infection in the pelvic area, in the uterus or the bladder. This infection can seek out damaged valves and produce a disease called infective endocarditis, which can lead to permanent heart damage or even death.

The woman is safer if her labor is normal, with all aseptic precautions. If she is expected to have a prolonged labor, the obstetrician is advised to give her antibiotics to prevent this infection to the heart's valves.

Ramona, a stunning woman of 36, had tried to conceive for years. She had mitral valve damage but was only mildly symptomatic before her pregnancy. She finally became pregnant during her husband's absence on a prolonged business trip to Italy. She was slim and vain about her figure, so for the first four months, she remained deceptively slender. Her husband wasn't aware of her condition until she was actually in her sixth month. By this time she was frantic for a double reason: her pregnancy and what effect her mitral stenosis would have on it.

When she confided the truth to her family physician, he referred her to us. Dr. Franklin examined her and felt she belonged in Class III. She told him that her husband was not the father of her child, and that he would, of course, know it. She said the natural father meant nothing to her. Dr. Franklin suggested that she and her husband come to the office and discuss the situation.

At first the husband was outraged at his wife's betrayal. He gradually quieted down when he learned she had no relationship with the other man, and perhaps he sensed that her previous sterility might be due to him. He did want children. Before they left the office, he had accepted the prospect of being a surrogate father.

But the tension and anxiety told on Ramona. She was admitted to the hospital with recurrent bronchitis. She had difficulty breathing, and we were concerned that she might not carry to full term without encountering problems that would harm the child.

We wouldn't catheterize her because of possible X-ray damage to the fetus. Based on clinical judgment, we advised her to have surgery to open the mitral valve. The operation was successful. She continued her pregnancy and delivered a healthy eight-pound boy.

There are several possibilities with mitral stenosis: A patient may be so ill that she requires an abortion in the first three months. Or she cannot carry to full term and requires heart surgery for a normal birth. Or she is able to make it without surgery and delivers normally.

Some years ago, it was believed that female patients with serious congenital heart defects wouldn't live to their adult years, and if they did, could not conceive. Very often these defects are recognized early in life by school doctors. And if the children have surgery, the girls can lead normal lives, reaching their 30s and 40s. Today they have care which wasn't available a decade ago. But even today, pregnancy in these young women is infrequent. A report from Montefiore Hospital in New York suggests that they require much stricter medical management, better control and supervision. They deliver earlier as soon as the fetus is viable, and its survival can be expected. The infant is usually four weeks premature.

Parents with congenital heart disease do not necessarily have children with the same problem. Although the incidence of heart disease in their offspring is slightly higher than normal, the difference is not significant.

A pregnant woman with nephritis, kidney disease or preexisting high blood pressure may develop toxemia. Control of her blood pressure is extremely important as it would naturally increase somewhat in childbirth. She must not gain excessive weight. Her urine must be checked frequently. She may be delivered earlier.

"I'll never get married," Helen thought as her thirtieth birthday passed and all of her girl friends already had their broods. She was 32 when she met Karl, a machinist in the manufacturing company where she was head bookkeeper. They were married and wanted to start a family immediately. Helen had no problem getting pregnant.

She carried her pregnancy well at first. She was big-boned but thin, watched her diet, took vitamins and drank skim milk. But around the fifth month, she began to gain too much weight and her blood pressure began to rise. By the end of the eighth month, she seemed swollen and her face was puffy in the morning.

Karl said, "Why don't you see the doctor?"

"I'm not due in his office for another week."

"See him anyway. I'll feel better if he checks you today."

Her obstetrician found her blood pressure elevated and albumen in the urine. He examined her eyes with the ophthalmoscope and found evidence of high blood pressure. When he pressed his thumb on her shinbone, a depression was obvious, and it stayed long after—pitting edema. Helen was developing toxemia. She needed immediate hospitalization and potent medicine to control her blood pressure. The situation was dangerous. Helen feared the loss of her baby. Karl feared the loss of Helen.

The obstetrician remained close at hand until Helen's blood pressure was controlled, and then he decided to perform a Caesarian. Allowing her to go full term would endanger her life and the infant's.

The doctor's verdict was too much for Helen and Karl, particularly for Karl. The threat of what might happen to Helen brought back the loneliness and anguish of his early years in war-torn Czechoslovakia when he had lived, like other lost children, in bombed-out buildings.

Biting his lip, he waited at the hospital while Helen was in surgery. When the obstetrician came off the elevator, Karl suspected the worst. He was already sunk in the agony of a bereaved husband when the doctor took his hand and shook it. "Karl, you have a son."

"Helen?"

"She's in good condition."

Their son is now ten years old, and they have adopted a younger boy.

"Karl's like a rock about most things," Helen said, when she continued to come for high blood pressure treatement, "but let something happen to me or the kids and before you know it, he is biting his lower lip until it bleeds."

A woman who is born with a narrowing of the aorta (coarctation) usually develops high blood pressure. If this condition is detected early in life and it usually is, it is corrected, and the result is a complete cure. If it has gone uncorrected for years and is discovered for the first time during pregnancy, it can produce the same problems high blood pressure would—toxemia and its complications. It also may cause rupture of the aorta and bleeding into the brain.

Pregnancy itself involves certain risks and can produce a kind of heart disease, a cardiomyopathy which is quite infrequent. We're not sure of the cause, but during pregnancy some women develop weakness of the heart muscle or congestive heart failure. There is no pre-existing valvular disease; there is no coronary artery disease; no previous evidence of high blood pressure; no manifestation of inflammation of the heart. Still, the muscle grows weak and flabby and the heart dilates. The young woman may change from normal to a severe cardiac patient. After delivery of the child and the six weeks post-partum, some young women return to normal. Others do not.

"Do you recommend natural childbirth for a pregnant woman with heart disease?" we are often asked.

It would depend on her health status and the physiologic capacity of her heart. The final decision on natural childbirth would depend on her family physician, her obstetrician, and her cardiologist. For a woman with "borderline" status as a heart patient, too much strain in natural childbirth may trigger congestive heart failure. For those less vulnerable, the risk can be minimized by the use of diuretics and salt restriction. Digitalis may also be needed. Then these women may come through natural childbirth nicely.

DR. KRAUTHAMER:
The call came when I was doing evening rounds at the hospital. A local physician was treating a 15-year-old girl for a case of intractable asthma. He asked that one of our group see his patient in order to rule out congestive heart failure or any other heart condition.

Cynthia was a pretty, carrot-haired girl, who was just growing out of the adolescent stage in which palomino horses are preferable to rangy boys. That night, as I entered her room, it was evident that she was in dire respiratory distress, breathing about 60 times to the minute, gasping for air. Her parents and a tall thin nice-looking boy in jeans waited outside in the hall while I examined her.

She was completely coherent, but at the moment was expending all of her energy in just trying to breathe. There was no wheezing, which made it bizarre.

I placed my stethoscope between her shoulder blades and heard a murmur in her back that I had not heard in the front. This is a very rare sign that is a tip-off to massive pulmonary embolism. These are the blood clots that look like long worms, and travel in the blood stream. When they hit the pulmonary arteries, they coil up on themselves. As the blood tries to flow past these clots, it must be forced through by the pumping action of the heart. This causes turbulence, and the turbulence produces a murmur, best heard in the back, between the shoulder blades.

I suggested to the family physician that Cynthia did not have asthma or any heart condition, but a pulmonary embolism.

"Impossible!" he exclaimed. Cynthia had no history of phlebitis or any disposing feature to cause such a condition. However, he decided to reevaluate the case.

By morning, she had suffered a cardiac arrest. We could not resuscitate her. The family doctor was close to the family and asked for permission to look through the medicine cabinet in her bathroom. He found nothing that would point to an answer to Cynthia's death. Then her mother went through Cynthia's suede-fringed shoulder bag, and there she uncovered a package of contraceptive pills.

The family agreed to an autopsy. Large wormlike blood clots found in the pulmonary arteries confirmed my diagnosis. We had to admit that in all probability The Pill contributed to Cynthia's death.

DR. FRANKLIN:

The Pill has liberated today's young woman. But it has caused side effects that are beginning to receive considerable publicity and many women are seriously concerned. To others, The Pill is worth the risk.

The Pill contains various female hormones. One of these can cause the release of another hormone from the kidneys which leads to high blood pressure. This can be a dangerous sequence of events.

Another hazard which can be caused by hormones in The Pill is fluid retention. A week before a woman's normal menstrual cycle, she is apt to have swelling in her ankles and around her abdomen, accumulating anywhere from two to five pounds. The same happens with The Pill. If she stops taking The Pill, the fluid leaves the body and the weight will drop.

For some women, The Pill acts as an appetite stimulant. As they put on weight, and perhaps become less interested in sex, they are apt to blame their condition on anything but the contraceptive measure. But no man, we have been assured, can appreciate the full value of The Pill not only on a woman's sexuality, but on her peace of mind.

Strokes have been related to the use of oral contraceptives, particularly cerebral thrombosis. Unfortunately, we have no adequate criteria for screening women who may be more susceptible to blood clots. But it would be advisable for women with family history of thrombosis to avoid The Pill and use other means of avoiding pregnancy. A young woman with a history of high blood pressure or migraine headaches should definitely not take oral contraceptives unless advised by her physician.

Why does The Pill cause trouble? It is related to the female hormone estrogen. The less the amount of estrogen in The Pill, the less danger of embolism and thrombosis (blood clotting).

Oral contraceptives also decrease the effectiveness of oral anti-coagulants, which may be taken as treatment for blood clots.

The fact that women with Blood Group O have been less troubled by thrombo-phlebitic disease may be a clue to a future evaluation of who should or should not use The Pill.

We all have a tendency to assume without question that anything new must automatically be good. At first, only suspicion suggested that oral contraceptives have such specific ill effects on some women.

Blood clotting is a highly technical phenomenon that is incompletely understood even by experts. Usually, blood doesn't clot within blood vessels. Small particles (platelets) which circulate in the blood stream of all normal people have a certain amount of "stickiness." This is extremely valuable when you cut yourself and you want the bleeding to stop. But it has been shown that oral contraceptives increase this stickiness of the platelets. They also promote clotting by other means.

These contraceptives contain the female hormone, estrogen, which seems to have an odd effect on the blood vessels, causing them to behave like an overstretched girdle. Thus, when the blood tubing system of the body is somewhat dilated, blood flow through the vessels will slow slightly. This effect has been found to be more pronounced in the legs than in the arms.

The combination of more widened blood vessels, reduced blood flow and increased stickiness of the platelets does result in some tendency to increase the danger of blood to clot in the legs. These clots can break off and travel to the lungs—pulmonary embolism.

What does this mean in terms of the average woman?

Obviously, thousands of women are taking The Pill without having blood clots form in their legs. Of significant interest is the fact that nine months' use of The Pill by a normal woman is perhaps no more and probably less hazardous than the normal pregnancy itself. The latter increases the clotting ability of the blood also. The pressure of the uterus and child on pelvic blood vessels impedes the blood flow from the legs. But the incidence of thrombophlebitis in women using oral contraceptives is twelve times as high as would be expected in an exactly comparable normal young female population. And embolism is eight times as high.

Women with a history of congestive heart failure or some other forms of heart disease, or of inflammation of the veins in the legs, would be wise to use other methods of contraception.

In clinics making a study of people with high blood pressure, the use of oral contraceptives has shown an additional rise in blood pressure which cannot be explained by any other cause. It has been found that blood pressure may not rise for the first six months after taking The Pill. Also, it returns to previous levels three to six months after The Pill is discontinued.

The present medical opinion is that women with high blood pressure should not take oral contraceptives. If they insist, then their blood pressure should be checked periodically. Should it elevate, the contraceptive should be discontinued.

Congenital heart defects and diseases

DR. FRANKLIN:
One of every 250 live births have some abnormality of the heart or blood vessels. 10,000 such children die in this country each year. The incidence is even higher in stillbirths while some defects are so severe that miscarriage occurs. The most common defects are compatible with life through childhood, though they may cause incapacity or death by middle age. They can usually be corrected by surgery with but little risk.

When one child in the family has heart trouble, the parents usually overcompensate at the expense of the other children, perhaps even unwittingly restricting the activities of the disabled child. Nothing makes a child more conscious of his affliction. It is better for the parents to allow the child to lead as normal a life as possible, within the limitations of his illness.

"What is a congenital heart defect?" asked the mother of a small heart victim.

"A defect you're born with," I answered. "The heart wasn't formed normally during its development in the fetus. All holes between left and right sides of the heart normally close by the first month after birth. In your child's case this did not occur."

The most common defects are holes in the muscular walls (*septa*) which separate the right from the left side of the heart. The result is abnormal circulation between the two atrial chambers (*inter-atrial septal defect*) or between the two ventricles (*inter-ventricular septal defect*). The higher pressure on the left side shunts blood from the left to the right side. This blood is then recirculated through the lungs.

However, if for some reason, the pressure on the right side increases to a high level, blood will be shunted right to left, *before* it passes through the lungs for oxygenation. This blood has a dark reddish color. When it circulates to the body and skin, it causes a bluish hue called cyanosis, and this is the condition that causes the child to be known as a "blue baby."

One of the causes of a blue baby is a complicated condition called *Tetralogy of Fallot*. There is a hole between the ventricles plus an obstruction to the flow of blood out of the right ventricle. This obstruction causes pressure to rise in the right ventricle, forcing its unoxygenated blood through the hole to the left side and out to the aorta.

It also decreases blood flow to the lungs, and if this flow is critically reduced, it can cause fainting. Today, surgery corrects this defect.

Most congenital heart defects can now be corrected. But some children are born with multiple abnormalities and these the surgeon's skill cannot save. If we feel after a careful evaluation, including if necessary cardiac catheterization, that there is a chance to correct the heart's defects and the small patient will be able to lead a fairly normal life, we recommend surgery. Heart surgery for the young patient is aimed at adding 20–60 comfortable years to an otherwise limited life expectancy. Rarely, the child fails to survive the operation. To bring this tragic news to the family is a physician's most difficult obligation.

Modern techniques of open-heart surgery guarantee little risk in children with a simple "hole in the heart" or valvular problem. The corrective surgery is usually done before the child starts nursery school. It is usually delayed until the child is physically fit. Sometimes parents decide to correct the defect when the youngster is seven or eight years old and a little larger and stronger. It is often done during the child's vacation.

Sometimes, a hole between the ventricles will close by itself.

Recently, a local physician asked Dr. Tai to check his boy. The pediatrician had detected a murmur.

"Sometimes, it's difficult to know if the murmur is innocent or indicates a hole in the heart," the cardiologist said.

When he examined the small boy, he found that the child did have a hole in the heart at the ventricular level. However, the child had no symptoms and it was decided to wait and see. The boy has thrived, has gained weight, and is so energetic that he wears out his parents. He was examined at the end of three years.

"The hole is closed," we were happy to inform the father. "Your son is now a perfectly normal child."

This miraculous closure happens in 10 to 12 percent of the children with this particular disease.

In the last 100 cases of hole-in-the-heart surgery done at a university hospital, the surgeons didn't lose a single child. The hole is patched with a Dacron graft or just sewed in. The little patients return to normal life. Once the hole is closed, the heart behaves normally. In our experience, we find that these children can go on to normal lives, active, busy; they reach adulthood, they can marry and the females among them can conceive and produce normal offspring.

DR. TAI:

Why do some babies have congenital heart disease?

There are various medical reasons but none can ever assuage the grief of the parents. For them, there is always the unspoken self-accusation. Is it because of our genes? Or the mother will worry that some medication she took during pregnancy was responsible. Or she may take the blame because she was careless about taking care of herself, and didn't see an obstetrician until the last months.

"Doctor, I have a heart murmur," a young pregnant woman asks. "Is my child likely to inherit it? Will my condition predispose him to any kind of heart disease?"

If one parent has congenital heart disease, the chance of his child inheriting it isn't significant. If both parents have heart disease, the incidence would be slightly greater. There are cases on record of children who have the same heart disease as their parents, but it is the exception rather than the rule.

Until they are five years of age, heart disease in most children has congenital origin. These children may have other associated abnormalities. Heart disease in twins is usually of the hereditary type. Mongolism is a defect of the chromosomes and is frequently accompanied by heart conditions. A chromosomal disease called the Turner's Syndrome is also associated with disease of the heart and blood vessels. Many chromosomal abnormalities are now recognized in patients with heart disease. Any defect in the chromosome may also involve the heart. Some types of congenital anomalies are seen more commonly in boys than girls, and vice versa.

There are, unfortunately, some diseases that affect the heart's muscle and nothing can be done for children who are born with this affliction. Their heart disease is progressive and their life is short.

Children born of mothers who have rubella (German measles) early in the first three months of pregnancy have a significant incidence of heart disease. They often have hearing and visual problems, too. So abortions are recommended for mothers exposed in this period unless the mother has been vaccinated with German measles serum. However, the heart and blood vessels of the fetus are completed by the third month, so if the mother has rubella after that period, the formation of the fetal heart will not be affected.

You haven't been feeling well, so you make an appointment with your doctor. He is not likely to ask you, "What did you eat the first year of your life?"

Not that you'd remember. What does any infant eat? Milk from a bottle or his mother's breast, orange juice, and finally all the canned fruits, vegetables and baby foods to be found on supermarket shelves.

But we know more about feeding babies today than a generation ago. Researchers are discovering that the eating habits of an infant's first twelve months lay the foundation for his future health.

Mary, a young woman, who works part time in our offices, has recently put her four months' old infant on skimmed milk, much to her own mother's horror.

"Mama raised us on homogenized milk, eggs, fat lamb chops, ice cream and thick milk shakes. When she sees what I give the baby, she says I'm starving her. Yet mother goes to her doctor for high blood pressure. I may have a predisposition to it, but I'm sure taking prophylactic measures. In our house, nobody gets more than two eggs a week, and nobody has rich, fatty meats—and my husband loves pork roast. We all drink skim milk and use corn oil margarine."

Would you believe that arteriosclerosis begins with the child's diet? Fatty substances can be deposited on the vascular wall from a very early age. Autopsies of children killed in auto accidents have shown lipid streaking—little streaks of fatty material—in the aortic wall. Small amounts of fat have already collected in children's blood vessels by the age of five. It isn't good to contemplate; mothers with such devotion, such good intentions, feeding their infants rich food which may shorten their lives.

For years, research on heart disease has focused on the adult. More recent studies have begun to put emphasis on the child. The consensus is that we must educate the child (and his mother) in proper nutrition and an early awareness of the importance of the right food in avoiding heart disease. What the child eats, how he exercises, how he fits into the family constellation, and his school and his friends, are all subtle indicators of his future cardiac health. The mother who feeds her infant high cholesterol foods, may be looking for trouble if her child has inherited a tendency to accumulate cholesterol.

The child who is free of this tendency can absorb more cholesterol in his feeding. Even later in life, on a high cholesterol diet, he will not have the first child's problem.

We do know that although you may have inherited the gene, if you discipline yourself and modify other troublesome factors, you can lead a normal life.

Which suggests a whole new life style for our children. When a child's taste buds are sensitized from childhood to a low cholesterol, low animal fat diet, he has no problem as an adult sticking to nutrition that will give him health and energy without ruining his blood vessels. Since arteriosclerosis begins at an early age, prevention must begin at the same time.

Premature deposits of cholesterol in the blood vessels may be due to environment, tension, eating habits. But the genetic factor is strong. Since we cannot select our genes, we must do the next best thing: modify the factors that cause heart problems. It is urgent that a newborn child of parents with a history of heart disease be tested. This is done by taking blood from the umbilical cord—placental blood—which can then be typed and will reveal whether the child is predisposed to heart disease at an early age. The doctor can do a complete fat and cholesterol analysis from this cord blood.

We still do not know positively that a child born with a high cholesterol count will be burdened with a high cholesterol all of his life.

There seems to be a variable pattern of a high or low cholesterol during certain seasons or months of the year. This is still a puzzle. But there is a definite seasonal pattern emerging in all disease, including heart disease. This is called *circadian rhythm*. The incidence of heart attack increases during the winter months. The incidence of heart attack is greater on Monday than on weekends.

There is a similar rhythm system in cholesterol and triglycerides. Once we solve its riddle, it will help us greatly in our fight against heart disease.

Mothers are asking: "How can I protect my unborn child?"

"By judicious feeding, particularly if there is a family history of heart disease."

The late Dr. Paul Dudley White had embarked on what he called a "Children's Crusade." He said, "We've got to start with the child at birth, to change his way of life, so he'll no longer be dependent on the automobile, on rich food, smoking. Heart disease before eighty is our fault, not God's, or nature's will."

If statistics bear us out and we recognize and change our life style, the generation ahead of us will have it over us. Not only in their kind of food but in handling the tension and stress that causes an excessive rise in cholesterol.

It isn't easy to educate your children to withstand the pressures of their peers. If their friends are wolfing hamburgers with French fries and thick malteds, and you insist your children eat a hamburger made of lean round steak with absolutely no fat, fresh finger vegetables and skimmed milk, they are apt to rebel. Particularly if it is a recent edict. But if you start them early on a low fat, low sugar, low cholesterol routine, they'll never feel deprived and will have good nutritional habits as adults.

One wise mother persuaded her three growing sons to stick to their eating habits by stressing the importance of proper food for athletes. Two were in the Little League and the third already was an outstanding swimmer. Indeed, they were soon boasting that their "health diet" was what gave them stamina and resistance.

Parents can also get across the idea of staying in good

physical condition. Some children are naturally active, others passive. It's good psychology for the family to participate in sports together, such as long interesting walks, bicycling, sailing, skiing. If started quite early, this kind of physical activity is usually pursued into the adult years.

If you think these are good habits, start them now. You could save a life.

Chapter 24

Dying and living

DR. FRANKLIN:
"I've had a heart attack. What is my future?"

The question torments all heart disease patients. "What about my job, my marriage, my children?" And they might add, "my fun, my special interests"—and that might be music or hunting or the PTA.

We often see the traumatic experience of people who lose their jobs through a merger of two companies. The young survive easily, but the able and experienced men and women cannot find comparable jobs. But as long as they command the respect, understanding and love of their families, they can maintain enough self-confidence to come through the crisis.

The same thing often happens to a middle-aged man whose coronary heart disease has curtailed his stressful job. Or a woman who cannot maintain her full role as wife, mother, hostess, community leader. The activity in which so much of life and health were invested suddenly is not there. What have they to offer the world now? The crane operator who earns $20,000 a year becomes depressed after an attack and thinks, "I'd be better off dead." And calculates how much insurance he carries to protect his family.

Many of our heart patients emerge from a financial and emotional crisis to turn to new jobs with the inner strength. Such patients are leading rewarding lives with a renewed appreciation of what it means to be alive.

The patient who causes us considerable concern is the

man who makes his living with his hands—the carpenter, the plumber, the house painter. If he is obliged to change his work, it becomes a serious problem. Here some of the retraining programs can be of help.

But sometimes we have a man who does heavy construction work, and at 42, he has a heart attack—we've got a real problem. Often, the only option for him is to go on welfare. For a proud man, this can be a dead end. In training programs for cardiac rehabilitation, we would like to see more thought given to the care of this type of patient, so that he, too, may have a chance to keep his options open.

DR. TAI:

My first experience with heart disease was in my own family. My father, Issa Tai, was a textile manufacturer and secretary of the Stock Exchange in Pakistan, a man who had become somewhat overweight. Fat is a kind of status symbol in our mother country, and food is rich, spicy and cooked with butter and fat.

A man whose days were full and demanding, my father also smoked constantly, as much as three packs a day. He found alcohol a form of relaxation, particularly during conferences that lasted into dinner and beyond.

One evening, as he was dining with business associates, he became aware of pain, then numbness in his left arm. His friends reassured him, but when his discomfort didn't ease, they brought him home. Still a boy at the time, I was greatly shocked at the sight of my father looking helpless and in obvious pain.

When our physician, a general practitioner, arrived, I sat beside him as he examined the patient who was half-sitting, half-lying on his bed. Nothing radically wrong, the doctor announced. A touch of indigestion, perhaps. He gave my father an injection of B-12, which he probably used in many crises. Such an injection couldn't hurt anyone and made the family feel that the doctor was doing something helpful. I stayed with my father for twenty-four hours, I remember. As the pain gradually disappeared, he became active again and soon went back to his office.

The arm pains returned. Finally a cardiologist in Karachi took an electrocardiogram and gave the family the sober news that my father had indeed suffered a heart attack.

"You must cut down your work load," the cardiologist advised.

So Issa Tai phased himself out of his textile mills and concentrated on the Stock Exchange. He never again complained of discomfort. I went on to complete my schooling at the University of Karachi and went to England to study in my chosen field: cardiology.

Four years later, in 1963, my father suffered another heart attack. "Now you must completely retire," his cardiologist advised. At that time, the medical consensus was that a sick heart made an invalid of the patient.

When I returned to Karachi for a vacation, I was astounded at the change in my father. The active, dynamic man had been replaced by a stoic, who accepted his lot as one of the living dead.

By this time, at the beginning of the 1960s, a revolutionary idea appeared in the treatment of heart patients after heart attack. Dr. Samuel Levine had advocated early activity of the patient for maximum improvement at Peter Bent Brigham Hospital in Boston. Dr. Herman Hellerstein advanced this idea with great enthusiasm. I heard him lecture on it, and found his data so convincing, his reasoning so sound and logical that I tried it on my father.

Although I had not done any studies on him, I advised my father to return to his activities, at least part time, for it was work and outside interests that had made him such a vital and compelling man. I also asked him to give up cigarettes and alcohol.

"I will listen to you, Razzak," my father said.

On a low cholesterol diet, Issa Tai lost 60 pounds, reducing from 210 to 150. He continued to function well for a while and back in London I received encouraging reports about him from the family.

Then Issa Tai began to notice extra beats in his heart. Tests revealed a hyperthyroid condition which could be controlled by drug therapy. During the following three years, Issa Tai lived a full life. By this time, I was practicing cardiology in the United States, and I returned to Karachi to spend a month with my family.

I treasure the memories of those days. Father and I walked each day for at least two miles. We talked and talked, and the generation gap which was part of our culture was warmly closed. As a young doctor, I saw my father in true perspective now, not only as my parent, but as a human being, and as a friend. I returned to the States, both happy and saddened, knowing that he now had extensive coronary artery disease. But by following the activity therapy that I had learned through reading Dr. Levine and Dr. Hellerstein's work, he had added four normal years to his long and useful life.

In 1970, Issa Tai developed a stroke, which was followed by pulmonary edema. He died quickly.

Patients often complain that their physicians are so detached. But the doctor who has suffered the loss of someone in the family from a major disease works not only with his knowledge and skill, but with empathy. And like a sixth sense, that empathy is communicated to the patient.

DR. KRAUTHAMER:
Some of our patients are victims of stress and tensions in their work. Others are happy, well adjusted, successful, yet driven by some inner force that is finally as destructive as a difficult boss or an unhappy marriage.

One of the most successful obstetricians in New York City recently suffered a myocardial infarction. This man had everything going for him. He is loved by his patients, admired and respected by his profession, handsome, with gray hair, blue eyes and a warm smile than can turn wintry if his patients are not properly attended by the hospital staff. Whoever manages his financial affairs has looked after him well. John M. no longer needs to produce a yearly income to live comfortably. Yet for him to think of renouncing his work was nearly as traumatic as his heart attack.

"Give up obstetrics?" he exclaimed when we first broached the idea. "Are you nuts? What's left for me?"

In the Coronary Care Unit, five days after his attack, he was more relaxed than he'd been in years and yet to the professional eye, he showed signs of restlessness and hyperactivity in spite of sedation.

His was a transmural—a full thickness—heart attack. It was average in size, with about 20 to 25 percent of the heart muscle involved. Ten days after the attack, when he was in the Intermediate Care Unit, his blood cells had cleaned out the destroyed tissue. However, the ingrowth of scar tissue was not yet at its maximum. This means that the area where the heart attack took place was still weak. From the tenth to the fourteenth day after a heart attack, the scar is fragile. This period always causes us some anxiety because the patient is under tension and the weakened area which is forming scar tissue could be stretched, leading to an aneurysm or bulge on the heart. Aneurysms of the heart rarely rupture but do cause irregular heartbeats or congestive heart failure.

Even though John was somewhat fretful about his future, there was no problem. His heart grew a firm scar. Starting from the edge of the infarction, the rate of scar formation is about one millimeter per day, so it takes about a month to fill in one inch. Before he left the hospital, he was able to discuss the life style that had brought him to this catastrophe.

"Smoking and hyperactivity did me in," he said.

His wife was afraid that once he went back to his practice, he would expose himself to more coronary problems. Because they were a well-adjusted couple, and their children were grown, they decided to make a drastic change in their way of life. They sold their New York cooperative apartment and their big Westport house, and bought a condominium in Sarasota, Florida. John made arrangements to teach at a medical school and he has a contract to write a textbook on obstetrics.

He discovered that he enjoys teaching. Naturally, he misses the excitement of obstetrics and the adoration of his patients, but he has learned to use leisure in a new dimension.

"I remember once reading that Lincoln's schedule was so arranged that he could have a half-hour for himself, just to ruminate. I understand that now.

"I think all heart patients should begin their new life on a different level," he said. "The past is behind. You use what you can of it to create a new way of living. It may not be as gratifying, but it sure beats being a cardiac cripple. In time, it has positive values, too. For me, now that I'm older, I find I like to teach. It's the *paterfamilias* idea, passing on to kids what you've learned at a pretty rough cost. I've got a good bunch of senior medical students. Their hair is long, and I don't know what they think of me, but they're sharp and they're motivated. It's not bad. As a matter of fact, at times it's pretty good."

The post-coronary patient who learns to adjust finds it easier to take his place again. At first, there is considerable compromise. But with the help of those close to him, he keeps his options open.

KEN WACHTER:
"Later," says Mary, when I announce I am going to mow the front lawn. "It's only a few weeks since your heart attack. There's a scar you can't see. There's a healing process going on."

I listen and pay heed. My wife doesn't nag. She just states facts and she is right. I get carried away with enthusiasm, feeling that since I have no pain, I have totally recovered. This is the tough part of my convalescence. If the understanding between my wife and me was less strong, I might have failed. Because there's a switch in roles which can play havoc between a man and wife, unless there is a broad base on both sides.

We go out for a short drive. Mary opens the car door for me. For 24 years, I have been holding open the door for her. She slides into the driver's seat. I sit in the passenger's seat. When we hit downtown traffic, I am unconsciously driving for her. She goes into the supermarket, and I remain in the car, reading a paper or a book. I see men and their wives coming out of the automatic doors, each carrying packages. Mary and I used to shop every Saturday morning for the week's supplies, and I would carry the bundles to the car, the heavy canned foods, leaving the lighter packages for her. Now she comes out of the market, trundling one of the wire carts, and when I get out to help her, she says, "No, no, you just sit there, Ken. No trouble."

It isn't exactly a reversal of roles because Mary and I always have shared household chores. Still, it makes me feel passive. My male ego, or whatever you choose to call it, rebels. I should be doing the heavy chores. I always have.

Maybe it's an outmoded way of looking at life. But Mary is no woman stevedore, nor are our three daughters. Mary and I both came from the Midwest. The man used to be the only breadwinner, and felt he was the head of the family. Mary has often worked, and we raised the girls to take care of themselves. Now Mary is working because she has to, with two college educations coming up, and one newly married daughter. But even so, we have an older established outlook and I can't change.

I work for a large corporation. In my department, men are still judged by their experience and capability, and I expected in due time to retire. And now I had to have a heart attack.

Dr. Tai was waiting when I got to the hospital. Mary came up in the elevator with me, and the nurses in the Coronary Care Unit met us. I started to take off my coat, but they said, "We'll do it." They took over completely.

My last day in the hospital, one of the local ministers dropped in to see me.

"Your heart muscle is the strongest thing you've got going for you," he said. "You treat it right and it'll give you years of service."

I wanted to treat it right, and my family was intent on doing it also, especially my daughters.

"I'm not an invalid," I told them. "I'm in the recuperative stage. The best way to help me is to help your mother."

The changes in our life style began with food. We were brought up in the dairy country, and from childhood on, we were accustomed to rich milk and cream, plenty of fresh eggs, bacon and ham. My favorite breakfast was a dish of bacon and eggs, well-buttered toast, coffee and a glass of milk. My favorite dinner menus were steak or roast beef with baked potatoes and plenty of sour cream.

And now—meat only three times a week, lean meat, with all the fat cut away. Lean meat, as anybody can tell you, is usually tough, and the best part of the steak or roast beef is the outside fat, crisp like cracklings. I used to look forward to meals.

I don't care much for fowl or fish, but I learned to tolerate them. Mary prepares a dozen varieties of broiled chicken, with the skin removed. Fortunately, I can have polyunsaturated oils, but I have removed fried foods from my diet. I was never one for sweets, which is good, I suppose.

My recovery began slowly, but I was so grateful to be up and around that I didn't complain. I would get up, have breakfast, watch Mary drive off to work and then face eight hours to fill until she came home. This was one of the bad times of the day. The first weeks of my recovery, I'd go back to bed in the morning. I read a lot. I did crossword puzzles. My attention span was considerably shortened and that worried me. I took up crewel work, which amused the girls no end. But I reminded them that the late Duke of Windsor was also an embroidery addict.

I stopped smoking the day of my heart attack, which made me somewhat restless. The first week I was allowed to move around the house. The second week around the yard. I took on small tasks, like filling the bird feeder or checking my new barometer. I watched television. It was a long day before Mary and the girls came home.

Two months after my heart attack, I began the exercise program that Dr. Tai had laid out for me. Now I work on the stationary bicycle for about twenty minutes and pedal five miles. If my pulse rate goes above 110 beats per minute, I stop and rest.

Dr. Tai levels with his patients. In the hospital, I went into a depression for a few days, but then came out of it. We talked about it, and he put me on a tranquilizer to help out.

At the end of two months, I returned to work. The men all wanted to know about my symptoms, the tests, the catheterization. The women showed a tendency to mother me. "Don't walk the steps. Take the elevator."

Lunch in the office cafeteria now is a tossed salad or cold roast beef. I haven't influenced the other men in my office, although one did cut out cigarettes, and another has made an appointment for a treadmill stress test. In time, I expect all large companies will include stress testing in their yearly checkups for their employees.

What I couldn't do, my fellow workers did for me, taking up the slack. I now go out of town for the company, but I space the appointments.

A heart attack, I've discovered, changes not only the patient but his family. You know how tenuous life can be, and somehow you find yourself enjoying every day with a new sense of reality.

DR. KRAUTHAMER:
We first saw Martha-Mary when she was 76, and a patient in a nursing home on the outskirts of Danbury. She was deposited there, at considerable financial strain, by her devoted family because of "cerebrovascular insufficiency and premature senility."

Strangely enough, it was through her grandchildren, long-haired youngsters in T-shirts and jeans, that we got a picture of Martha-Mary before her cardiovascular system betrayed her.

"It's not fair," one granddaughter often burst out. "Grandma—it wasn't so long ago—she was like a ball of fire!"

Martha-Mary had a slow heart beat due to complete heart block. Her doctor, a conservative old gentleman, had been trying to persuade her for the last two years to have a pacemaker.

Martha-Mary said tartly: "I won't hear of it."

Her family agreed. To their staunch Vermont souls, there was something wicked about inserting a machine to help your heart work for you. A person's heart is his soul, and if the soul is being operated by electric wires attached to a battery placed under the skin of the chest, why it's no longer a soul at all!

"Besides," Martha-Mary had said with a wicked gleam in her steely blue eyes, when she was still coherent, "What woman wants three breasts?"

Nevertheless, Martha-Mary's heart beat was phasing out. It was a critical decision now. Her family, remembering Martha-Mary as she had been a year before, so dynamic, so tart, and so full of humanity, simply couldn't bear to watch her disintegration and suffering. Finally, they all agreed that she deserved that chance.

We put in a temporary pacemaker. It did increase her heart rate, but she was no more alert mentally than before. Nevertheless, the temporary pacemaker wire remained in her heart, sewed in place where it entered the vein and attached to a battery pack strapped to her chest. We decided to leave it there for four weeks and observe her reaction before putting in a permanent pacemaker.

One of her sons-in-law was dubious about the procedure. "Why keep her heart beating when her mind's gone?

She is now a complete burden to her family. I'm sure if she were aware of it, she'd prefer to be dead."

But we decided to extend the therapy and after three weeks in the hospital, she was driven back to the nursing home with the temporary pacemaker. During her entire stay in the hospital, Martha-Mary had never once recognized us clearly. She had not walked around the room or in the hall. She was never really coherent.

One morning, several weeks later, we got a call to see her. Something was wrong with her pacemaker. We arranged to meet her in the Emergency Room, and since all three of us were in the hospital, two of us were waiting when she arrived by taxi.

She walked into Emergency without any help, a tall spare woman, with an erect bearing and a pleasant expression on her face. Her eyes lit with recognition as she shook hands with us.

"I've seen you before," she said crisply. "You are—yes, your name is Dr. Franklin. And you—you are Dr. Krauthamer. You both worked on me while I was here."

We couldn't believe the change in her. We and the nurses in Emergency wanted to cheer. We were so excited that we called up to the Special Procedures Room where Dr. Tai was about to start a cardiac catheterization and insisted that he come down to see her.

Her problem was easily remedied. We then arranged for a hospital admission and implanted a permanent pacemaker.

We wish everyone who has an infirm parent could see Martha-Mary. We're not saying that what worked for her would work for all elderly people. But it would for some. And what a joy to see life and interest restored, to see a human being who is again treasured by her family. Martha-Mary spends four months of each year with one of her three daughters, who vie for her visits. As a matter of fact, her 18-year-old grandson, who lives in a commune in Massachusetts, has put in a bid for her to come and visit. It seems that Martha-Mary knows a great deal about organic foods and wild-growing things like ferns and mushrooms. She is a great walker and the vitality of her spirit makes her invaluable and dear to those she comes in contact with.

We keep in touch with Martha-Mary for our own selfish satisfaction. We're so proud of her.

The pacemaker is one of the great successes of modern cardiology. In some cases, it can restore a human being to human status.

DR. TAI:

Taylor W., age 51, was referred to us because of increasing shortness of breath, swelling of the ankles and pronounced fatigue. Three years ago, a cardiologist at a university-connected hospital had examined him and performed a cardiac catheterization that showed no coronary blockage.

Taylor never experienced chest pains but his shortness of breath was a distinct handicap in his work as a master carpenter. He was a big-boned man, over six feet tall, devoted to his family, a good provider and a strict father. Recently, small matters had begun to upset him. He felt that people were picking on him or were sympathizing because he was sick. If his wife tried to save him steps, he regarded it as a sign that he was incapable of doing the task, and this upset him even more.

After tests, we came to the conclusion that he had a cardiomyopathy with congestive heart failure—weak heart muscle. It may have been caused by a virus infection in the past. His heart wasn't working as an efficient pump.

Since his heart failure was related to progressive disease of the heart muscle, his life expectancy would be shortened. Unfortunately, such patients require repeated hospitalizations until they die from their ailments.

His family physician wanted confirmation of the diagnosis. Taylor underwent another cardiac catheterization which verified that he had normal coronary arteries and a very weak heart muscle.

I was given the responsibility of talking with the patient and giving him the grim news about his future. It has taken a number of years for me to learn how to be honest and objective with a patient. The truth can be cold and cruel or merciful and gentle when hope is preserved. Speaking the truth and explaining to a patient what the outcome may be while telling him the plans for treatment and keeping him comfortable (without pessimism, yet without excessive optimism), is usually well accepted by the patient, and he is encouraged to cooperate.

When Taylor and his wife arrived at our office, I sat

down with them and carefuly outlined the whole disease process. "Your treatment is medical," I told him.

"So, it's hopeless?" he said, half a question and half a statement. "I'm going to die."

"Don't talk nonsense, Taylor," his wife chided him. "You're in the hands of good doctors."

It was evident to me that this denial on his wife's part and her anxiety were not only about Taylor's death, but about her own future.

One thing I have learned about Western culture. To many, death is final, the door that closes everything off. In my own culture, it is a door that opens on everything. In other Eastern cultures, death is a transition to another kind of existence on earth. Belief in reincarnation is strong. While in the Western culture, many believe death is the end of life on earth.

I was obliged to explain to Taylor and his wife that the disease was progressive. We would do our best to keep it under control and not allow it to progress rapidly. We would make his life as comfortable as we could.

"Doctor—" Taylor looked across the desk into my eyes, "am I going to die within a year?" As I hesitated, he added, "I'm not afraid of dying. I just don't want to talk about it, not even with my wife."

"No one can foretell another's life span. With so much viral infection around, there is a possibility that the pills may become less effective and you will be spending more time in the hospital. We will always be around to help and keep you comfortable."

An American writer who recently did a study on the reaction toward death found that there are actual emotional steps in dying that prepare the patient for his fate:

1. The initial denial: I'm okay, nothing wrong with me, I'll live to be a hundred; then

2. Anger: why should this happen to me? Is it true, the good die young?

3. A kind of bargaining: God, if you help me come out of this sickness, I will be good; then

4. Depression: and finally,

5. Acceptance: Thy will be done—and a kind of leave-taking from dear ones.

Although it doesn't always happen this way, we have found this kind of sequence in a number of patients.

Interestingly enough, 80 percent of the physicians in a study wanted to know the truth if their illness was terminal. Yet 80 percent of the doctors questioned would not give this news to their own patients. Their reasons: The family will be upset. The family doesn't want the patient to know. They are afraid that by giving this sad news to the patient, his condition will deteriorate more rapidly.

The patient himself, with his own personality and approach to life, helps the physician decide what and how much to tell him. Patients have told us, "If I know I am very sick, it is possible for me to treasure each day that I am still alive and able to relate to my family, and even to the nurses and doctors."

The fact that a person is going to die can be, as I've said, either cold and cruel or merciful and compassionate. It depends greatly on the communication between patient and doctor, the bond of trust between them.

After I finally talked to Taylor and his wife, tactfully but with truth, there was an initial period of sorrow. Gradually they began to accept it. We have found that when patients are given the facts, they develop a greater capacity for acceptance than we give them credit for. Perhaps some inner strength takes over that we do not recognize or understand in our normal everyday procedures. Perhaps what initiates the beginning of life comes, unseen, to ease us towards its ending.

Taylor came to the office frequently in the next twelve months. Several times we readmitted him to the hospital for treatments to help make him more comfortable. I would try to arrange my rounds so that I could spend some time in Taylor's room, and sometimes we talked, and sometimes we just sat in a kind of comforting silence. His wife told me that he looked forward to my visits. Even when all of us realized there was nothing more we could do for him, even though he knew that each day brought him closer to the end, he was hopeful, and the fact that he trusted me added to his strength. He was honest with me, too. At first, he would tell me he felt fair, later on that he knew he wasn't improving. Because of our relationship, it seemed to me his wife was adjusting better, too.

On his final admission to the hospital, Taylor had severe congestive heart failure which became refractory to all treatment. In spite of medication, he was almost incoherent and he was developing side effects to the medication.

"Isn't there anything more you can do?" his wife pleaded.

"It is possible that we may prolong his life for a week or two more, by kidney dialysis," I said. "This would help eliminate excess salt and water from his body and allow his heart to work better. We can give drugs to lower the work load of the heart. It might give him a temporary improvement. But it's not going to reverse the process."

"Do what you can to make him comfortable—" her words came out with a long in-held sigh, "but don't prolong his life and make him a vegetable. He'd hate that."

On a short-term basis, we reduced the work load of his heart. Taylor improved. But the treatment couldn't be continued indefinitely and he had a relapse. An infection developed in his lungs and then broncho-pneumonia.

The following day when I saw his wife, I told her that I was not in favor of treating him vigorously with antibiotics. I would rather take this opportunity to allow him to lapse into a coma. She agreed staunchly. We gave Taylor treatment to make him comfortable and in thirty-six hours, he passed into death.

Three months later, when the shock of his death had eased and she was able to show her feelings, she wrote us, thanking us, the hospital, the medical and nursing staff for their kindness.

"We are content not with the fact that he was mourned so much but that he was loved so much," she wrote, "and before Taylor drifted off into the final coma, he said, 'We have to remember that not even God can keep everybody alive.' "

I have learned a great deal about life and death from our dying patients.

There is more to life than surviving. A young patient of ours was destined to die before his time. He told us he intended to savor every day of his shortened life, rather than brood about his fate.

Life forces pain and unhappiness on all of us at one time or another. No invitation is required. Love and happiness can be all around, but they *cannot* be forced on us. We must reach out or invite them into our lives in order to enjoy them.

We in the medical profession are constantly looking at death. Death is our challenger. We aim to help the patient before he gets too sick, and death grabs him. You can't look at the glare of the sun all the time. It can make you blind. If we looked at death constantly, it would depress us. But if we learn to regard death in a very objective way, not with guilt for our inadequacy, nor as a token of failure of our ability, and if we accept the gratitude of patients and their relatives as the glasses that save us from the blinding sun, then life becomes bearable for us, as physicians.

DR. FRANKLIN:
A 42-year-old man was brought into the Emergency Room by his friends. Jeremy F. had complained of a headache but had sought no medical help for a week. Fifteen minutes before he was brought in, he told his friends that his headache was growing more severe. He suddenly became comatose. His breathing was harsh. Friends carried him to the hospital where he had a cardiac arrest. He was resuscitated. I was on call and received the summons at 5 A.M. After brief questioning on the phone and making sure that adequate resuscitation was being maintained, I asked the resident-in-charge whether the patient was salvageable or not.

He told me he could not make this judgment. I dressed and hurried to the hospital. Meanwhile the resident and nurses continued resuscitation.

I analyzed all the data. The patient had massive bleeding in the brain. I called in a neurosurgeon who confirmed my findings. I asked him bluntly, "What are the chances of his getting better?" The neurosurgeon felt they were nil. The patient was being kept alive by the respirator, and a temporary pacemaker to overcome the slow heartbeat (bradycardia) which he was developing. The overall statistics were totally against him. We knew the patient was dead for all practical purposes, but we had to be sure. His vital signs were maintained for the next two days but the patient remained the same. The patient's family would come and sit, and look at an unconscious man attached to tubes and wires. They waited in fear and anxiety for the final news. The two days were torture for the family but verified that he could not survive.

I talked to the family and told them what the situation was: that the patient's brain was in fact dead. I looked at them, and they nodded without speaking, and left.

I turned off the pacemaker, disconnected the respirator. In three minutes, he was gone. This was a hard decision for his family, and for me as his physician.

Sometimes the fight for life is touch-and-go, and we have a better chance with a young patient or one in early middle age. A 41-year-old man had been seen by his physician on a routine physical examination and was told that he was normal. But Gabe A. had a strong family history of heart disease. His father and brothers had died prematurely of heart attacks. Gabe was a heavy smoker, overweight, with high blood pressure. He drank excessive amounts of coffee and was under constant stress. His blood cholesterol was over 300 mg. His risk factors were high for coronary artery disease. And as president of a large manufacturing company, he had no time to take care of himself.

Gabe had gone bowling with friends one night and during the first set he complained suddenly of chest pain and collapsed. Fortunately, the local firemen were also in the bowling league and they were able to resuscitate him, continuing it with mouth-to-mouth breathing and external cardiac massage, while rushing him to the Emergency Room. At 8:30, I received a call. Gabe was in ventricular fibrillation. He was defibrillated. He had acute pulmonary edema. An intravenous line had been inserted. Resuscitation was continued, and drugs to control arrhythmia were given. After stabilizing the patient, I re-evaluated him.

I was told he was a man who wanted to live. I felt everything must be done to keep him alive.

He was transferred to the CCU after he was stabilized. The first six hours were very critical. For two days the patient was in a coma. Blood pressure was regulated and the work load of the heart was reduced by proper medication.

Every parameter or detail of body function was measured. The three of us contributed almost 'round-the-clock service to keep this patient alive. On the third day, we saw a chance to win. Gabe began to respond. For the first time he could communicate. We were able to remove the endotracheal tube, warning him it would hurt. With the cooperation of his physician, the residents, and nurses, Gabe gradually improved.

He was out of CCU in ten days, and onto the general floor. Four weeks later he was discharged from the hospital to recuperate at home from his massive heart attack. We knew he had developed a weakness and scarring of a large part of his heart, possibly a ventricular aneurysm. We recommended that he be evaluated completely now so that a similar catastrophe could be avoided. He was catheterized three months after the heart attack.

One artery was totally blocked and had resulted in a ventricular aneurysm. The other two arteries were severely narrowed. If nothing was done, Gabe's life expectancy was short.

Here was the chance to get Gabe back to normal life. We talked to his physician. He was reluctant to subject his patient to surgery. He felt that he could treat Gabe on a medical program and asked him to retire from business.

I objected, tactfully. Keeping the patient from his work would not necessarily prevent further narrowing of the coronary arteries. Reducing the tension might alleviate symptoms, maybe even delay another attack. But I felt that Gabe had to be considered for surgery. His family physician allowed me to discuss it with Gabe and his wife. The wife was rather reluctant to have me discuss it openly with the patient, which is our habit. I told Gabe that if he went through surgery, he would be a high-risk patient. And if he did not go through surgery, his chance of getting a second and fatal heart attack would be very great.

Gabe and his wife, even though anxious, accepted the verdict and agreed to surgery. He has done extremely well. He is still head of his company, though now he delegates some responsibility to other people. He has stopped smoking, has modified his hectic life style, lost weight and is getting more satisfaction out of his family life. Gabe is one of our most optimistic patients.

DR. KRAUTHAMER:
Our story would not be complete without Jimmy Fitz. Whenever we get depressed, we think of Jimmy and our spirits lift. Needless to say, he's been lifting spirits—Kentucky bourbon, no less—for a considerable portion of his seventy-five years.

Jimmy Fitz is a living example of how to defy all the rules of nature and live to a ripe old age. He sold bottled spring water, but he never used the stuff, except to dilute his bourbon slightly. He smokes two packs of cigarettes a day. He is a cardiologist's nightmare. How can you keep on preaching moderation to young men when they look at Jimmy, living the good life of steaks, bourbon and branch water, and cigarettes. They think: "If Jimmy can get away with it, why can't I?"

And who can blame them. Jimmy had a heart attack five years ago. But he's been doing well on a very intensive medical program including digitalis and diuretics (and of course, bourbon).

Recently, Jimmy Fitz slowed down somewhat. His legs were swollen, and he puffed a bit if he walked too fast. Otherwise, he said, "I'm okay, my boy," making a hand gesture reminiscent of W. C. Fields.

With a slight change of medication, he said he was "One hundred percent better." No question about it. His cerebral function was markedly improved and his legs were not as swollen.

We're convinced that hardening of the arteries won't get Jimmy. In a way, he's kind of a mascot. Every holiday that it is possible to celebrate, he has a toast for us and goes right on doing everything we ask him not to.

JACK READY:
I always had a great deal of energy, the kind of energy that only physical work could burn up. As a kid, I wrestled and boxed for the fun of it. I was short and not all that rugged, but I developed good muscles. I suppose I was trying to prove something to myself, because I always suggested to the coaches that they match me with someone bigger.

Our family doctor used to say, "Jack, you're in the wrong profession. You should be working in a gravel bank or with a construction gang rather than teaching."

There are so many things I want to see done on my job. Schools are a busy place and there are numerous details that need my attention.

My actual heart attack came after I was discharged from the hospital for an attack of chest pain and had had coronary arteriograms. I was at home, waiting for the surgeon to schedule me for open heart surgery. But this was the real thing. A myocardial infarction.

Dr. John Sacco admitted me to the Coronary Care Unit Wednesday evening. My heart stopped Friday at 3 P.M. When I went into cardiac arrest, everyone who was needed was there. Dr. Sacco, the nurses, technicians, backup people. It was uncanny. This is where the Hand of God comes in. I happen to believe in Him, and that I am alive for a lot of reasons.

When I came out of the arrest, I said to a man in white, "What are you doing to me?"

"We can't get proper readings," he said, "so we're putting more wires on you."

"Man, you've got me wired up like a power plant now."

Later, he told me I was going to make it because no one coming out of cardiac arrest can act like that. During my hospital stay, everyone worked hard to help me make it and I suspect I was a difficult patient. The nurses said that when I saw Dr. Franklin after the cardiac arrest, I said, "My, God, you're young."

My wife, Carroll, was there almost constantly. Her buoyant spirits were so important to me in my lucid moments. My son and a lot of other people were pulling for me spiritually and some of them spent long patient hours in the waiting room with Carroll.

I remember needing a sense of security. Those first few nights in the Coronary Care Unit, I'd hold on to Dr. Franklin's hand. He seemed always to be there.

Friends have asked me what happened during my cardiac arrest. I really don't know. If I had dreams I don't remember them. Maybe it's because I have no feeling of having trespassed on the brink of death. Maybe it's because I have no fear of death. What I do fear is the danger of total incapacity. And fear for my family.

There have been changes in my life since my heart attack. Have you ever kept running mentally? I still do that. But I now pace myself physically, and while I work as hard, I do it in moderation. Dr. Franklin made me pace my home routine at first.

"All you may do is dust with a cloth. Don't look quizzical, Jack. Eventually, you will be allowed to run the vacuum."

"Thanks," I replied, "Carroll will love you for that."

As the days progressed, I did the laundry in the washing machine, provided, Dr. Franklin said, "You lift out one piece at a time and put it in the dryer."

I follow orders. I try to cover five miles a day. I walk at the beach and around the yard, in addition to the walking I do at school.

I was a chain smoker, but I quit. By the time you're out of the hospital, you've lost your taste for it.

There is no difference in our marital relations.

I returned to work three months after my heart attack. Life isn't greatly different, except that I don't do as much physically taxing work as before. Dr. Franklin approves of work, provided I rest *before* getting tired.

I am more stoic than fatalistic, although both attitudes probably work in parallel. I happen to have a tremendous belief in God. I feel that when the time comes, it does. If you want to stand in front of an onrushing locomotive, you can make that choice. But He has given you the reflexes to get off the tracks.

The same philosophy applies to anyone who's had a heart attack.

APPENDICES:

Appendix A is a basic cardiac classification to aid the physician in deciding functional and therapeutic limitations. It was originally compiled by the New York Heart Association.

Appendix B tells how much energy is expended in normal everyday activities. It is given the patient as a guide for the amount of energy (indicated in METs) which he can safely expend with his doctor's permission.

Appendix C. As exercise is a crucial part of rehabilitation, this chart serves as a reminder for the cardiac patient exactly how he may advance in his program of increasing physical endurance. It is a good guide also for non-patients who desire to build up a healthy heart—as are the following cardiac diets.

Appendix D is an important classification used to indicate types of people who are susceptible to arteriosclerosis.

Appendix E is the low and high cholesterol food list, a highly recommended guide for all of our heart disease patients. It would be well if all of us, beginning with our children, would heed the diet suggestions in this list.

The triglyceride food list of Appendix F is equally important, as sugars and starches are now suspected as significant in the cause of arteriosclerosis.

Low salt (*Appendix* G) foods help to prevent the retention of fluid in the body, which causes an extra burden on the heart. The diet is often suggested for other conditions as well.

Foods high in potassium (*Appendix H*) are necessary for the proper function of the heart, and are recommended for patients on some diuretic medications.

Appendix I lists both chemical (generic) and brand names of common cardiac medications.

Appendix A

Classes of cardiac patients, physical limitation (New York Heart Association functional and therapeutic classification)

• *Functional Classes:* Class I: No limitations of physical activity. Ordinary physical activity does not cause undue fatigue, palpitation, shortness of breath, or anginal pain.

Class II: Slight limitation of physical activity. Patients are comfortable at rest. Ordinary physical activity results in fatigue, palpitation, shortness of breath, or anginal pain.

Class III: Marked limitation of physical activity. Patients are comfortable at rest. Less than ordinary physical activity causes fatigue, palpitation, shortness of breath, or anginal pain.

Class IV: Unable to carry on any physical activity without discomfort. Symptoms of cardiac insufficiency or of the anginal syndrome may be present even at rest. If any physical activity is undertaken, discomfort is increased.

• *Therapeutic Classes:* (Exertion limits imposed by the physician) Class A: Physical activity need not be restricted in any way.

Class B: Ordinary physical activity need not be restricted, but patients should be advised against severe or competitive efforts.

Class C: Ordinary physical activity should be moderately restricted, and more strenuous efforts should be discontinued.

Class D: Ordinary physical activity should be markedly restricted.

Class E: Complete rest, confined to a bed or chair.

• *Definition of ordinary activity:* Those exertions most of us meet in an ordinary day. We consider climbing two ordinary flights of stairs or walking three city blocks at a reasonable pace as the equivalent of ordinary activity.

Appendix B

Activity Energy Expenditure (in METs) (see page 258)

METs	*Rehabilitation Activity*	*Occupational*	*Sports & Recreation*	*Household*	*Garden & Farm*
1–2	Supine rest Sitting or standing relaxed Eating Walking to 1 mph	Watch repair Typing Electric business machine operation Desk work	Playing cards Auto driving Flying (passenger) Motorcycling (cruising) Painting while seated	Sewing—hand or machine Sweeping floor Knitting	
2–3	Level walking 2–2½ mph Level cycling 5 mph Dressing & undressing Propel wheelchair Washing hands & face	Auto repair Radio-TV repair Manual typing Bartending Janitorial Light woodwork Play musical instrument	Canoeing 2½ mph Billiards, bowling Skeet shooting Shuffleboard Golf (riding cart) Powerboat driving Horseback (walk) Sex, gentle	Washing small clothes Potato peeling Kneading dough Scrubbing (standing)	Riding lawn mower

METs	*Rehabilitation Activity*	*Occupational*	*Sports & Recreation*	*Household*	*Garden & Farm*
3–4	Level walking 3–3½ mph Cycling 6 mph Showering Bedside commode	Plastering Wheelbarrow (100 lbs.) Bricklaying Drive truck-trailer Moderate load welding Machine assembly Rock or jazz musician	Non-competitive: volleyball Badminton Golf (pulling cart) Horseshoes Sailing Boat Archery Sexual intercourse (with spouse)	Cleaning windows Scrubbing floors Making beds Standing & ironing Mopping Hang wash Wringing by hand	Tractor plowing Pushing light power mower
4–5	Level walking 4 mph Cycling 8 mph Using bedpan Walking downstairs Some calisthenics	Light carpentry Paperhanging Masonry Painting Wheelbarrow (115 lbs.)	Golf (carrying clubs) Fox trot dancing Ping Pong Badminton (singles) Tennis (doubles) Swim 20 yds./min.	Beating carpets	Gardening Hoeing Raking leaves

METs	Rehabilitation Activity	Occupational	Sports & Recreation	Household	Garden & Farm
5–6	Walk 4 mph Cycling 10 mph	Carpentry	Canoeing 4 mph Non-competitive singles tennis Ice or roller skating Stream fish in mild current		Digging in garden Shovel light ground Horse ploughing
6–7	Walk 5 mph Cycle 11 mph Walk with braces or crutches	Shovel 100 lbs./min.	Trot on horseback Competitive Badminton Tennis (singles) Water skiing Light downhill ski Cross-country ski @ 2½ mph in loose snow		Cutting down tree Hand mow lawn Split wood Shovel snow

METs	*Rehabilitation Activity*	*Occupational*	*Sports & Recreation*	*Household*	*Garden & Farm*
7–8	Jog 5 mph Cycle 12 mph	Saw hardwood Carry 80 lbs. Planing Carry 17 lbs. upstairs @ 27 ft./min.	Horseback (gallop) Touch football Canoe 5 mph Paddle tennis Basketball Climb mountain Ice hockey		Shoveling or spading Ditch digging
8–9	Run 5½ mph Cycle 13 mph	Shovel 140 lbs./min. Tend furnace	Social squash or handball Competitive basketball Ski: Vigorous downhill Ski: Cross country @ 4 mph in loose snow Fencing		

METs	*Rehabilitation Activity*	*Occupational*	*Sports & Recreation*	*Household*	*Garden & Farm*
10	Run 6 mph	Shovel 160 lbs./min.	Competitive: Handball Squash Ski: Cross country @ 5 mph in loose snow		

NOTE: The energy expenditures listed do not include any emotional overtones. This must be taken into consideration in certain activities, especially operating a vehicle or in activities in competition, or sex.

Comment: The schedule for the average patient recuperating from acute myocardial infarction is as follows (days [d] into recuperation/METs allowed): 0–7d/1 MET; 7–14d/1–2 METs; 14–21d/2–3 METs; 4–8 weeks/3–3½ METs. METs values are obtained by stress electrocardiogram (see chapter 14, Testing, testing). Intermittent activity can safely be performed up to 75% of this value. Continuous action should not exceed 60% of this value.

Appendix C

Exercises, according to expenditure of energy (in METs)

These calisthenics are recommended by the Colorado Heart Association and exclude any movements which could add to the burden on the heart of the cardiac patient.

They are also of course suitable for normal people.

They must be preceded by warmup exercises. The cardiac patient must undertake them only on instruction of his cardiologist.

Combining and increasing the energy output is essential for the patient or normal person to increase stamina and well-being in accordance with age.

The patient's symptoms (angina, shortness of breath, palpitation or fatigue) are the gauge for the exercises he may do. It is advisable for the patient to start his exercises at a low level beginning with number 1. If an exercise precipitates more than minimal symptoms, then he should go back to the next lower levels on the chart.

The column on the right indicates energy requirements, in METs, for each exercise, per minute of exercise.

Times/minute indicates how many times each entire sequence is to be performed each minute.

Start with a three-minute period of exercise. Then a rest period for two minutes, then back to three minutes of exercise and two of resting. In the beginning, the patient may not be able to do more than ten to thirty minutes.

As tolerance increases, he may decrease the rest period until he is able to do fifteen minutes of continuous exercise without any symptoms of angina, shortness of breath, palpitation or fatigue.

Then he can cautiously progress to the next higher level of exercise again with three minutes of exercise, two minutes of rest for ten to thirty minutes and repeat the progression.

EX. NO.	*Times per minute*	METs
1)	*16*	1.1
2)	*16*	1.2
3)	*16*	1.3
4)	28	1.4
5)	28	1.5
6)	*16*	1.5
7)	20	1.6
8)	28	1.6
9)	28	1.7
10)	*10*	1.8
11)	28	1.9
12)	*16*	2.0
13)	28	2.1
14)	*16*	2.1

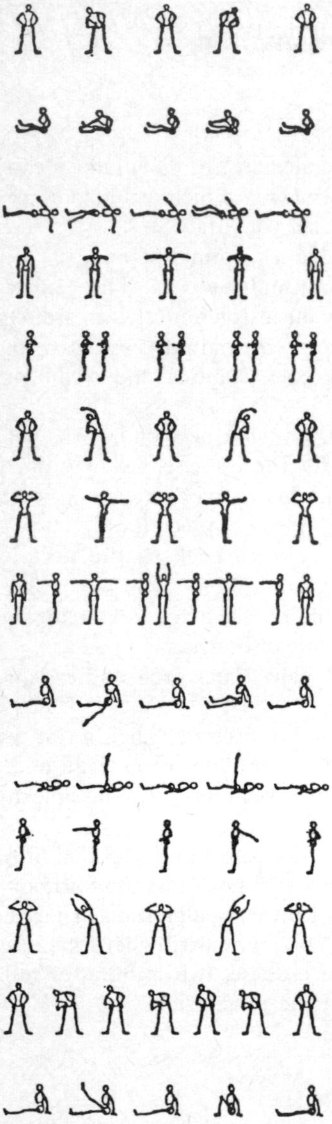

EX. NO.	*Times per minute*
15)	*16*
16)	20
17)	*10*
18)	20
19)	*16*
20)	*16*
21)	*16*
22)	*16*
23)	*16*
24)	*10*
25)	*12*
26)	*16*
27)	20
28)	*16*

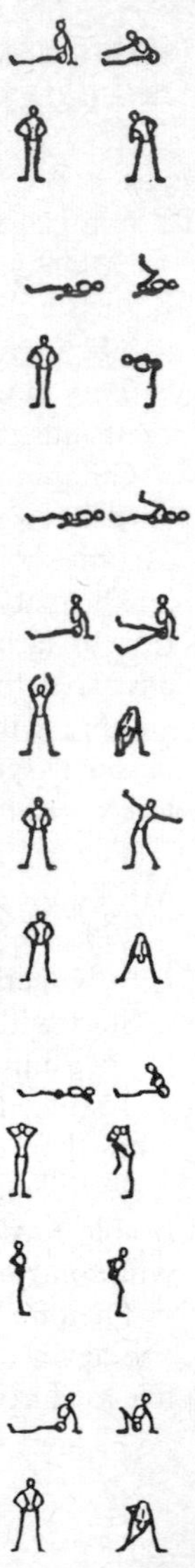

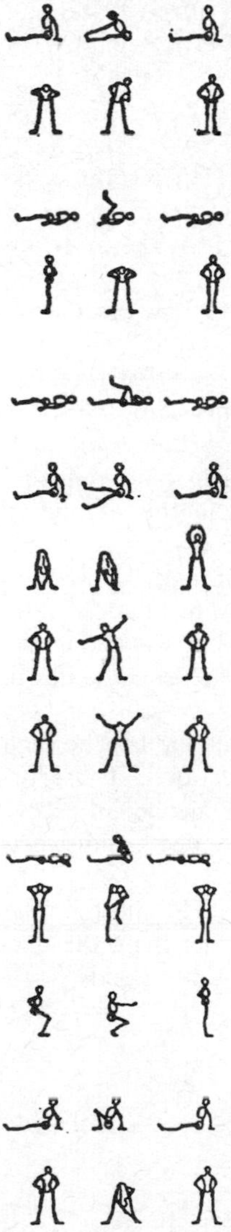

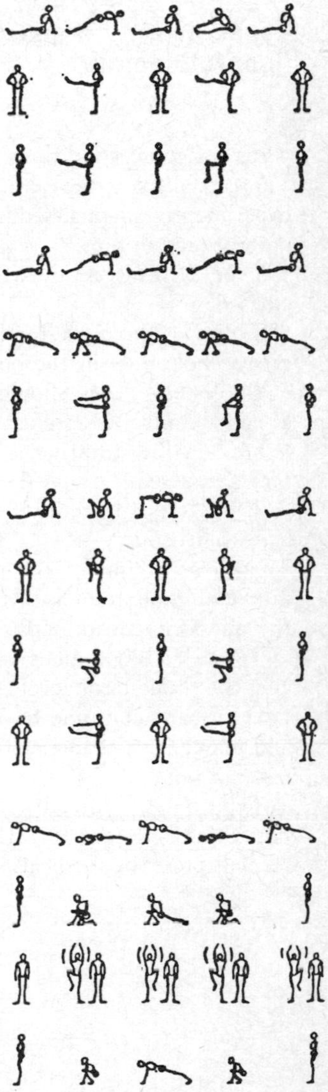

	METs	EX. NO.	*Times per minute*		METs
	2.1	29)	*16*		3.1
	2.2	30)	20		3.2
	2.3	31)	20		3.2
	2.4	32)	20		3.3
	2.4	33)	*16*		3.3
	2.5	34)	20		3.5
	2.6	35)	*16*		3.6
	2.8	36)	*16*		3.6
	2.9	37)	*16*		4.0
	2.9	38)	20		4.8
	3.0	39)	*16*		6.6
	3.0	40)	*16*		5.1
	3.1	41)	20		5.6
	3.1	42)	*16*		6.0

Appendix D

Types of fatty blood conditions, Hyperlipoproteinemia

Three of these conditions (Types II, III, and IV, see pp. 139–144), predispose the patient to arteriosclerosis. In all types of hyperlipoproteinemia, reduction to normal weight is the most important prescription.

Type I: This is always genetic (inherited). Low-fat diet is advised.

Type II: The cholesterol count is high. The gene that produces excess cholesterol in the body may have been inherited.

Cholesterol level should be reduced by low-cholesterol diet. Weight control is essential. Medication can help bind the cholesterol in the intestine, so it is not absorbed in the circulation but is excreted.

Type III: Apparently combines elevation of both cholesterol and triglycerides. It is a familial trait, but is fortunately rare. Treatment is simple: the patient must lose weight, reducing the intake of cholesterol and triglycerides. If levels fail to come down, the physician can prescribe medication.

Type IV: Blood analysis shows the triglyceride level to be high and the cholesterol level normal or slightly elevated. These patients usually consume too much sugar or drink alcohol in excess, and may have a tendency to diabetes. This type must avoid sweets and alcohol.

Type V: A combination of Types I and IV. The most important thing is weight loss. If a patient needs further help, the doctor will prescribe medication. See chapter 11, "Killer Foods."

Appendix E

Foods low and high in cholesterol

FOODS ALLOWED	FOODS TO BE LIMITED
Fruits	
Any fresh, frozen, canned or cooked fruit or fruit juice	Avocado
Cereals	
Any cereal with skim milk Rice.	
Soups	
Vegetable soups made without meat stock	Cream, chicken and meat stock soups
Meats, Fish, Poultry, Eggs and Cheese	
Medium portion of lean baked, broiled or boiled beef, lamb, veal, chicken, turkey or fish daily except inner organs listed opposite. Liquid shortening. Margarine, if not hydrogenated. Egg substitute. Cottage cheese, Mozzarella. Synthetic cheese	All pork, mutton and duck. Fish roe, shrimp and oysters. Inner organs, as sweetbreads, brains, liver and kidney. Eggs and food prepared with egg. All cheese, except those allowed. Animal fats, lard and solid shortening. Butter, solid margarine, and margarine hydrogenated
Vegetables	
At least two servings of fresh or frozen vegetables daily, either raw, cooked or as a salad. Potatoes	Sweet potatoes

FOODS ALLOWED	FOODS TO BE LIMITED
Breads	
Any breadstuffs not containing egg yolk, solid shortening, dried egg, lard or cream	All breadstuffs containing egg yolk, cream, solid shortening, dried egg or lard
Beverages	
Skim milk, tea, coffee and coffee substitutes	Whole milk, cream, malted milk and any drink containing egg yolk
Desserts	
Gelatin desserts, fresh or cooked fruits. Sherbets and ices. Puddings made without egg yolk or cream. Angel food cake and fruit pie made with egg white and liquid shortening	Chocolates, cakes, pastries, puddings and desserts containing solid shortening, egg yolk, dried egg, cream lard. Ice cream
Miscellaneous	
French dressing, macaroni, spaghetti, sugar, syrups and nuts allowed	Gravies, mayonnaise and noodles. Cashew and macadamia nuts. Cream substitutes made with coconut oil

Appendix F

Foods low and high in carbohydrates or triglycerides

FOODS ALLOWED		FOODS TO BE LIMITED
Diet jams, jellies, candies		Jams, jellies, honey, candies
	Cereal	
Oatmeal, rye, barley		Spaghetti, noodles, pastas
	Soups	
All clear soups, consommes, bouillon		Cream soups
	Salad	
Any salad. Use spices, herbs		Dressing with cream
	Meat	
Trimmed of all fat. Fish, lean meat, lamb, chicken. Liquid oil (polyunsaturated)		Animal fat, pork, ham, duck, butter, solid fat, shortening, solid margarine, coconut oil
	Breads	
		Egg breads, cheese bread, muffins, pancakes, sweet rolls, butter rolls, biscuits, cookies
	Vegetables	
All except potatoes, lima beans (limited allowed)		All fried vegetables
	Beverages	
Diet soft drinks, unsweetened juice, unsweetened canned juices		Soft drinks, coffee, cocoa, sweetened juice, alcohol
	Desserts	
Gelatin, fresh fruit, tapioca prepared with skim milk		Ice cream
	Miscellaneous	
Nuts, olives		Sugar, candy, chocolates, icings

Appendix G

Low sodium foods

FOOD	FOODS ALLOWED	FOODS TO BE LIMITED
Beverage	No more than 1 pint of milk daily; coffee, tea, cocoa, decaffeinated beverages	Milk & milk drinks, dutch process cocoa, instant cocoa, fountain prepared beverage mixes
Bread	No more than 4 servings of commercially prepared breads or rolls (with unsalted tops) unlimited amounts of unsalted bread & unsalted crackers	Salted crackers, soda crackers, graham crackers; breads & rolls with salted tops. Quick breads made with baking powder, baking soda and salt
Cereal	At least 1 serving of whole grain or enriched cereal	Flavored crackers

FOOD	FOODS ALLOWED	FOODS TO BE LIMITED
Meat, Fish, Poultry, Cheese	Rabbit, bass, bluefish, whitefish, diet canned tuna & salmon. Beef, veal, lamb, chicken, turkey, liver, duck, quail. Low sodium cheese	Canned, smoked or salted meat as: balcon, bologna, ham, frankfurters, kosher meats, sausage, luncheon meats, smoked tongue, frozen fish fillets, canned, smoked or salted fish as: anchovies, caviar, dricd cod, herring, salmon, sardines & tuna. All other cheese except those allowed.
Egg		Egg fried in bacon fat Synthetic eggs high in sodium
Potato or substitute	One serving daily of fresh, frozen or canned artichokes, asparagus, broccoli, brussel sprouts, carrots, cabbage, cauliflower, chive, chicory, cucumber, eggplant, endive, escarole, green beans, kale, lettuce, mushrooms, squash, onions, peas, pumpkin, rutabaga, white turnips, frozen lima beans & peas. Potatoes	Spinach, beets, celery, sauerkraut or other vegetables prepared in brine.
Fruit	At least 2 or more servings of fresh frozen or canned fruit or fruit juice daily	Crystallized or glazed fruits. Maraschino cherries.

FOOD	FOODS ALLOWED	FOODS TO BE LIMITED
Fat	Butter, cream, margarine, vegetable shortenings, salad dressings & oils	Bacon, bacon fat, salt pork
Dessert	Fruit; gelatin desserts, water ice, fruit whips; fruit pie, cake, cookies; tapioca & cornstarch puddings and junket made with allowed milk, ice cream & sherbet if using milk from allowance.	Canned fruit
Soups	All homemade soups without salt made with allowed foods, salt free bouillon	Cream soups or commercial canned soups; bouillon and consomme
Sweets	Sugar, syrup, honey, jelly, jam, marmalade, hard candy, sugar wafers	All chocolate preparations
Miscellaneous	Low sodium baking powder, spices, unsalted nuts and popcorn, yeast, cocoanut, tapioca, unsalted peanut butter, salt substitute	Salt, monosodium glutamate, salted nuts, garlic salt, prepared mustard, horseradish, onion salt, celery salt, soy sauce, Worcestershire sauce, catsup, chili sauce, chives, salted popcorn, salted peanut butter, meat tenderizers, pretzels

Appendix H

Foods high in potassium

Fruits: (per portion)
- Apricots—6
- Banana—1 medium
- Cantaloupe—½
- Prunes—7 large
- Dates—8
- Raisins ½ cup
- Figs—4

Juice:
- Orange juice—½ cup
- Orange-grapefruit juice—1¼ cup
- Prune juice—1 cup
- Tangerine juice—1¼ cup

Vegetables:
- Brussel sprouts—10 cooked
- Lentils—⅓ cup
- White potato—1 large
- Squash, winter—¾ cup
- Sweet potato—1 large

Appendix I

Medications

The following is for the convenience of the reader and is not to imply approval or disapproval of particular items. Only the most commonly used cardiac medications are included.

GENERIC (CHEMICAL) NAME	TRADE NAME
Digitalis preparations	
Digitalis Leaf	Digitora
	Pil-Digis
	Digifortis
	Crystodigin
Digitoxin	Digitaline Nativelle
	Myodigin
	Purodigin
Acetyldigitoxin	Acylanid
Digoxin	Lanoxin
	Davoxin
Lanatoside C	Cedilanid
Anti-arrhythmics	
Procainamide	Pronestyl
Quinidine Gluconate	Quinaglute
Quinidine Sulfate	Quinidex
	Quinora
Quinidine Polygalacturonate	Cardioquin
Lidocaine	Xylocaine
	Seracaine
Diphenylhydantoin	Dilantin
Propranolol	Inderal
Isoproterenol	Isuprel
Vasodilators	
Nitroglycerine	Nitroglycerine

GENERIC (CHEMICAL) NAME	TRADE NAME
Nitroglycerine-Time release forms	Nitro-bid
	Nitro-cels
	Nitroglyn
	Nitrospan
	Vasoglyn
Amyl Nitrite	Amyl Nitrite
Erythrityl Tetranitrate	Cardilate
Isosorbide Dinitrate	Isordil
	Sorbitrate
Pentaerythritol Tetranitrate	Peritrate
	Duotrate
	El-Petn
	Kaytrate
	Neo-Corovas
	Pentafin
	Pentritol
	Tetrasule
	Tranite
	Vasodiatol
Propranolol (not a vasodilator but used for angina—see text)	Inderal
Diuretics	
Chlorthiazide	Diuril
Hydrochlorthiazide	Esidrix
	HydroDiuril
	Oretic
Benzathiazide	Aquatag
	Exna
Hydroflumethiazide	Saluron
Bendroflumethiazide	Naturetin
	Bristuron
Methyclothiazide	Enduron
Trichlormethiazide	Metahydrin
	Naqua
Polythiazide	Renese
Cyclothiazide	Anhydron
Chlorthalidone	Hygroton
Quinethazone	Hydromox
Ethacrynic Acid	Edecrin
Furosemide	Lasix
Spironolactone	Aldactone
Dyrenium	Triamterene

GENERIC (CHEMICAL) NAME	TRADE NAME
Anti-hypertensives	
Rauwolfia Serpentina	Raudixin
	Rauval
	Hyperloid
	Rauja
	Raulin
	Rautina
	Wolfina
Reserpine	Serpasil
	Lemiserp
	Rau-Sed
	Resercen
	Reserpoid
	Sandril
	Serfin
Alseroxylon	Rauwiloid
	Rautensin
Deserpidine	Harmonyl
Rescinnamine	Moderil
Syrosingopine	Singroserp
Guanethidine	Ismelin
Methyldopa	Aldomet
Mecamylamine	Inversine
Hydralazine	Apresoline
Pargyline	Eutonyl

Multiple combinations of diuretics, anti-hypertensives with and without sedatives and tranquilizers are available as a single tablet. Space prohibits listing them.

"Anti-cholesterol" agents	
Cholestyramine Resin	Cuemid
	Questran
Clofibrate	Atromid-S
Dextrothyroxine	Choloxin
Niacin, Nicotinic Acid	Niacin, Nicotinic Acid
Anti-coagulants	
Heparin	Heparin
	Depo-Heparin
	Hepathrom
	Lipo-Hepin
	Liquaemin
	Panheprin

GENERIC (CHEMICAL) NAME	TRADE NAME
Acenocoumarol	Sintrom
Bishydroxycoumarin	Dicumarol
Phenprocoumon	Liquamar
Warfarin Sodium	Coumadin
	Panwarfin
Warfarin Potassium	Athrombin-K
Phenindione	Danilone
	Eridione
	Hedulin
Anisindione	Miradon
Diphenadione	Dipaxin

INDEX

(Page numbers in italics refer to illustrations.)